Dr ANDREW STANWAY

Prevention is Better...

An A-Z of
Common Illnesses
and Problems
and How
to Prevent Them

CENTURY
London·Melbourne·Auckland·Johannesburg

Acknowledgement
I have been greatly helped by the self-help groups
and organisations listed on pages 387–394.

First published in 1986 by
Century Hutchinson Ltd,
Brookmount House, 62–65 Chandos Place,
Covent Garden, London WC2N 4NW

Century Hutchinson Publishing Group
(Australia) Pty Ltd,
16–22 Church Street, Hawthorn,
Melbourne, Victoria 3122

Century Hutchinson Group (NZ) Ltd,
32–34 View Road, PO Box 40–086, Glenfield,
Auckland 10

Century Hutchinson Group (SA) Pty Ltd,
PO Box 337, Bergvlei 2012, South Africa

Design & typography by Tony Fahy

Set in 10½pt on 13pt Palatino Roman

Printed and bound in Great Britain by
Butler & Tanner Ltd, Frome, Somerset.

British Library Cataloguing in Publication
Data:

Stanway, Andrew
    Prevention is better . . . : an A–Z of common
    illnesses and health problems and how to
    prevent them.
    1. Health—Dictionary
    I. Title
613'.03'21   RA776
ISBN 0 7126 1211 4

CONTENTS

PART ONE
Prevention and Health: The Arguments

THE HISTORY OF PREVENTIVE MEDICINE

Every society, no matter how primitive, has demanded some kind of curative medicine but a society has to be fairly sophisticated before preventive medicine is possible or even attractive. First, the members of the society have to be sufficiently stable to be able to see beyond immediate survival; second, there must be a positive attitude towards health because if health is not seen as an asset for the individual or the society then the prevention of illness is irrelevant; and third, there must be sufficient pulling together in the community to make the concept of 'every man for himself' less important than the concept of the common good. The history of preventive medicine then starts when a particular society can act on these goals and is ready to make them a part of everyday life.

Concepts of preventive medicine as we think of it today started with the Greeks, although undoubtedly there were simple forms of prevention being practised worldwide before this. In Ancient China the Yellow Emperor spoke about wholism and preventive medicine:

Sages here do not treat those who are already ill; they rather instruct those who are not yet ill . . . The superior physician helps before the early budding of disease. The inferior physician begins to help when the disease has already developed. He helps when the destruction has already set in.

Two thousand years later Huai-nan Tzu wrote:

The good doctor pays constant attention to keeping people well so that there will be no sickness.

Such concepts were adopted by the Greeks—the first western culture to take prevention seriously. From the very beginnings of Greek medicine efforts to preserve health seemed more important than those to cure diseases. Health, they maintained, was a state in which the various elements and forces of the body were in balance. Disease in this way of thinking was a disorder of this equilibrium. It seemed fairly clear that external (environmental) factors were important in causing a poor balance and the Greeks talked a lot about poor nutrition and physical factors. To the Greek the ideal life was one in which nutrition, exercise and rest were properly balanced. Other important factors were the person's age, sex, type of constitution and the seasons.

This ecological approach to medicine, which seems so modern today, led the Ancient Greeks to strive to balance their diet, exercise and environmental factors to keep the mind and body in good health. Unfortunately, because this meant a change in lifestyle, few could actually afford to go along with such elegant theories and as a result it was only the middle and upper classes who had the incentives, money and leisure to pursue these goals. Even though few Greeks actually lived like this the concepts continued to influence medical thought for centuries.

In the Middle Ages people began to realise that there was another major dimension to health which had to be taken into account in addition to the Greek notions. This realisation came about with the appearance of leprosy as a serious health hazard in Europe. The primary need to do something about leprosy led the society of the day to band together to isolate people with the disease and to clean up the environment, not just for the benefit of individuals but for that of society as a whole. Preventive public health could be said to have been born at this time.

The Church led the way with its insistence that spiritual and physical uncleanliness were linked. The Old Testament, and especially the book of Leviticus, puts great stress on processes such as menstruation and urethral discharges as being unclean and holds that people with such afflictions should be isolated from the rest of society until they have been purified. So leprosy was treated by the Church in a very literal Old Testament way and sufferers were isolated from the community to protect the healthy. Because this

disease was untreatable the individuals became socially dead as they were cast out from life.

The principle of breaking the chain in the transmission of an infective illness became the king-pin of the measures taken to fight the next major health hazard to hit Europe – bubonic plague. By this time there were laws that made it an offence not to report plague to the health authorities. Many public health measures were adopted to control this killer disease but from the preventive medicine point of view perhaps the most important was the introduction of quarantine regulations. The pandemic of plague in the middle of the fourteenth century forced the public officials of Italy and southern France to create *cordons sanitaires*, observation stations, isolation facilities and disinfection procedures. By the seventeenth century these procedures were widely accepted throughout Europe.

All this effort effectively removed plague as a scourge and as England approached the eighteenth century it was a far healthier place to live than at any time since the Romans left 1,300 years before. At least the upper classes could look beyond the problems of immediate survival. It was from this group that the first real preventive medicine was to appear. In 1662 John Gaunt, a haberdasher, was the first to show that more boys were born than girls and that more births occurred in urban than rural areas. In 1676 William Petty wrote a book on *Political Arithmetick* which asserted that health and education were as much a part of a nation's wealth and power as were its trade and manufacturing. This was something of a bombshell at a time when society simply didn't think of health as a valued commodity. You were either healthy or sick. Petty, valuing the worth of a King's subject at £20 a head, estimated that a 25 per cent reduction in natural death rate would add £4 million per year to the wealth of the nation. He estimated that it would take a century to achieve such a vast change in death rate but suggested that in the meantime the State should use the knowledge of illness rates to work out how many health-care professionals it needed.

Unfortunately, both of these far-sighted men were all but ignored – if only because they were centuries ahead of their contemporaries. Remember, this was a time during which people mainly accepted ill health as inevitable and during which the majority of society lived and worked with an overall condition of health that would appal most of us today. Chronic illness and early death were considered normal and diseases such as scurvy blighted the lives of millions yet did not kill them.

It was not until the eighteenth century that attitudes to health and disease began to change for the better – if only among the middle and upper classes. The concept that disease was simply divine retribution was being seriously questioned by the discovery that certain diseases at least had specific and provable causes. In 1757 James Lind proved that scurvy could be cured if sailors ate fresh fruit and vegetables, and environmental hazards such as lead poisoning were shown to be responsible for certain, hitherto mysterious, conditions. In 1798 Edward Jenner proved that smallpox could be prevented by vaccination and John Snow clearly proved the link between cholera and infected drinking-water supplies. Remember that all this was occurring long before bacteria were discovered.

The next significant step forward in preventive medicine came with the alarming realisation that health was not just a middle-class luxury. In other words the middle and upper classes began to realise that whether they liked it or not their own health and wealth was deeply involved with the health of the ordinary working people. It is perhaps surprising that industrialists did not see the economic link between the poor and unhealthy working classes and low productivity earlier, but they did not and in 1848 when parliament was debating the first Public Health Bill even the *Economist* magazine did not see the connection between the two. As we have seen, Petty had been talking about exactly this link over a century beforehand but an Austrian, Johann Peter Frank, was the first to make the assertion that governments were strengthened by healthy, happy workers. His thinking produced the world's first government medical system, in Germany in 1883.

The growth of preventive and public health measures in any industrialised country appears to follow a fairly predictable pattern as the country becomes industrialised. First, there is a rush for power, then an increase in exploitation which is difficult to control. Along with this, rural people and even those from outside the country migrate to the major cities, become separated from their own food supply and depend on cash as wages. At the same time death rates rise dramatically and the value placed on individual life is low. But such a system, whether it occurs in nineteenth-century England or twentieth-century Third World countries, produces wealth and makes money available for those who want to spread it around. Historically, individual philanthropists started creating better conditions for their workers and indeed for whole communities and this, combined with the new egalitarianism born as a result of the French and American Revolutions, made the upper classes more aware of the value of keeping the masses healthy.

At the turn of this century another truth began to dawn. About 60 per cent of all the men who volunteered for the British army's fight in the Boer War were unfit for service. This appeared to shake people's long-held attitudes almost more than any other single factor and led Sidney Webb to write:

We have become aware, almost in a flash, that we are not merely individuals but members of a community, nay, citizens of the world. . . . In short, the opening of the twentieth century finds us all, to the dismay of the old-fashioned, individualist, thinking in communities!

Slowly, the notion that society was a collection of communities began to

develop – rather more slowly in the US than in the UK, partly because of the individualistic frontiersman thinking in the former. But things were on the move and the time was ripe for the second phase in the development of preventive medicine – the scientific approach.

Until this time facts and figures about health were poor, so few lessons could be learned. Simple 'Bills of Mortality' had been collected in London since 1603 but it was not until the establishment of the office of the Registrar General in 1837 that guesswork was replaced by real statistics. The availability of verifiable facts now made it possible to enact regulations to prevent frankly harmful behaviour and to promote healthy behaviour and practices. Ordinances to abate noise, control sewage and dispose of decayed matter, dead bodies, filth and stagnant waters go back as far as 1388 and in colonial times several American communities enacted laws to quarantine ships and isolate smallpox. Baltimore organised America's first board of health in 1793. But effective public health administration was impossible in either country because local parishes and communities overruled national goals. As so often occurs in history, the activities of one man changed all this.

Edwin Chadwick (1800–1890) was a barrister who came to the same conclusion as Petty had done two hundred years before. He promoted the notion that disease amongst the poor was the major reason they couldn't look after themselves. He

11

maintained that the enormous level of government expenditure on Poor Law relief would be dramatically reduced if the poor were healthy. In this rather roundabout economic, as opposed to medical, way he became the father of British and American public health. His report, *The Sanitary Conditions of the Labouring Population of Great Britain* (1842), made the awful conditions of working people so apparent to the upper classes that they simply had to listen. He showed that, while the upper classes lived on average to the age of 44 and while only one in ten of their children died in the first year of life, the comparable figures for the working classes were 22 years and one child in four. He maintained that a cleaner environment with decent water supplies and adequate sewage disposal were the answers.

Chadwick proposed the formation of a centralised public health authority with a full-time staff, and after several years of debate the Public Health Act of 1845 established a three-man General Board of Health. But even once water and sewage systems were widely introduced it was still clear that these weren't the total answer to health, and slowly it became apparent that housing, food, working conditions and personal health services were just as important.

Chadwick's influence didn't stop at sewage and water mains though—he pushed for an even greater link between 'health' and 'welfare'. Even though there was already a definite move towards community services

and the realisation that health was a national asset, the puritan work ethic still ruled supreme and the fear was that anyone and everyone would rather receive welfare than work. This meant that welfare benefits put the person in a position lower than 'the situation of the dependent labourer of the humblest sort'. It is ironic that even today 'health' and 'welfare' are still bound together in the same bureaucratic machinery both in the UK and the US even though they are uneasy bedfellows much of the time.

But in spite of often conflicting pulls, public health made great strides in the last quarter of the nineteenth century. The work on bacteria by Pasteur and Koch took scientific endeavour a giant leap forward and placed the whole of disease on a different plane from supplying clean water and the disposal of sewage. Quite quickly it became apparent that public health measures were far more effective in controlling almost all common infectious diseases than was curative, personal medicine, and the seeds of medical discontent were sown that are still with us to this day.

When public health officials were making such an enormous impact on the nation's health doctors were relatively powerless to achieve much. The emphasis on sanitation, the absence of doctors from major decision-making bodies and the link between public health and 'welfare' made public health unattractive and unrewarding to doctors.

Unfortunately, there were more

fundamental problems too – problems which we still have today. In the nineteenth century voluntary hospitals were preoccupied with treating disease and they had a monopoly of medical education dating back a century. Clinical medicine, then as now, attracted interventionists whereas what preventive medicine needed was people who were happy with an absence of disease. Prevention seemed dull by comparison with the glamour of effecting cures, and even today when so many of the medical profession pay lip-service to the importance of prevention only a tiny fraction (1–2 per cent in the UK) of any westernised nation's health budget is spent on prevention – mainly because medicine has become almost entirely an active, interventionist profession.

Interestingly, the Hippocratic Oath itself could also be said to be an enemy of public health and prevention, insisting as it does that doctors put the needs of their patients before anything else. Doctors from the Middle Ages onwards (until the advent of the National Health Service in the UK, and still in the US today) have been private entrepreneurs selling their skills on a one-off basis to anyone who could afford them. So it was at the turn of the century in the UK. Doctors were wedded to a group of individuals who provided their personal income and it was clearly in their interests to ensure that nothing they did professionally jeopardised their patients' health and their own livelihood. Patients felt that in such a system they were

paying for highly personalised care and didn't want to hear about 'bad news' outside this one-to-one doctor/patient contract. This contrasts sharply with medicine in Eastern Europe where the physician's first duty is to strengthen the State by maintaining the health of its people. Everything in the doctor/patient relationship is secondary to this. Although most of us in the West find this approach unpalatable the benefit is that public health measures are more easily accepted and acted upon.

From public health to preventive medicine

As we have seen, the vast majority of preventive medicine in the nineteenth century was done by way of public health measures, but preventive medicine is really a link between environmental health on the one hand and personal medical care on the other.

True preventive measures probably started with diseases of children. In 1892 Pierre Budin, a Parisian obstetrician, asked women to come back when their babies were 6 months old for a post-natal check-up. He was amazed at the number of children who had already died by this age and started to think about what could be done to prevent this awful toll. Preventive and health-maintenance services for children started in Britain in 1908 and the Boston Lying-in Hospital started an ante-natal programme in 1912.

Once the idea of prevention caught on it spread rapidly, and industrial and occupational medicine quickly became a valued part of the system too. But popular though they were, there was (and still is in the US) a reluctance on the part of preventive services to do anything creative, for fear of treading on the toes of the curative doctors. In the US, for example, community health centres sprang up before World War I but confined themselves to education and prevention and many were in slum areas. They were almost always separate from hospitals. In fact many such clinics had a motto:

No prescriptions given; no sickness treated.

Preventive medicine then became associated with the business of keeping people healthy while 'real' doctors got on with treating the sick.

As the years went by it became apparent that public health and preventive medicine had chalked up some remarkable successes and reluctantly the medical profession accepted that prevention had a place. Much of this is still lip-service though, as can be seen from the curriculum of any teaching hospital on either side of the Atlantic. Preventive medicine and its concepts rank so low as to be almost invisible. Over the last twenty years or so doctors have realised that whilst *they* can do little for many of their patients, detecting disease early *can* produce truly dramatic results in conditions such as: glaucoma (a person's sight can be saved if the condition is caught early); obesity; depresssion (suicide deaths can be greatly reduced by treating the depression); hypertension (treatment reduces the incidence of strokes); and so on. The examples are numerous.

Some historical achievements of preventive medicine

It is all too easy in our cosy world to forget just how hostile life was as recently as a century ago and so to belittle what preventive medicine has achieved so far. A hundred years ago, only six babies out of ten survived to adulthood and the life expectancy of a British boy born between 1871 and 1880 was 41 years, and that of his sister 45 years. If they managed to survive the first year of life this improved to 48 and 50 years respectively. Today this has totally changed – mainly because of preventive rather than curative measures.

Generally speaking we all accept that when we have a baby it will be born alive and will survive to see old age – but this is a very recent assumption in the history of the human race. Childbirth itself was extremely hazardous for both a mother and her child only a century ago and then the child had to survive all the childhood infections, in addition to smallpox and TB. Nutrition in Victorian England was so poor that children's resistance was low and they were likely to pick up anything that was going. The majority of the population of Victorian England lived in urban slums, water was often unsafe and few houses had piped water at all. In the environment of cities diseases spread and took hold of whole communities, causing thousands of deaths in any one epidemic. Over the last hundred years, though, the death rates from TB, enteric fever and the main infectious diseases of childhood have been reduced by more than 99 per cent.

In western countries mortality in every age group up to the age of 35 is now one tenth or less of what it was a hundred years ago and among children aged 1–9 it is now one twentieth of what it was then. In fact mortality has fallen by 88 per cent.

Let us look briefly at the major preventive medicine achievements if only to give encouragement to show what can be done. After all, we are facing just as big a problem in preventive health care today but now the degenerative diseases are the scourge and not the infectious ones.

Cholera

We have seen how Chadwick pioneered the concern with water, drainage and sewage disposal, but it should not be thought that the battle was won without a fight. Years of opposition and debate were centred around the vast sums of money involved in the engineering needed. Such measures were also seen by some as infringing the liberty of the individual and when all is said and done the value of the whole exercise was unproven at the time. The result of these measures, though, was to eliminate cholera–a disease that killed tens of thousands every year in great epidemics.

Enteric fever

This was another major killer of the nineteenth century that was almost totally controlled by improved sanitation, although it wasn't realised that this would be the case at the time. Things improved further as measures to ensure the safety of milk, shellfish, ice-cream and other foods were brought in. Enteric fever is relatively rare today in the UK (200–250 cases a year in England and Wales) and in three-quarters of the cases the infection is acquired abroad. Today's regulations for food handlers and food preparation are safeguards against outbreaks of this killer disease.

Diphtheria

This, together with measles and whooping cough, was one of the frequently fatal diseases of childhood. It has been virtually wiped out and is so rare that most doctors wouldn't recognise it if they saw it. Yet only 35 years ago it was a killer that terrified every parent. Between 1916 and 1925 there were well over 50,000 cases every year and more than 4,000 children died annually. After 1940 and the introduction of active immunisation the death rate from diphtheria fell dramatically. This vaccine is now given to children routinely as part of their 'triple vaccine' (diphtheria, tetanus, whooping cough) with a booster on entry to school. Today there are almost no deaths from diphtheria in Britain.

Measles and whooping cough

More than 90 per cent of all cases of these diseases are in children below the age of 10. The main danger is that if they go on to pneumonia the child can die. Measles vaccine has been available since 1968 but it has not penetrated public awareness in Britain as it has in the US where the disease is now uncommon. As a result there are more than 250,000 cases of measles reported each year in the UK and doubtless many more go unreported.

Death rates from both these conditions were beginning to fall even before effective vaccines and anti-biotics (to prevent the complications) were available. Either the organisms were becoming less virulent or perhaps children were more resistant to infection because of better housing, nutrition and smaller family size.

Scarlet fever

In 1900 scarlet fever was so virulent that three out of every 100 children who caught it died. By 1973 there were only three deaths in 11,000 cases in the UK. Certainly children are better able to withstand the effects of the organism today but scientists are also sure that the organism itself has changed in some way.

Tuberculosis

In 1855 13 per cent of all deaths were caused by TB, and once again the young suffered most. TB is a classical example of a disease falling in the mortality league long before specific cures were available. Less over-crowding, better food, better personal hygiene and sanatorium treat-ment—all helped to reduce the illness and death from TB long before the drugs to cure it were discovered. Since the early 1950s, with mass X-rays, drugs and BCG vaccinations, there has been a rapid fall in the number of cases and deaths. New cases today are confined almost entirely to very old men and certain immigrants. But even today when the disease is virtually eradicated it causes the loss of 2.3 million working days a year in the UK. Just think what things were like a century ago!

Poliomyelitis

About thirty years ago polio reached its peak incidence. In 1947, 7,984 cases were recorded and 10 per cent of these died. Between 1952 and 1954 nearly another 1,000 died of the disease and many more were left paralysed. Today there are about 12,000 people in the UK suffering from the after-effects of polio.

The first vaccine was introduced in 1957. The result is that in the years 1972–4 only twenty-two cases of polio were reported in the UK and none died. But because not everywhere in the world has a similar record on this disease it still makes sense to be vaccinated before going abroad to certain countries.

Smallpox

Once the scourge of whole populations, this disease is now officially
extinct in the world.

Maternal mortality

We have seen how the outlook has
improved for babies and young
children but so too has that of
mothers during pregnancy and childbirth. A century ago maternal
mortality in childbirth was at epidemic proportions, and even as
recently as 1935 between forty and
forty-five women died for every
10,000 pregnancies. This totalled
about 2,500 women every year.

The establishment of the Royal
College of Obstetricians and Gynaecologists, and the Midwives Act of
1936 helped raise professional stan-
dards, and the care of pregnant
women and the confinement in
hospitals under specialist care has
reduced the maternal death figures
to one in every 10,000 births. There
are suggestions that even this can be
improved upon.

The history of preventive medicine,
then, is largely that of public health,
but now the challenges are different.
Certainly we have combated the
infectious illnesses to the point where
they no longer pose a fraction of the
threat they once did, but today we
face new threats from degenerative
diseases such as cancers, stroke, and
heart disease – the big single killer of
western man.

Can modern preventive medicine
do for these diseases what public

health so successfully did for the
infections? The problems today are
fundamentally different. The last
century's illness epidemics were
caused by poverty and shortage. This
century's are being caused by wealth
and excess. No one much minds
giving up poverty and shortage but
persuading people to give up 'the
good life' is much more difficult.

The three phases of prevention in the western world

Historically, as we have seen, the
prevention of disease has been the
greatest and most important contribution to the health of the western
world but simply to think of preventive medicine in terms of public
health is far too narrow a perspective
today.

The first phase of preventive
medicine was indeed this rather
authoritarian, organisational public
health approach. It was based on the
need to control infectious illnesses
using environmental control im-
posed on people 'for the good of the
community'. In this way clean water
became the norm, sewers took away
waste, food was inspected and its
quality improved, and pest-infested
slums were cleared. All of this did
wonders for life expectancy. In white
women in the US life expectancy
increased from 40 years in 1855 to 55
years in 1920. Almost all of this increased life-span came about because
of the reduction in infant death rates.
Little, if any, change was made to the

longevity of those who survived to middle life. In 1855 a 45-year-old American could expect to live another 24.6 years and in 1910 the figure was 25.5 years. Hardly a stunning advance!

As well as the giant steps forward being taken in sanitation, immunology began to blossom as a medical growth area and diphtheria, whooping cough, measles, polio and smallpox came under control.

Initially this era of prevention was characterised by individual heroism and leadership together with more health laws. The amount of voluntary action on the part of the public was minimal. Certainly immunisation required the individual to turn up to be vaccinated but otherwise preventive medicine was a 'painless' procedure that was done *to* an individual.

The second phase in the development of preventive medicine actually started before the ending of the first and came with the discovery of anaesthesia and antiseptics. Phase two, then, was that made possible by increasing technology and financial investment. Undoubtedly the greatest triggers to the growth of medical knowledge were the two world wars in this century. Knowledge of anaesthesia and antiseptics lay dormant until the vast number of operations done in World War I made advances necessary on an unprecedented scale. By World War II sulpha drugs (1935) and penicillin (1940) had been developed and the modern pharmaceutical industry as we know it was born. This opened up for the first time the idea of mas-

sive capital investment in the health field. In the first phase of the growth of prevention, public health measures were seen as a way of improving the nation's strength and wealth and a way of maintaining a vigorous population which could produce goods and services in a fast-growing capitalist society. In the second phase the goal of a healthy population became obscured as the health industry took on a life of its own. Today, doctors make the financial decisions which control this vast industry and often they make them in splendid isolation – thinking only in the context of their relationship with an individual patient.

This has led to the enormous sickness industry we now see. Yet for all this so-called advance and expenditure the life-span of a five-year-old has increased by only 2.9 years since 1940. The limits to this kind of medicine are all too apparent. It has been calculated that the elimination of all cancers of the cervix, for example, as a cause of death would add only three-tenths of a year of life to that which the average woman currently enjoys. If after fifty years of screening and gynaecological examinations her fate is that of many old people – to live alone in relative poverty – just how valuable are these extra three and a half months to her anyway?

The third phase of preventive medicine is now with us, as we start to consider health in the context of our environment – in short, man in his ecological setting. The excitement and drama of the last forty years' growth in medicine is beginning to wear thin and people are beginning to look at prevention in personal terms – as something they actually have a hand in and for which they have a responsibility.

It has been calculated that more disease, disability and premature death could be prevented by eliminating alcohol and tobacco abuse and by restricting the use of cars than by *any* foreseeable increase in expenditure on health. But it is *not* true that individuals are solely to blame now that doctors can do so little to help. The medical profession can't shrug its shoulders and say, 'Look what we've done for you, you should be grateful.'

It is no new concept that the choice as to how an individual uses his or her life rests with him or her. But the fact that there is a personal responsibility for health does not absolve doctors, nurses, politicians or administrators from responsibility, nor does it free them to ignore prevention on the grounds that it is something the individual ought to be doing for him or herself.

Phase three of the story of prevention involves the individual taking the dominant role – and this is what this book is about: personal prevention.

2

WHAT IS HEALTH?

Before we start to think about prevention we need to consider what we mean by health, if only because we have to know what we are aiming to prevent — presumably ill health.

Here are some definitions from various learned sources:

Oxford English Dictionary Soundness of body: that condition in which its function is duly discharged.

Collins Dictionary The state of being bodily and mentally vigorous and free from disease.

World Health Organisation A state of complete physical, mental and social well-being.

Parsons The state of optimum capacity of an individual for the effective performance of valued tasks.

Rossdale The product of a harmonised relationship between man and his ecology.

Dubos A modus vivendi enabling men to achieve a rewarding and not too painful existence while they cope with an imperfect world.

Illich A process of adaptation. It is not the result of instinct, but of an autonomous yet culturally shaped reaction to socially created reality. It designates the ability to adapt to changing environments, to growing up and to ageing, to healing when damaged, to suffering and to the peaceful expectation of death. Health embraces the future as well, and therefore includes anguish and the inner resources to live with it.

It is easy to see how different these approaches are. Some stress an ideal state and others a more practical approach. Some focus on physical conditions and others have the widest possible perspectives.

Various researchers on the subject quite understandably express very different views, but it is increasingly accepted that health involves far more than simply physical and even mental well-being or the absence of disease. Vibrant health and terminal illness are the extremes of the spectrum but modern thinking increasingly stresses the need to be nearer the 'vibrant health' end than midway between the two.

This broader view of health sees it as a state in which the individual is energetic, integrated, productive and self-actualised. This begs all kinds of questions though about what a particular person's ideas of fullness of life are for him or her. Obviously this sort of definition will vary from person to person and will depend on what individuals see as important in their lives. To some, physical wellness will be the most important part of their definition of health and to others psychological, emotional or spiritual factors will be of most value.

To some extent the way each of us defines health for ourselves depends on how we perceive illness. Some see illness as an intrinsic part of being a person—all human beings are destined to be ill in one way or another at some time in their lives—and to others it is only the way that we behave that makes us ill: perfect behaviour produces perfect health. The first group of people see health as a kind of battle and illness as some sort of evil spell that is put on mankind. This sort of thinking has very ancient roots going back to pre-Biblical times but it has been crystallised for Judaeo-Christian societies in the story of Adam and Eve. By going against the will of God, the story goes, they brought eternal suffering and illness on themselves. This line of thinking removes any personal responsibility for health because ill health becomes part of the divine plan for mankind and by definition can't be influenced.

By now the reader will be able to see how difficult it is to define health and illness but it is essential to be aware of what we mean by these terms or we will not be able to think intelligently about prevention.

Health and illness are not just personal matters though—they occur in a social setting and reflect a particular society's values, traditions and structures. We shall see in the next section how different illnesses are dealt with in different cultures.

Of all the symptoms that people have, only a fraction are mentioned to other members of the family and even fewer are taken outside the family. Only a small proportion of all symptoms are taken to health professionals, so clearly there is a hidden mass of 'disease' which, like an iceberg, lies submerged within society. Illness usually starts in the family context and most diagnoses are made by people in their own homes, sometimes helped by family and friends. Often, professional help is sought in order to get reassurance that the diagnosis is correct, or to get a prescription for a drug. The health professional's response is then relayed to the 'social-medical advisory system' of family and friends and action is taken that the person considers appropriate. At this stage the individual with the problem often comes to a different conclusion from that of the health professional—possibly because the individual has different perceptions of the problem and because he or she knows more about him or herself than the doctor does.

A subject that is very little discussed in medical circles but which is very important in this context is what makes an individual decide, on a particular day, to see a doctor, when the symptoms may have been present for some time without this decision being taken. In other words, few people in the illness iceberg see their doctors at the very first sign of illness, so what makes them go for professional help at a particular time? An understanding of this can often enable the doctor to get to the heart of the *real* problem very quickly.

Health and illness behaviour

'Illness behaviour' is the term used to describe the way we respond to abnormal body signs and symptoms. Obviously this involves concepts such as how a particular person monitors his or her body and its functions, defines or interprets his or her symptoms, takes action and uses the health-care system.

'Health behaviour', in contrast, refers to patterns of response to health, when the person has no specific symptoms. This is an especially useful concept when thinking about prevention because a lot of prevention is done by an individual who is well at the time. Examples of such activities are regular medical and dental check-ups, screening and so on. A lot of research has been done on people's views and beliefs in this area but the best is the Health Belief Model, which looks at the way an individual assesses the likelihood of a problem having serious consequences. It is really a sort of psychological cost-benefit analysis in which people do things according to how

important they consider the consequences of not doing them. So it is that we weigh up the advantages and disadvantages of factors as different as wearing a seat-belt, exercise, nutrition, medical check-ups, clinical examinations, careful driving, sanitation and personal hygiene. According to the effect we perceive each factor as having on our lives (for good or bad) we make decisions about how to maintain our health.

Unfortunately, doctors and their patients tend to see health and illness rather differently Doctors are trained to identify illnesses and to treat them as individual entities, whereas their patients see health as a more global matter which governs their overall sense of well-being. Symptoms and other frank signs of illness are seen by patients in the context of how they interfere with the business of living. In other words, illness to most people has a lot to do with feelings.

Many studies show how people's feelings influence their sense of physical well-being. People who complain of poor physical health are often depressed, feel neglected, have a low morale, feel alienated and are less satisfied with life than those not reporting poor physical health. Also, it is clear from many studies that psychological ill health and distress lead to a very much greater use of all kinds of health services. So psychological factors influence not only people's views of their health but also how much they actually use health services.

The way we react to illness varies considerably with our personality type and from culture to culture. Some people are stoical in the face of illness, others matter-of-fact, and yet others hypochondriacal. Some people go straight to the doctor with the most minor of symptoms and others are reluctant to trouble him or her with even quite severe problems. The same person over quite a short time-span can react and behave in very different ways. Most studies of illness show that women go to doctors more readily and more frequently than do men. Just why this should be is not known. Perhaps there are real sex differences in many diseases (i.e. they are in fact more common in women); or women may have a lower threshold of tolerance to symptoms; they may be more likely to accept a symptom and seek help for it; they may be more interested in health; they may be more concerned that they keep well because of the considerable pressures on them to run and maintain family and home life; or they may be culturally conditioned to running (in a little-girl-like way) to an authority figure to sort out problems quickly. Whatever the reason–and it might be that none of these is correct–the difference is apparent very early. Studies have found that young girls use child-driven school health-care systems more than do young boys.

Wherever the truth lies, repeated research has shown that much of the disability associated with physical and mental illness is not the result of illness itself but rather the way the person responds to the condition and the way it is managed. For example,

a lot of the aggressive behaviour previously seen with schizophrenia has been shown to be a result of the way that schizophrenics were dealt with by the authorities rather than as a part of the disease itself.

There are quite dramatic social and cultural differences in the way individuals and groups define illness and respond to it. Studies carried out in the US have shown that Jewish and Italian patients, for example, have been found to respond to pain in an emotional way–tending to make much of it–whilst the English and 'Old Americans' are more stoical and clear-headed about it. Irish patients more frequently deny pain. Whilst Jews and Italians appear to react similarly to pain, their underlying cultures are different. Italian patients seek relief from pain and seem satisfied when the pain is relieved, but Jewish patients seem to be more concerned about the significance of the pain for their future health. So pain relief may be what Italians need most but reassurance about the future may be what is most needed by Jews. Clearly this kind of information is essential if one is to plan any kind of preventive health programme.

The large differences in health and illness behaviour between groups and cultures suggest that it must be learned. Research shows that Jews and Italians claim that their mothers were over-protective and over-concerned about their children's health and participation in sports and that they were constantly warned to avoid colds, fights and other threatening situations. Perhaps this kind of upbringing fosters a type of personality which is particularly concerned and even anxious about illness

First-born and only children are more likely to want the company of another person when they face stress in adult life – probably because they are so much more psychologically dependent than later-born children. This is interesting in the light of studies which show that early-born children use more medical services than do later-borns (in whatever size of family).

We have already seen that psychological manoeuvres that are going on, usually quite unconsciously, are much more complex. Illness behaviour is part of a well-defined social pattern and we all have our views of how doctors (them) and patients (us) behave. I firmly believe, to paraphrase Shakespeare, that, 'All the world's a surgery and all the doctors and patients merely role-players.' It is my view that many of those going to their doctors are quite unconsciously playing a role – the sick role. Studies suggest that only about four out of ten people going to a general practitioner have anything physically wrong with them and that about 80 per cent of all ailments are self-limiting. So what are we all playing at?

Illness behaviour (adopting the sick role) is a very effective way of being relieved from social expectations, and is an excuse for failure, a way of obtaining privileges and sympathy, and so on. For those who

have few social ties, poor support and feel isolated, the medical system is a well-recognised and comfortable way of obtaining at least some of these. Thirty or more years ago perceptive doctors realised that what their patients came to them for was often quite unimportant but what it did was to establish a relationship with the doctor who would then confirm *them* in the sickness role. Doctors need people like this to make them feel wanted so that they, the doctors, can live out their role as health-givers. Unfortunately, many doctors do not understand this role-playing and as a result go along with their patients' endless demands for medical care. This results in numerous return visits, many if not most of which would be unnecessary if the patient's real problems and motivations had been perceived and adequately dealt with by the doctor at the first consultation.

Just as certain people unconsciously retreat into the sickness role because it is a release from unpleasant or unacceptable situations, others sacrifice their health to ambition, expediency or the good of others. Young parents overwork in the full knowledge of what they are doing, sometimes also going without things 'because of the children' and so on. The health of general practitioners is perhaps a good example. British GPs have alarmingly high rates of alcoholism, drug abuse, broken marriages, coronary artery disease and suicide, yet they presumably know all the answers. To some extent at least, they are choosing to sacrifice their own health in favour of that of their patients.

But closely allied to all this illness and sickness behaviour is society's concept of what is normal, and how it defines ill health. Mental illness for example, has been seen, at different times over the centuries, as demonic power, witchcraft and madness. The labels, the treatments and the social attitudes are all different and yet the 'reality' of the illness in question may well have been the same. Alcoholism is another example. When does social drinking become an illness? Sexual deviations and hypochondriasis or malingering are especially difficult to define yet somewhere along the line is a point beyond which sufferers could be said to be 'ill'. Certainly fashions and fads are all-important when trying to define behaviour of any kind, let alone illness behaviour. Forty years ago oral sex was a 'perversion' – today it is a fashionable pursuit that raises few eyebrows. Today we accept the fact that 30 per cent of the population have backache – it is 'normal' – and that thousands are killed on the roads every year. In developing countries parasitic diseases, infectious diseases, civil war or poverty may be similarly accepted as 'normal'.

The line between health and illness, then, can be somewhat arbitrary, and it is here that the real problems begin because it is not obvious whose responsibility health is. In our society we do not blame people for being ill – even if they themselves have played a part in the onset of illness. We have more ambivalent

feelings when it comes to VD and suicide attempts but even then most people do not come down too harshly on the 'ill' person.

Although we as a culture do not blame individuals for their illness we do expect them to do simple things to help themselves, and most of us think that ill people should co-operate with doctors to make themselves better. When looked at from a purist's point of view, much illness is preventable – indeed this book is about what we as individuals can take responsibility for – yet as a culture we have not yet arrived at the stage where we condemn people who do not co-operate, though there *are* signs that this is starting to happen with smoking-related diseases. Indeed, the anti-smoking campaign in certain western countries has taken something of a dramatic turn recently. But treating smokers as if they were lepers may not be the answer. It could, arguably, push those who would have smoked into other equally dangerous pursuits which fulfil their needs in the circumstances. In the final analysis everyone has the right to kill themselves in the way they choose. The truth is that most will almost certainly do so irrespective of government regulations and social prohibitions.

Perhaps the most influential work about health and the medicalisation of modern society is Ivan Illich's book *Medical Nemesis: The Expropriation of Health*. In Illich's view:

Health has ceased to be a native endowment each man is presumed to possess until proven ill, and has become the ever-distant promise to which one is entitled by virtue of social justice. . . .

In a morbid society the environment is so rearranged that for most of the time most people lose their power and will for self-sufficiency and finally cease to believe that autonomous action is feasible. The result is a morbid society that demands universal medicalisation and a medical establishment that certifies universal morbidity.

In a morbid society the belief prevails that defined and diagnosed ill health is infinitely preferable to any other form of negative label. It is better than criminal or political deviance, better than laziness, better than self-chosen absence from work. More and more people subconsciously know that they are sick and tired of their jobs and of their leisure activities, but they want to be lied to and told that physical illness relieves them of social responsibilities. They want their doctor to act as lawyer and priest. As a lawyer, the doctor exempts the patient from his normal duties and enables him to cash in on the insurance fund he was forced to build. As a priest the doctor becomes an accomplice for the patient, creating the myth that he is an innocent victim of biological mechanisms rather than a lazy, greedy or envious deserter of a social struggle for control over the tools of production. Social life becomes a give and take of therapy, medical, psychiatric, pedagogic or genetic.

In a sense we all control our own health–at least to some extent. We decide on certain health activities (even if they are as simple as cleaning our teeth) and avoid dangerous or illness-promoting situations (by driving carefully, for example), but the level at which we do this depends on all kinds of things, such as our perception of the amount of control we have over our surroundings (and thus our health), our personalities and our social class. Because class is a factor we as a society *can* influence, perhaps we should look at it in more detail because it has important implications for preventing disease.

Socio-economic status and health

However we define health, illness and prevention, it has to be said that health and disease are very unevenly spread throughout society. Put bluntly, people lower down the socio-economic scale have more disease and illness, and die younger, than those higher up. Analyses show that since 1910 those at the top of the social scale have consistently lived longer and are healthier, both mentally and physically. Not every disease is less common or causes less mortality among those better-off in socio-economic terms but this is generally so.

One of the best illustrations of health differences between socio-economic groups is the infant mortality rate. In 1975–7 the infant mortality rate in the world was 99 per thousand live babies, ranging from 11–20 per thousand in advanced countries to 100–200 per thousand in less developed countries. Within advanced countries, though, the variation between the figures for different socio-economic groups is remarkable, with those lower down the scale having three times the infant mortality of those higher up. Whilst British and US statistics show a consistent overall fall in infant mortality the differences according to position on the socio-economic scale still persist.

In the US socio-economic group is clearly related to racial composition since a large proportion of the non-white population lives in poverty. This is less true of the UK but there are close parallels. Infant mortality rates amongst the US black population are still double those amongst the white population – in fact the gap has widened over the last thirty years.

The crucial questions when thinking about prevention are to do with trying to understand why these discrepancies occur. Factors such as the mother's age, nutrition, literacy and use of the health services greatly influence the risks for her baby. 'High-risk' mothers are more likely to be at the extremes of reproductive age, to be unmarried, to have had several babies, and to have had miscarriages and still-births. There is also a higher incidence of prematurity and low-birth-weight babies in the less advantaged socio-economic groups. These two conditions carry an increased risk of infant mortality and of physical and intellectual handicap in the baby. Women from these groups also have two behavioural factors that act against the best interests of their babies – they are more likely to smoke, and to have below-normal weight-gain during pregnancy.

I have used infant mortality as an example, but there are many other sets of statistics that show how much more commonly diseases occur in the less advantaged sections of society. Infectious diseases are more common, possibly because the poor may be living in conditions which make infections more likely and lower their resistance to them. As recently as 1972 the mortality rate for TB among British men was ten times as great lower down the social scale as it was

at the top. Better environmental conditions do not always act in favour of the rich though. People living in poor sanitary conditions acquire antibodies against poliomyelitis and hepatitis A virus early in life, whereas those living in clean conditions are vulnerable unless they are immunised.

When we look at chronic illnesses such as heart disease and cancer – the two biggest killers in the western world – the story is more confusing. The relationship between socio-economic group and heart disease, for example, has changed with time. A position towards the bottom of the scale seemed to 'protect' men from heart attacks in 1960 but today this advantage has largely disappeared. One UK study found that the direct relationship between socio-economic status and heart disease (those at the top of the scale having more heart disease) disappeared when each category was analysed for physical activity. Once, the kind of work a person did was what determined his or her level of physical activity, but with the coming of jogging, squash and other leisure-time sports this is no longer so.

There is also a relationship between socio-economic group and psychological well-being, whether one is rating subjective happiness, psychiatric symptoms, or first admissions to mental hospital. Studies show that certain neurotic conditions are commoner among those lower down the socio-economic scale. These groups are less likely to feel well in themselves, physically and psychologically. In a major US survey, groups lower down the socio-economic scale (mostly members of racial minorities) were consistently (60 per cent) more likely than those higher up the scale to report their health to be 'fair' or 'poor'. Reports of 'excellent' health increased with income–and people in the highest income group were more than twice as likely as those with the lowest incomes to report 'excellent' health.

The factors influencing these differences are very complex and far from completely understood. It is clear, though, that the influences determining an individual's health are many and varied, and are not always within his or her own control.

3 WHAT IS PREVENTION?

Preventive medicine is very difficult to define and today it is no longer acceptable to think simply in terms of preventing the occurrence of specific disease processes. With current trends to whole-person health there is a more wholistic approach which involves a more positive approach to preventive health care. Most people understand preventive medicine in terms of public health activities such as immunisation for children, the control of fresh water supplies, safe sewage disposal, an assurance that foods and drugs are safe and the detection and control of infectious diseases. These activities are routinely and effectively carried out by local health authorities in most western countries, and we tend to take them for granted. Today we face new problems of prevention, with chronic diseases and self-induced environmental hazards causing a substantial proportion of all illnesses and deaths.

Partly because of the way that preventive medicine has grown out of public health and sanitation, and partly because of the way that health care is centred on after-the-fact procedures, preventive medicine is poorly regarded within medical and health circles and most doctors simply pay lip-service to the concept. This statement is borne out by the fact that only 4 per cent of the total US medical expenditure goes on prevention and only 1.5 per cent of all that country's doctors are involved in full-time preventive medicine! The figures are not much better in other western countries.

The influence of preventive medicine is also obstructed by the fact that it needs little that modern technology has to offer and therefore appears to be outdated and simplistic. All of this limits its appeal to those doctors and other health-care professionals who are looking for drama in medicine rather than what is best for society as a whole.

Unfortunately, prevention also tends to be handicapped in another way. Because of the difficulties already mentioned those who do go into it become so frustrated at the small resources and slow progress that they tend to become somewhat evangelical in their zeal to get things changed, so that they alienate even some potential allies. As one expert put it: 'If there is one thing more difficult than submitting oneself to a regime, it is refraining from imposing it on other people.'

Preventive medicine can be divided

into three categories. *Primary prevention* involves the removal of causes so that the condition doesn't occur in the first place. Diseases related to smoking are obvious examples here: stop people smoking (primary prevention) and the smoking-related diseases disappear. *Secondary prevention* picks up disease before symptoms occur. This is the essence of health screening which, by detecting disease early, can prevent the development of more serious manifestations of the disease. Detecting previously undiagnosed high blood pressure is a good example of this kind of prevention. *Tertiary prevention* involves the management of diagnosed disease in such a way as to prevent or limit the development of a disability or to prevent the person dying prematurely. The best example here is diabetes. Diabetics with good tertiary prevention can now live long and near-normal lives.

But what are we aiming for with all the prevention–eternal life? No. Most people, when asked, are happy to settle for a reasonably long lifespan spent in good health. In simple terms medicine over the last hundred years or so has shifted deaths in early years to later life. However, despite a four-fold increase over the last century in the number of men living to be 100 and a nine-fold increase in the number of women living to that age, the proportion is still only one in 1,000 and 5 in 100 respectively. Suggestions that we could all live to 130 or more are as yet somewhat fanciful but we can now reasonably aim to live to about 85 or 90, with few

of us dying of disease under the age of 70. If we are to achieve this we have to attack cancers and heart disease, which account for more than half of all life lost under the age of 85, and those few diseases that stand out as special cases. These include diseases associated with the excessive use of alcohol, addictive drugs, motorcycles, cigarette smoking in women and large numbers of sexual partners.

But being healthy is not just a matter of what you do or do not do. It seems that health and long life are often a gift bestowed on a person at conception when they inherit good genes. With the combined effects of healthy habits and good luck many people's health can be maintained for years with good medical care taking the edge off diseases and accidents.

Until fairly recently, living longer usually meant accumulating more and more disorders, diseases and disabilities which, together with social isolation, poverty, failing memory, a loss of purpose, reduced family contacts and other limitations, have led to a vast increase in the numbers of elderly people living out the last years of their lives in residential care.

Younger people, seeing this as a depressing future for themselves, are beginning to get concerned–and rightly so. A questionnaire in a Swedish magazine in 1971 asked readers how they most wanted to die. A large majority said they wanted to pass away quickly and without worrying. So, ironically, what we are all trying so desperately to prevent–heart disease–appears to be exactly what, in one form, many of those 'at risk' most want to die from. But as in the old monk's prayer–'Dear Lord, give me patience; but give it to me *now*'–we can't choose when this sudden and quick form of death will take us. None of us would mind dying like this in our seventies or eighties but the tragedy is that increasing numbers of men in their forties or fifties are losing their lives in this way.

Some people worry about the long-term effects of a population with an ever increasing proportion of ever older people, and they have a point which has to be taken seriously by those who try to prolong life at almost any price. Viewed in the widest possible socio-economic perspective, the gradual move from a three-generation society to a four-generation one is likely to produce increasing strain between the productive and reproductive groups and those who are mainly 'takers' from society. Our industrial society cannot find enough jobs for its working-age people, let alone the elderly. So we could soon see countless millions of pensioners in the western world with many years of life to live but with nothing to do.

No one would dispute the benefits preventive medicine has brought in the earliest part of life but, some people are asking, should it be allowed to do the same for the other end of the life scale–at least in those societies where already those who reach middle age tend to live into their eighties? All of this may appear somewhat pessimistic but it could

well be that within the reasonably near future the elderly will be taking up so much of the nation's resources that curative medicine for the productive sector of society will be seriously put at risk. There are those who would say that this is already happening, at least to some extent.

What can be done to prevent disease?

The opportunities for prevention can be classed under eight headings.

1 Social improvements

As we saw earlier, the sober truth is that the poor are much less healthy than the more advantaged socio-economic groups and do not benefit nearly so much from medical advances. A book like this is no place to go into this in any great detail but suffice it to say that the resources that would be needed to make an impact on the health of poor families are so great that they could not come solely out of the 'health' kitty.

2 Modification of lifestyle

If no one smoked, death from all cancers would fall by a third; almost all long-term lung diseases would disappear; several diseases of the arteries would be eliminated; about one quarter of heart attacks would be prevented and there would be a small reduction in perinatal mortality. Some of these benefits can be obtained by switching to low-tar cigarettes. Preventive measures include better health education, further restrictions on tobacco advertising, the restriction of smoking in public places, and increased taxation of tobacco. All of these have been proved to work both alone and in combination.

Eating a more healthy diet understandably has beneficial effects and we look at this in more detail on page 70. Any diet that helps people slim, increases dietary-fibre intake and reduces calorie and fat intake will reduce the risk of cancer of the endometrium and gall bladder, may reduce the risk of breast and colon cancer, and may reduce the risk of cancer generally in a number of ways. There is little doubt from several studies that being overweight makes it more likely that you will get *a* cancer. The avoidance of obesity also reduces the risk of high blood pressure and diabetes, and can reduce the risk of having a heart attack. It reduces the likelihood of suffering from a hiatus hernia, other hernias, degenerative arthritis of the knees and many foot problems. Most people say that when they lose weight the quality of their lives improves dramatically because they feel better, look better and enjoy life more.

Alcohol produces effects not only on the drinker but on those whom he or she influences while drunk. Alcohol consumption is rising and although a little alcohol has been claimed to protect against heart disease most people who drink find it difficult to draw the line and end up having too much.

Too little physical activity results in obesity, high blood pressure, high cholesterol and too much insulin. The benefits of regular, controlled physical activity are now beyond doubt. Perhaps the most valuable is the effect it has on weight loss. People who take regular exercise find it easier to lose weight and to keep it off. This occurs because the body's metabolic rate continues to remain high even after the person stops taking the exercise. There are also suggestions that the sense of well-being that exercise produces means that people who would otherwise have eaten because they felt 'low' now have no urge to do so.

3 *Protection against injury*

Death rates on the roads are now below the levels of the 1930s despite the vast increase in traffic, but car accidents are still far too common. Worldwide the traffic death toll is calculated to be 250,000. Given that there are about forty times as many injuries as actual deaths it is easy to see how big a problem road-traffic accidents are.

But injuries don't just take place on the roads. Accidental injury, which includes homicide and suicide, is the fourth commonest cause of death in the US and is the commonest cause of death under the age of 35 in the UK. In the US more people are killed as a result of accidental injury under the age of 40 than by all other causes put together. About one in three of the population of the US each year has a non-fatal injury bad enough to cause them to lose a day or more of normal activities and a fifth of these injuries put the person in bed for at least a day. In the developing countries also, injury is a very common cause of death.

We shall look at accident prevention in more detail on page 108.

4 Control of infections

Many of the most common infections around the world can now be prevented by vaccination. The notable exception is malaria. Public health programmes, if strictly adhered to, can prevent epidemics of almost all the childhood and most adult infections. It is almost impossible to prevent new influenza-virus epidemics, and genital herpes, gonorrhoea and AIDS are proving a problem to prevent, but almost certainly vaccines will eventually be developed for these conditions. While the scientific world seeks pharmaceutical answers to these sexually transmitted diseases a return to a less sexually promiscuous lifestyle would help control the epidemics of some of them. There are signs that this is already happening – especially in the US.

With the shrinking world we now live in it is hardly surprising that quite exotic diseases are seen in westernised countries from time to time. TB is still commonplace in many areas of the world and can easily be caught by a non-immune person and brought back home.

5 Control of pollution

There are relatively few areas in which pollution could be more rigorously controlled than it is now. Air-pollution controls would save some lives; reduced cigarette smoking in public would reduce the risk to the non-smokers present; and the elimination of certain food colourings and additives would almost certainly be beneficial; there is some evidence of carcinogens in certain western water supplies and so on.

It is easy to list the many possible pollutants, but Sir Richard Doll, the distinguished British epidemiologist, has estimated that pollution of all types probably is not responsible for more than 1 per cent of all total cancers, for example. The cost of eliminating *all* such pollutants would, he claims, be too high. The effects of lead on mental activity in children are difficult to assess, but it makes sense to take the lead out of petrol as many countries have already done.

6 Mass screening of populations

One of the most successful stories of modern prevention has been the reduction of perinatal mortality. This has come about by persuading mothers to go for ante-natal care. But there are still mothers who receive little or no ante-natal care and thus are at greater risk of losing their babies, and in the UK the perinatal mortality rate is nothing to be proud of when compared with other developed countries. The screening of pregnant mothers for fetal abnormalities is a powerful preventive tool, but only if the mothers are prepared to have an abortion if the baby is abnormal. We shall look at screening in more detail on page 49.

7 Preventive medication

For decades now iodine has been put into table salt (to prevent thyroid disease), fluoride into drinking water (to prevent dental decay) and vitamins into margarine (to prevent rickets). This kind of mass medication is open to debate if only because it exposes the majority of the population who do not need the medication to its, often unknown, hazards. The provision of preventive medications or vitamins for specific groups at risk (such as those mothers who have a history of spina bifida children) is quite another matter because the individuals are strongly motivated to do something positive and have the choice whether to do so or not. Trials are now under way in many such areas of preventive medication including the prevention of bone thinning and fractures in post-menopausal women (by giving oestrogens and/or calcium), dietary supplements to act as anti-cancer agents, and aspirin to reduce the risk of heart attacks and strokes in everyone over 50.

8 Stress reduction

There is no doubt in any doctor's mind that stress plays a crucial role in many of today's illnesses, both physical and mental, though just how big a role stress plays in any particular disease is difficult to assess. Undoubtedly the link between 'type A' behaviour (competitive and aggressive) and heart attacks is real enough and the links between stress and high blood pressure, certain bowel disease, asthma, eczema, migraine and many other conditions are all too obvious to many people. We look at stress control in more detail on page 80.

Each of these eight headings points to what the preventive medical world calls 'risk factors'. If you want to reduce your chances of getting a particular disease, or indeed of being unwell at all, you have to be aware of what you personally are at risk from. Only by knowing what your risk factors are can you understand the causes and set about possible risk-reducing activities.

Risk appraisal generally depends on the study of probability tables. The Robbins-Hall method of risk-factor analysis (probably the best devised so far) looks at the top twelve to fifteen causes of death, because between them they account for about two-thirds of all deaths. By comparing treated and untreated groups of people in any specific disease category a doctor can find out which intervention produces results, and can work out a 'health appraisal' age to compare with the patient's actual chronological age. Let's look at an example.

Take a 41-year-old man with a blood pressure of 180/94 mmHg and a cholesterol level of 220 mm/dl who is overweight by 15 per cent and is a non-diabetic. He also smokes twenty cigarettes a day, has eighteen drinks a week, drives 15,000 miles a year, wearing a seat-belt 75 per cent of the time, and exercises moderately each week. He has no family history of heart disease and his parents are both over 60 years old. Using the Robbins-Hall method this man's total personal risk is 9,680. This means his chances of dying during the next 10 years are 9,680 in 100,000.

If he stops smoking, has his mild blood pressure treated and cuts his drinks to six per week, he can reduce his risk from 9,680 to 4,992. This large reduction is possible because by changing his behaviour in this way he can reduce his risk of heart attack considerably. It would also reduce his risk of cirrhosis, lung cancer, stroke and car accidents.

This man's total personal risk before he starts his personal preventive programme translates to a risk age of 46.5 years compared with his actual age of 41 years. By using personal preventive measures he can reduce his personal risk age to 40. The Robbins-Hall printout would show that this man's level of high blood pressure elevates his risk of heart attack by 150 per cent, and that his smoking plus his raised blood pressure increase his stroke risk. His drinking increases his chances of both liver cirrhosis and of having a car accident.

Most people know that if they stopped smoking, drank very moderately, ate the right food, exercised regularly and got enough sleep they would live longer and be healthier. Yet most of us continue to do all or most of the things we know we shouldn't. We see why this should be on page 41. True, *mortality* rates for heart disease and strokes have been falling in the US (heart attack deaths have fallen by 30 per cent over the last 10 years), but the number of people having heart attacks has not fallen as dramatically. Clearly at least some of these improved statistics are the result of better medical care, once a heart condition is apparent.

In the face of unhealthy pressures all around us it would be surprising if self-help methods unfailingly succeeded in improving the health of the individual. But how reasonable is it to place the burden on the individual when cigarette and alcohol advertising continue to bombard him or her from all sides? Can children be brought up to take control of or responsibility for their health when they learn so soon that what they try to do has so little impact? And supposing our man described above did cut out all his vices, what would he do instead – and might it not be even more hazardous?

So if individuals often cannot help themselves, how about the State lending a hand? This only works if the public is ready for the legal restrictions. Prohibition in the US did not work because people weren't ready for it, yet penalties for driving when under the influence of drink and for not wearing seat-belts are apparently acceptable in the UK and elsewhere. Increased taxation on illness-producing habits works at least to some extent but research shows that real devotees simply give up other things (a healthy diet perhaps) to fund their addictions. Anyway, how far does a government have the right to impose its will on the masses? In other words there is a considerable ethical dilemma involved in preventive medicine. Should I be allowed to behave in any way I want, even if it affects others adversely? We all want to see laws such as those that prevent drunken driving, but a balance must be struck between measures like this, which benefit us all, and the reasonable liberty of the individual And then there is the question of individual freedom to act in ways that *don't* directly affect others. It could be argued that the man who smokes heavily in private is doing society a favour in several ways. First, he is relieving the society of the cost of the drugs that might otherwise be consumed if he were not smoking and being tranquillised by his cigarettes. Second, his habit will kill him younger, and relatively quickly, by lung cancer (the average lung cancer victim lives only eight months from the discovery of the tumour) or heart attacks–the other major smoking disease. Both kill very quickly, so reducing his capacity to be a burden on society and its medical facilities. Lastly, he will probably not live long enough to collect his old age pension–another saving to society.

Looked at coldly, then, a case could be made for allowing people to do what they want if it kills them quickly and prematurely, if only because we have so many old people and too large a burden of chronically ill already.

My approach to prevention, then, is not a dictatorial one, mainly because after fifteen years of preventive medical experience I know that forcing it on people does not work. In the last analysis everyone must be free to choose his or her way of death–and most of us will do so whatever governments or health educators do. Some kill themselves with overwork, some on the road, some through their hobbies, while others smoke themselves to death, and so on. What I as a health educator can do is to make them aware of the dangers of these harmful pursuits so that they have a choice. I never tell a patient to stop smoking. That's his or her choice. I don't expect patients to tell me to stop driving my car–and that could kill me. What I *do* do is to lay before them the facts as they are currently understood about the harmful effects of smoking. The choice is then theirs.

The difficulties come when another person's behaviour affects my life and health adversely, and most of us agree that the State should step in here. But here again the problems are formidable. Should the State, for example, pass laws to prevent any form of extramarital sexual activity on the basis that it harms innocent third parties? Such a suggestion seems preposterous yet we happily go along with similar laws that stop people polluting the air of innocent third parties with cigarette smoke on far flimsier evidence.

Occasionally the forced introduction of one preventive measure has unexpected beneficial effects elsewhere. The best example was the introduction of the 55 mph speed limit in the US in 1974. During the 1970s life expectancy went up by 2.7 years in the US and much of this was the result of the slower driving and reduction in car accidents. In 1973 the death rate was 4.17 deaths per 100 million miles travelled; by 1976 this figure had dropped to 3.3 – an all-time low. So what started as a way of saving fuel because of the oil crisis ended up substantially reducing road deaths.

Unfortunately, not all illnesses and diseases are as clear-cut as are accidents. The vast majority of modern illnesses are still poorly understood. This makes preventing them difficult, if not impossible. It is probably this confusion within the medical profession over the causes of many conditions that has held back so many preventive efforts in the past. These debates among the professionals have confused the public who, in turn, have often wished a plague on all their houses and gone on living as normal until the facts are incontrovertibly established.

All of this has given prevention a bad name but the medical profession is not wholly to blame. The 'simple' diseases have all been conquered and we are now left with highly complex conditions which involve many factors – the majority of which are beyond the influence of medicine in its present sense. Almost any real advance in preventive medicine now involves major social rethinking on a scale every bit as adventurous as the major sanitation programmes of the last century. The difference is that no one wanted foul drinking water and open sewers but convincing people they don't want junk food, cigarettes and alcohol is a task of a very different order – because they *do* want them. The complexity of the modern world is now so great that any mass change in public behaviour would have repercussions on employment, social structure and many other areas as well as simply health.

As the prevention of many conditions is so difficult because of a lack of knowledge of how to achieve it, it has been very difficult to get the ball moving in much simpler areas such as screening for disease. In the current tight economic climate no one wants to waste money on preventive programmes that do not in fact prevent anything. Decision-makers and consumers would rather carry on with curative medicine they know works, even if it is obvious that this is a second best to preventing the illness in the first place. Money is cheerfully allocated to curative services but not to preventive ones. This attitude is commonplace throughout the western world and is especially obvious in the US and other countries where health insurance pays most medical costs. It has arisen mainly because modern medicine sees itself as being about curing people or at least dealing with their symptoms, but also partly, as we have seen, because the effectiveness of many preventive measures is difficult to prove. This situation will almost certainly change in the next decade or two as costs of this kind of 'health' care spiral out of most societies' abilities to pay for them. There is also growing interest among ordinary men and women in a more wholistic approach to living generally and this too will hasten a serious interest in prevention. But until the medical profession accepts this approach, no real change will occur.

There are, fortunately, signs that this is happening. With the present interest in 'alternative' medical practices such as osteopathy, acupuncture, herbal medicine, homoeopathy and healing, increasing numbers of people are by-passing the orthodox profession to go straight to an alternative practitioner. Many, if not most, of these stress the importance of prevention so it cannot be long before this rubs off on orthodox doctors. The current fashion for all things 'natural' and the growth of interest in do-it-yourself health all favour a growth of preventive medicine and a reduced reliance on the medical profession as suppliers of health. The current medical system in the West is a sickness service not a health service, but things could change very fast. Medical unemployment is now a serious problem in almost every western country so doctors are having to make greater efforts and change their ways of thinking about prevention, or more people will go elsewhere.

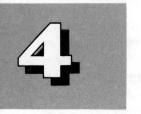

WHAT CAN INDIVIDUALS ACTUALLY ACHIEVE?

Preventive medicine is probably imbued with more rhetoric and noble ideas than any other medical speciality, but amongst all the high-flown talk one assertion stands out—that people ought to be more responsible for their own health. This argument suggests that if we were all more 'responsible' and 'pulled ourselves together' we could prevent much illness both in ourselves and others. I personally find this a naïve and unhelpful way of looking at prevention because it puts too great a burden of responsibility on millions who can't cope with it. If they then 'fail' they are double losers—not only do they have the health problems to deal with but they are deemed to have brought them upon themselves.

The idea that personal lifestyle has implications for health is very old indeed. It underlines many of the injunctions of the Old Testament. The golden rule formulated by Juvenal (a healthy mind in a healthy body) was intended to achieve both physical and psychological well-being simultaneously. Even during the eighteenth and nineteenth centuries when real strides were being made in preventive public health measures, novels of the day suggested that it was the responsibility of individuals to look to their own well-being.

The idea that an individual can prevent the occurrence of illness is not new, then. What we now understand better is that human behaviour is not simply a matter of what people can will themselves to do—it is the combined result of forces acting from within (many of which are unconscious) and without. So today we can look in a very different way at how human behaviour affects health. No longer can we condemn people on 'moral' grounds for their lack of control, or whatever, and punish them, however unconsciously, with ill health. Also, the almost total control of mass infectious illnesses and the increase of chronic diseases as a cause of death makes the whole business of prevention even more important because the latter are so difficult or even impossible to cure.

This has all led to a generally held assumption that the next great milestone in medical advances will be a wholesale change in personal health-related behaviour brought about by a better understanding of human beings as a result of the behavioural sciences. If this is so and if it is to form the basis of preventive medicine for the future we ought to look at it more closely.

We have looked at health and illness behaviour in some detail already (see page 22). Obviously an understanding of the subject is crucial if we are really to make any progress in preventing anything. The key study in this area has resulted in the Health Belief Model which attempted to explain how and why people used preventive services such as TB screening, dental check-ups and vaccinations. Since this model was first developed in the US in the 1950s numerous studies have classified areas touched on by the Model.

The Health Belief Model, simply stated, proposed that in the presence of certain triggers to take health action the likelihood of action actually being taken depends on the person's belief about the seriousness of the health condition, his or her susceptibility to it, the efficiency of the proposed action and the difficulties he or she might encounter in attempting to carry out the action. This, then, is a rational model of human behaviour in which people respond to given situations with thought and with some knowledge.

Unfortunately, even this simple analysis of what happens is fraught with problems, and when we look at a specific example it begins to fall apart. For example, studies have found that women who are relatively young and well educated and have higher incomes are more likely to hold beliefs that are appropriate to taking action to have a cervical smear

test than are women with less education and lower incomes. It is obviously not satisfactory to rely on any particular group's own perception of health risks and the advisability of preventive action. The facts, alas, are often that the very groups who are least able to perceive the value of a preventive measure are those most at risk.

The next challenge then is to understand why people believe what they do and to try to find out how their attitudes can be changed to their advantage. In a free society this is a complex business because the people concerned have first to be convinced that a particular health goal is worth achieving. Many approaches are possible and an oblique one often works better than a full-frontal one. For example, many men happily take exercise because it makes them feel good yet they are blissfully unaware of the positive health benefits of their actions. These are purely a bonus to their sporting activities.

Obviously there are many factors that influence what we believe about preventive health and our behaviour when we do decide to act. Many of these factors can be related to socio-economic status. For example, studies have repeatedly found that people from the less advantaged sections of society receive less accurate health information and have more difficult access to health facilities, as well as being less inclined to take prevention seriously, defining illness differently, delaying longer in seeking health care and participating less in community health programmes. When they do approach the health-care system they are more likely to select sub-professionals, and once under the care of professionals are likely to be treated differently from middle and upper socio-economic groups. This is partly to do with definitions of health and disease. If a condition is not seen as a disease in a particular sub-fraction of society then the individual in that sub-fraction will not react to it as a disease. If everyone you know has tooth decay or dentures you come to see these as normal, just as some people see back pain as normal – and do nothing about it.

Millions of people are simply not tuned in to thinking about health as something that is, to a significant extent, within the control of the individual. In a major study in Wales in 1982 the researchers did in-depth interviews with forty-one women to find out what their views were about the causation of diseases and who was 'responsible' for illness. When asked for the main reasons for illness the top five categories the women gave were all essentially outside their individual control and included environmental factors such as: the weather; heredity; individual susceptibility; germs, bugs and infections; and stress and worry. Most of the women were clearly thinking about short-term illness. (Indeed most people *do* think like this when asked to think about disease.) They put low down on the list causes such as diet, hygiene, and 'way of life'. When questioned about individual behaviour they stressed the importance

of being 'run down' and thus vulnerable to illness. Illness was something that attacked from outside, and people who ate well, exercised and didn't abuse their bodies were in a much better position to 'fight off' germs effectively. For many, this was the extent of the link between their behaviour and resistance to illness.

Because it became evident that some of the women felt guilty for having allowed themselves to become ill the researchers looked at their willingness to accept blame for their illness. The researchers found that readiness to accept blame varied with the emphasis placed on the role of the individual behaviour in the theory of illness causation. The women fell into two main groups on the subject of blame. The first thought that one could be blamed if one didn't go to the doctor or delayed too long, and the second group thought that blame was reasonable if one put oneself into dangerous or risky situations through carelessness, stupidity or lack of forethought.

Perhaps the most interesting finding of the study was on responsibility. A 'responsible individual' according to the Department of Health is one who 'avails himself of the various preventive and screening measures offered by the health services; leads a healthy life and doesn't bother his or her doctor unnecessarily with trivia'. The reader will have noticed that this definition is all from the service-provider's point of view – the consumer's point of view is almost totally ignored. So failure to act responsibly is the patient's fault;

is the result of his or her ignorance, personality shortcomings, or whatever. The authors of the study point out how strange it is that so great an emphasis is generally put on encouraging people to lead a healthier life when they by and large (according to this research) perceive germs and other outside factors to be the cause of their illness. Because germs can affect anyone and presumably are not malicious, such people argue, the sufferer is by definition blameless. Another researcher in this field claims that the amount of personal responsibility people feel for their illness has declined (certainly for colds and chills), and thinks illness has become more social.

An interesting finding from the original study was that even those women who said that they thought lifestyle was the main cause of illness stressed the germ theory of illness when talking to their children about disease. Very few made any link between behaviour and illness to their children and not one used the opportunity to discuss the implications for health of different lifestyles. In another study of students asked about 'communicating their last illness to a five-year-old' it was found that very few accepted moral responsibility for the illness – a situation that has changed dramatically over the years. An earlier study had found that 'nearly every level from getting sick to recovery was a moral battle ground'.

One of the problems with the Department of Health's definition of a responsible individual quoted above is that it assumes that everyone has the ability and the resources to make the changes necessary to ensure a healthier life. This simply is not so. One study of family life in an urban setting found that there was very little in the way of perceived flexibility associated with the events of the working day and that there were also very high levels of routine. The researcher found that for the average working-class inner London family routine was strict and choiceless. People in this study described about 70 per cent of their day (excluding sleep) as routine and over 90 per cent as characterised by the absence of any real choice.

The Welsh study detailed above proves what many of us with experience in health education had already realised from bitter experience – that a substantial sector of society is resistant to change partly because the people in it do not share the authorities' view of personal responsibility for health. It is also clear that, attitudes apart, a certain sector of society lives in socio-economic circumstances that make the adoption of suggested healthier lifestyles impractical or irrelevant. Remember that in Ancient Greece, with all its lofty ideals of wholistic health, only the most privileged section of society could afford to subscribe to them.

So how can one go about changing personal health behaviour, especially among those whose motivation is low? One way is to control everything by law. Although many of us would resist this idea, our lives are already controlled far more than we often realise. Laws already control certain health behaviours, as we saw on page 35, but where legal regulation is not possible or advisable progress will depend on individuals altering their behaviour and the provision of skills to enable them to do so. Beliefs, however well founded, are not enough in health care and prevention. The individual needs to be motivated or he or she will not be able to make anything happen. The classical gag is that of the man who is so convinced that his smoking will kill him that he continues to smoke to relax him when he thinks about it.

Studies on persuasion show that beliefs usually precede motivation in the change process and that it is important to know the stage of knowledge any target group has reached before trying to persuade them to do something. Almost everyone knows that smoking is harmful to health yet millions are not sufficiently motivated to stop. Such people need to be convinced that the future health reward is worth the short-term pain of stopping smoking; that the unpleasant consequences of stopping smoking are not as bad as they think; and that there are advantages in the present to stopping smoking that they had not even thought of. Once such people realise these things they become motivated to *do* something about their smoking.

But many people are well-motivated yet haven't the behavioural skills to do anything about it. They need to learn skills to bring their smoking behaviour under conscious control.

Wherever we look around the world, and whatever the health practices we look at, the diffusion of information, ideas, beliefs and behaviour follows a predictable pattern that is roughly S-shaped. At first only a few people take up the new beliefs or practice while those around them discuss them and look out for the consequences. Soon others take them up at an increasing rate. Perhaps the major factor that determines this acceleration is the intensity of communication within the population. Self-help groups and other consumer networks are very powerful agents of change and research has found that people who make a public commitment to a health goal are far more likely to make the change required than those who don't. This is because we live within social networks in which we share beliefs, attitudes and behaviour patterns, and once groups become at all formalised people's loyalty to the group overrides almost any other consideration. The evidence that this is so has come from stop-smoking and weight-loss groups that have disbanded. Members backslide very quickly. Viewed this way, it seems that few of us act truly independently.

Whether in groups or in individual cases, fear is often used as a way of changing people's attitudes, motivation and behaviour. Making people afraid of certain consequences of their actions is cruel, though, unless at the same time they are told how to protect themselves from the feared result. Some so-called sex education, especially in schools, has in the past done little more than induce in the recipients a terror of VD. This sort of scare tactic alone obviously isn't enough–it does nothing to tell youngsters about how to handle their emerging sexuality, being limited to stressing the horrors of what might happen if they do have sex. Similarly, showing people pictures of lung cancers has only the most temporary effect on smoking habits.

Persuasion methods, whether they are face-to-face or through the mass media, are really only successful if they are accompanied by specific opportunities for putting more beneficial behaviour into action. Various studies have shown that mass media campaigns can alter beliefs and to some extent motivation but changing behaviour involves building up skills in people, and this can be difficult whatever their social class or level of education.

So far we have looked mainly at rational and conscious behaviour. It is in this context that we can understand, for example, why for many of us turning on the TV is a signal to eat and drink. The relaxing behaviour of the TV watching triggers another relaxing (self-pleasuring) activity– eating–and the two are seen as enhancing each other.

However, there is another whole side to human behaviour–the unconscious mind. And this plays a vital role in understanding the prevention of illness. Much of my description of illness behaviour lower down the social scale arises from the study of unconscious attitudes. Few people,

in any socio-economic group, rationally argue through such things–they are simply an intrinsic part of their behaviour handed down from the unconscious minds of their parents. All of us are far more controlled by our unconscious minds than we realise. A good example I shall use to illustrate this point is the one of unwanted pregnancy.

To the logical, rational thinker there is no reason why, in the 1980s, any baby should be born unwanted, but the Family Planning Association estimates that about 200,000 of the 648,000 babies born in the UK in 1984 were 'unwanted', or at least unplanned. Contraception is available to all so why and how does this major preventive health programme fail so dismally? Surely someone who doesn't want a baby, doesn't have to have one, and can take steps to ensure that he or she doesn't? It is true that no method of contraception is absolutely 100 per cent successful (though the combined pill, properly used, is virtually so), but it is quite wrong to think of the majority of unwanted pregnancies as simply due to bad luck.

Some research shows that women having abortions are psychologically just like other women but have simply taken more risks or have used inefficient contraceptive methods. Other research suggests that this is too simple a view and that most of the women got pregnant to prove their love for their man, to add satisfaction to a relationship, or to secure a failing one. Some women were found to have got pregnant to punish themselves for sexual mis-demeanours or for a previous abortion. Sometimes it was to replace a dead child or a lost boyfriend. On investigation most of the 'bad luck' category can be reallocated to other causes. These include:

Depression

This can lead to carelessness over contraception and a hope that a baby will improve things.

Uncertainty over sexual identity

A few women have to prove that they are really female by having a baby.

To punish parents

A teenage girl often wants to punish her repressive parents, especially if they have implied that she is promiscuous when she is not. Some of the girls also see having a baby as a way of getting away from home.

Trying to trap an unwilling or hostile partner

This is much less common than it was.

Wanting some fun and freedom

A final 'fling' before 'settling down to middle age' is not an uncommon story in older women who have an extra-marital pregnancy.

Deliberate non-contraception

A conscious failure to practise effective contraception is remarkably common. Many women either don't like the method of contraception they are using, or really want to get pregnant, however unconsciously, or follow a moral or religious code that bans contraception.

Personality problems.

Women who seek abortions are found to have different views on sex compared with those who go through with their pregnancies. Abortion-seekers often don't see themselves as instrumental in their unplanned pregnancy.

Changes in circumstances after conception

An example of this would be the collapse of a relationship.

Partner factors

These are not all that common but must be considered. Some men deliberately get their partner pregnant to test their own fertility; to try to secure the relationship; to give themselves added personal status; to give the woman something to worry about; because of an inability to keep away from intercourse during unsafe periods; because of a weak personality; or because of a refusal to let the woman use oral contraception (a virtually 100 per cent safe method), supposedly on religious or medical grounds but sometimes really because they fear her fidelity or the demands for sex she might make on them, and so on.

Psychosexual problems

Sexuality is simply one aspect of a person's personality and women who get pregnant when they know they shouldn't often have some kind of psychosexual problem of which they may be unaware. The types of psychosexual disorder involved are numerous. An example of one of the commoner ones is a woman who believes that reproduction is the only justification for sexual pleasure. Such women may have had several babies yet deny that they are interested in sex. A second category includes those women who unconsciously believe that sex is sinful and that pregnancy is a punishment for their sin. This means that there must be a risk of pregnancy if they are to enjoy sex. Other women believe that sex is something done to them by a man and is therefore something for which they have no responsibility, so they don't bother with contraception because to do so would be a contradiction. Many young women who believe that love is the only justification for sex refuse contraception until they are sure of the man (as a kind of denial that they are having sex) and get pregnant in the intervening time. Some women who don't accept their sexual drives deny them consciously yet unconsciously try to indulge them (by getting drunk, losing control and then getting pregnant, for example). A small proportion of women cannot tolerate any sort of contraception because they feel guilty enjoying any form of sexual pleasure. Some women are so filled with shame about their sexual drives that they don't seek contraceptive advice. Another common fear is that to accept effective contraception is to open the floodgates to promiscuity. Such women (especially when they are unmarried) refuse all contraception and then get pregnant. Some women are unconsciously incited to pregnancy by their mothers (who want a baby for themselves) but then regret the conception when it has occurred.

Lastly there is the teenage girl who has just started having intercourse. Such adolescent girls frequently refuse to accept that their status has changed and even though they are not virgins can't bring themselves to accept the fact and continue to live with the fictitious belief that they are virgins. Many such 'part-time virgins' say that they are better able to keep up the lie to their parents and themselves that they *are* virgins if they don't use contraception. Such a girl believes she is still a virgin (albeit a part-time one) and for this reason doesn't really need contraception. Such a delusion in a part-time virgin unfortunately leads, all too often, to unwanted pregnancies.

Clearly an apparently simple thing like an unwelcome pregnancy is in fact enormously complex, and the unconscious mind plays a substantial part in almost all the mechanisms I have outlined. Consciously the woman says she doesn't want to be pregnant. Contraceptive services are one of the most widely publicised and available of all the preventive services, yet still unwanted pregnancies abound.

Similar situations operate in all kinds of other health areas–not just those to do with sex. At certain times in our lives we might have an unconscious need to be ill as an escape from something or as a way of gaining attention or being cared for. A smoker may have quite unconscious needs for oral gratification, as does many an over-eater and no matter how good the preventive medical information is, nor how good his or her motivation, little progress can be made until the individual can confront and understand the underlying psychological drives that make him or her smoke or eat. Similarly, a man with a poor sense of his male self-esteem who smokes because he considers it manly to do so may be quite unable to stop smoking until this part of his personality can be satisfied in other ways.

It is only by confronting the psychological realities outlined in this section that it is possible to begin to understand why it is that even in the face of good information and motivation, most of us find it difficult or impossible to modify our behaviour in a way which prevents disease. And in this respect social class has little or no part to play–we are all ruled to a variable extent by unconscious motives and drives over which, by definition, we have no control until they are brought into the conscious mind and confronted.

Whilst we frequently hear that 'prevention is better than cure' hardly anybody behaves as though he or she believes it and it has now become such a piece of fashionable cant that

it should be relegated to the waste-bin along with 'health is better than wealth' and other such empty phrases. Not until the medical and health educational fraternity come to terms with the reality of people's health needs will prevention ever be anything other than a subject of lofty rhetoric.

What people do about their health depends more on what needs they feel they have than upon what they know. So the best doctor-patient relationship stems from a real understanding of the patient's needs and perceptions of the situation rather than from a doling out of knowledge from one who 'knows' to one who 'doesn't'. So it is that in the medical profession as currently organised health-*directed* needs can be coped with but health-*related* needs can't. As we move away from the essential interventions of crisis medicine towards prevention, the importance of attaining health diminishes for the individual and other more pressing everyday needs take over; doctors, because they are health-*directed*, appear to be of less value because what is needed is someone who is health-*related*. Both epidemiological and clinical studies show that there are almost no areas of human behaviour that are not related to health, so in this sense preventive medicine takes in all of a person's life; yet doctors are trained to see the person through a narrow slit–that afforded us by his or her symptoms. A lot of health education has tended, often with moralistic overtones, to convert health-related to health-directed behaviour. The answer to the prevention of diseases is not to medicalise life but to be more aware of the un-healthful aspects of it and to modify them.

Unfortunately, the sickness-centred health-care system of the western world has produced a love-hate relationship between professionals and the end users. Few people choose to go to their doctor unless they have what they perceive to be a problem. This makes the medical profession moppers-up of ailments and dealers in 'problems'. Doctors and the allied health professions are thus seen as an unfortunate necessity that one keeps away from until absolutely necessary.

This kind of thinking does nothing to generate positive preventive health behaviour. It is an ironic but predictable conclusion to say that doctors are almost the worst people to be saddled with the responsibility for preventive services. What is needed is a new profession which would be much less illness-centred and much more alive to the realities of the needs of the community in which they work. Individuals know what is important to them and their community, yet so much of the time preventive efforts have tried to superimpose some quite alien behaviour or perception on them.

We have seen in this section how important group influence is, and experience shows that people don't see themselves as potential 'road accident victims', 'VD sufferers' or whatever. What appear to work better are programmes aimed at groups, such as teenagers, pregnant mothers, the elderly or whatever. Within these cohesive groups, peer-group pressure can be used creatively to implement changes, and change is more likely to occur as one piece of preventive behaviour interacts with others to produce a lifestyle that tends to prevent disease rather than produce it.

5 SCREENING

Screening specific groups of people who are either totally without symptoms or who have symptoms that prompt a search for disease in its earliest stages has been a part of preventive medicine in the UK for about seventy years, since the regular examination of schoolchildren was first introduced on a national basis. Shortly afterwards – during World War I – pre-natal care for mothers and the medical examination of young babies were recommended and soon became commonplace. In 1943 mass X-ray screening for tuberculosis started nationally. The idea behind this was not only to find people with the disease and treat them but to remove them from contact with others, so limiting the spread of the disease. Today, the importance of infectious diseases has lessened and most screening programmes are on the lookout for degenerative or potentially chronic conditions. But why should people want to be screened for diseases they don't have?

Perhaps the most widespread form of general health screening in the adult population is the insurance medical for a job, a mortgage or a life-insurance policy. Naturally the insurance company wants to try to reduce the odds in this gamble. Put simply, the policy-holder is betting the company that he or she will die and that it will have to pay up. The company, on the other hand, is betting that the policy-holder will live – at least until all the premiums are paid. This kind of screening protects the insurance company and ensures that they win more 'bets' than they lose. It does nothing for the health of the individual.

The second reason for screening is to protect other people in the com-munity. The control of infectious diseases and the health screening of people who work dangerous machinery are two good examples. Again the main intention is not to protect the individual screened.

In the USA, and to a lesser extent in other westernised countries, screening has become a fashionable alternative to personal health services. Millions of people every year go through a broad batch of screening tests and procedures *instead* of seeing a doctor. Abnormal results then ensure that they get to see a doctor. People in the US have been brought up to think of the 'annual physical' as an essential part of preventive health care but the mood of experts is changing on this. It is now thought that healthy young people (under 40) need only have a thorough medical check-up every five years – not yearly as was recommended in 1947 by the American Medical Association. The concept of even a five-yearly check-up from this age is alien to most British people. After the age of 40 more frequent checks are recommended in the US, and the table on pages 58–9 summarises the age and frequency recommended for different screening procedures by various experts in the field of health screening.

The fourth reason for screening someone is to obtain a 'healthy' baseline of data so that should anything go wrong with the person in the future better clinical judgements will be made. The best example of this kind of screening is an electrocardiogram on a middle-aged man.

The final reason for screening an apparently healthy population is to detect conditions that are not apparent and which the medical profession can hope to influence in a positive way. But screening large populations is very expensive and time-consuming, and has an effect on the people being screened, so it behoves us to ask some tough questions before deciding to spend vast amounts of money and other resources on what is at first sight unquestionably a 'good thing'. The first important question that has to be asked is:

Are screening procedures likely to pick up the diseases that really matter?

This is difficult to answer but an examination of the results of ten major industrial health examination programmes in the US found that less than half of the people who subsequently died from cancer had the condition diagnosed at a screening examination, and slightly fewer than two-thirds of those who died from heart disease were identified prior to developing symptoms of lethal heart disease. Even if we do agree that picking up some people who are at risk from such serious disorders, and treating them ahead of time is valuable, regular screening appears to be a rather insensitive tool for the early detection of serious diseases.

Will the treatment of a risk factor really have an impact on the development of the disease?

It is all very well knowing that someone has an increased likelihood of, say, having a heart attack or stroke if he or she has high blood pressure but prevention is more complicated. Reducing blood pressure brings a marked reduction in the risk of having a stroke but, it seems, a much smaller reduction in the risk of having a heart attack.

Will people act on the results of screening?

Results from screening procedures are of no value in themselves – they have to be acted upon by someone. Any smoker knows how difficult it is to stop and every fatty how difficult it is to slim.

The results of the many studies

that have examined how reliably patients take medication are sobering. Studies in Canada, for example, have found that 'ambulatory patients are unlikely to take more than 50 per cent of the prescribed medications they receive from clinicians and the amount of knowledge which a patient possesses about his or her illness has almost no relation to that patient's degree of compliance with therapeutic instructions'. So if people won't or don't take their medication or the advice the doctor gives, why bother to tell them what's wrong in the first place? A study of high-blood-pressure patients found that those who were told they had the condition, following screening, had more sickness absence from work than those who weren't told.

Do screening programmes really alter the outcome of disease?

Interesting research has come from the Kaiser-Permanante Group in California who randomly divided several thousand patients into two groups. The first group were encouraged to have regular health screening whilst the other used the medical services as and when they needed them. After seven years of study the results showed no advantage to those who were screened regularly – or rather no advantage for women and only a small one for men. Only men aged between 45 and 54 when they entered the trial showed differences in illness and absenteeism from work.

Perhaps of most significance is that of the 400 deaths occurring in the control group (those not given regular screening) during the experimental period only 15 per cent were judged to have been 'potentially postponable' with the best possible application of preventive medical treatment!

Are we evaluating screening tests properly?

Every disease has a natural clinical course and to a great extent the success doctors have with treatment depends on where in this process they catch the disease. Early diagnosis through screening will always appear to improve survival because screening will tend to detect patients in whom the disease has a long hidden (pre-clinical) stage. As a result conditions picked up during screening can expect to have a better outcome even if the treatment they receive has no effect at all.

Could screening actually be harmful in any way?

In our understandable desire to detect everything as early as possible it is easy to forget that screening has a potential for harm too. First, it costs an enormous amount in terms of both money and other resources to screen thousands or even millions of people, and the ratio of positive discoveries to cost can be very low indeed. This is closely linked to the fact that in a free society we cannot force people to be screened for most things. So it is that in certain conditions (notably cervical cancer) the people who come forward to be screened are the least likely to be at risk, while those who stay at home would be the most cost-effective group to be screened. In a society with finite resources for medical care – which is now the case in almost every country – such a 'waste' of money and resources must be a serious cause for concern.

Money spent on screening obviously has to come from somewhere and often it is diverted from curative services. This is all very well for those whose diseases are picked up early and successfully treated but what about those who are not treated for diseases only identified later? This raises all kinds of moral dilemmas for the medical profession and for society as a whole.

Next, it is worth considering the emotional, social and occupational harm done to people who think they are healthy but who are subsequently labelled 'ill' as a result of a screening procedure. Labelling someone with a disease has profound effects on his or her life. This would not be so bad if doctors could be sure of their labels but they often cannot because such labels are difficult to apply. Doctors disagree profoundly, for example, over significant levels of raised blood pressure, cholesterol and many other apparently straightforward parameters of body function. This means that one doctor will expend time and his or her patient's emotions investigating further a laboratory result which another would consider 'normal'. And none of this takes into account the false positives and false negatives that occur in any screening programme and which cause worry and complacency respectively. So it can be clearly seen from all this that simply detecting disease early is not necessarily enough. A World Health Organisation Report, recognising this as a real problem, says the following about screening programmes:

1. They must lead to an improvement in end results in those in whom a diagnosis is made (or in those around them in the community).
2. The therapy for the condition must have a favourable effect on its normal course – not simply bringing forward the date of the diagnosis but improving survival or function (or both).
3. There must be sufficient health services to ensure that diagnosis raised at screening can be properly confirmed and to provide meaningful medical care for the person.
4. People who have been diagnosed as having an abnormality must be prepared to go along with medical advice about what to do about it, or the whole procedure is a waste of time.
5. The long-term beneficial results must outweigh the long-term disadvantages.
6. The procedure must be cost-effective.
7. The problems produced by the disease that is being screened for must be large enough to make it worth while doing all the above. Clearly an extremely effective and cheap screening method for a trivial condition, however common, would be difficult to justify.

Having now injected a note of caution into the subject of health screening, we can ask what *is* worth doing in a preventive health context. Opinions vary, as you would expect, but there is little doubt that it is worth screening for the following seventeen conditions:

1. Abnormalities of growth and development in children.
2. Hearing loss.
3. Visual problems (acuity, squint, glaucoma).
4. Scoliosis (curvature of the spine).
5. Cardiovascular risk factors: hypertension, hyperlipidemia (high blood fats), diabetes, sedentary lifestyles, smoking and obesity.
6. Cancer (cervical, breast, large bowel, testicular).
7. Anaemia.
8. Kidney disease.
9. Sexually transmitted diseases (syphilis and gonorrhoea).
10. Menopause problems.
11. Alcohol and drug abuse.
12. Various diseases of the chest other than lung cancer.
13. Various conduction and rate abnormalities of the heart.
14. Sickle cell trait in the black population.
15. Rubella immunity in females.
16. Phenylketonuria in newborn babies.
17. Hypothyroidism in newborn babies.

Let's now look at how these can be screened for:

Physical examinations by a doctor

Many – if not most – people believe that they should have 'a thorough check-up' now and again. There is a widely held misconception that a doctor (usually a general practitioner) can do a kind of 10,000 miles service of everything that really matters and do it in a few minutes. This is totally untrue. Even a very lengthy clinical examination by a highly expert physician might well miss even quite obvious disease which cannot be picked up by his or her bedside diagnostic skills. The problem with such examinations, even if they are very well done, is that if given an 'all clear' patients imagine themselves to be well and may as a result actually take *less* care of themselves because their current lifestyle, they argue, appears to be doing them no harm.

Young children and the elderly need more regular professional examinations because they get ill more often and can go downhill very quickly once something starts. Physical examinations in middle age are more worth while than in younger people because of the higher rates of heart disease and cancer.

Obviously it makes sense to limit physical examinations to those periods of life at which they are most likely to produce results. A thorough physical examination at birth and periodically throughout early childhood makes good sense because so much is going on developmentally that it is reasonable to try to pick up abnormalities so that they can be dealt with quickly. It is probably sensible to have a physical examination every five years after this up to the age of 40 and then every other year up to 65.

Growth screening

The regular weighing and measuring of children enables certain conditions to be detected early and treated. Measuring a baby's head circumference is also a valuable screening procedure because it can alert the doctor to preventable conditions developing inside the skull.

Developmental screening

Used on babies and older children this appears to produce good results, but too little attention is usually paid to emotional and other non-physical parameters.

Blood pressure checks

Abnormal blood pressure is worth screening for from the age of 10–15 onwards. When it comes to adults, some experts recommend that every GP should use each occasion he or she sees a patient as an excuse to check the blood pressure and others claim every two years is enough.

Pap smear

This test for cancer of the cervix in women *is* valuable but the evidence about when it should be done is very confused. Most experts agree that the first test should be done when the woman becomes sexually active

or at 20 and should then be repeated within the next year. The various cancer and health bodies around the world have different recommendations but once every five years until the age of 65 or 70 seems to be a workable suggestion. To be really sure of not missing a treatable cancer a smear should be done every year but this is considered unworkable by most people, and most women seem loath to have one done this frequently. A sensible compromise would be every other year.

Pelvic examination

The American Cancer Society recommends a pelvic examination every three years from 20–40 and then annually after 40.

Breast examination

The American Cancer Society recommends a breast examination every three years between 20 and 40 and then annually after 40.

Mammography

X-rays of the breast for cancer are still the best method of detecting a lump that cannot be felt but they are expensive and expose the breast to radiation. Because of these disadvantages it is sensible to have a baseline mammogram done between the ages of 35 and 50 and then annually or every other year after the age of 50.

Hearing tests

Hearing should be simply tested for

at birth and then by audiology in older children. Hearing tests have been recommended every five years in adults until 65 and then every two years after that, but testing during middle life is usually a waste of time.

Vision testing

This is done as part of the pre-school examination and at regular intervals during childhood. Adult screening is recommended every five years to 65 and then every two years after that, but visual testing during the middle years is unnecessary unless the person complains of reading or visual difficulties.

Looking for squint

This is needed only for children and is done at 18 months of age and repeated several times up to the age of 6.

Tonometry

This is a simple, painless method of measuring the pressure of the fluid in the eyeball. It is valuable to be aware of this pressure because an early rise, if caught, can be treated and can save the person's sight. It is a test worth doing every two to five years after the age of 40.

Sigmoidoscopy (Looking inside the rectum or back passage)

Most cancers of the bowel lie within the view of a special instrument, called a sigmoidoscope. It is generally

considered sensible to have a sigmoidoscopy every three to five years following two negative examinations a year apart at age 50. Other experts recommend one examination at age 56 because this is the peak age for this cancer, which is the second commonest.

Testing the stools for blood

Because microscopic amounts of blood can be lost in the stools in people who have bowel cancers this can be a very good way of detecting such cancers early and certainly long before they start to produce symptoms. It is probably sensible to have such a test done every year after the age of 50.

Testing for anaemia

Recommendations for the screening of adults for anaemia range from every two to every five years. Women are particularly at risk because of having periods and childbearing. Many millions of people, women especially, are walking around sub-clinically unwell with anaemia yet remain unscreened. This is an easy and cheap test to do and the treatment is straightforward and inexpensive.

Blood sugar tests

Whether or not it is worth screening populations for their blood sugar levels to see if they are undiagnosed diabetics is controversial–mainly because there is no evidence yet that the early detection of diabetics without symptoms does anything to alter the long-term outlook. Some experts think that as the test is relatively cheap it is worth doing every five years until 65 and then every two years. Others feel that looking for sugar in the urine (another sign of diabetes) every five years is quite sufficient.

Screening for sickle cell trait

Certain high-risk populations (mainly black) should be screened prior to childbearing so that they can receive genetic counselling about the likelihood of having an affected baby. Some experts recommend that the test be done at the age of 10 years.

Checking for German measles (rubella) immunity

This disease, whilst not serious during normal life, can produce terrible handicaps in the baby of a pregnant woman who catches it. It is estimated that even with rubella vaccinations being widely available, about 15 per cent of women get to childbearing with no immunity to the disease. The most logical time for screening is just before childbearing age. Pregnancy should not be allowed to occur for three months after the immunisation. A girl who is not immune can be vaccinated in her early teens. Many authorities think that every pregnant woman should be routinely tested for antibodies to rubella.

Testing blood fat levels

High blood cholesterols are clearly associated with a risk of heart attack but blood triglycerides (another sort of fat) are not. Screening for cholesterols is recommended every five years from the late teens. They are not worth screening for past 65.

Syphilis tests

Three-quarters of all cases of undetected syphilis will eventually develop incurable 'tertiary' complications which are very severe indeed. The 'at-risk' group is the 20–50 range. Recommendations for screening vary greatly but it is probably sensible to do one test when the person becomes sexually active and every five years after that to age 50. Pregnant women should be screened for syphilis as a routine

Gonorrhoea tests

This is a disease without symptoms in 75 per cent of women and 10 per cent of men. Some people feel that screening is not warranted because the disease is relatively easy to treat, and because however well we screen we shall never be able to eliminate the disease from the population most at risk. Others recommend that yearly screening be done from the time a person becomes sexually active. Perhaps a good compromise is a test at the time of the first pelvic examination and then every five years to 44.

Screening for phenylketonuria

This disease, which can cause mental handicap if not detected and treated very early in life, is already routinely screened for at birth.

Chest X-rays

Because of the low cure rates of lung cancer (8 per cent survive 5 years, regardless of the stage of the tumour at detection), it is now no longer thought reasonable to do chest X-rays as a screening procedure. 'At-risk' populations should still be screened for tuberculosis though. Perhaps a baseline chest X-ray at 35 or 40 is sensible with a repeat at five- or ten-year intervals.

Electrocardiograms

It is useful to have a baseline ECG done at about age 35–40 with repeats every five to ten years.

Screening procedures that are definitely *not* worth doing routinely are barium enemas; barium meals; looking for cells in the sputum (spit); stress testing; lung-function tests; and biopsies of the lining of the uterus. All of these are, of course, useful diagnostic procedures in specific individuals.

Screening can be carried out in the community in general or it can be focused on specific sub-groups who are thought to be 'at risk'. As we have seen, when screening for cervical cancer, money is best spent on screening women from lower down the socio-economic scale because it is much more common in this group.

Families are population sub-groups ripe for screening. The predisposition for many diseases (as well as truly hereditary disease, of course) runs in families. Common examples are breast cancer, diabetes, asthma and high blood pressure. Doctors have always considered screening families in the context of infectious diseases in the past but few do this kind of intra-family screening for chronic conditions.

Screening, especially the sort that involves paying a fixed sum for a batch of tests and examinations, is currently enjoying something of a revival. One of the attractions of screening programmes is that they can often be inexpensive and can be implemented by relatively low grade personnel rather than doctors. But, as the price has come down, fewer questions tend to be asked and screening is now–with the coming of interactive computer systems–set to become even more popular, after a decade of apathy and serious questioning of its worth. Another reason for an increased interest in screening recently is that, with the setting-up of new health maintenance and prevention-orientated medical organisations, screening equipment and personnel can be used with the curative staff on hand. A major criticism of screening centres in the past has been that they left the patient high and dry with his or her findings from the screening. These new ways of working enable responsible follow-up to be a part of the whole picture. This is essential in the light of the numbers of false positives that occur with certain screening procedures.

Much more research needs to be done before we can be absolutely

Advisability of Various Health Screening Techniques throughout Life

Age: 16 17 18 19 20 21 22 23 24 25 26 27 28 29 30 31 32 33 34 35 36 37 38 39 40 41 42 4...

Technique	Age pattern (dots)
History & Physical	• (19) • (21) • (29) • (35) • (40)
Breast Exam by doctor	• • • • • (21–25) •• (27) • • •• (29–31) •• (33) • •• • (35–38) •• (40) •• • •• • (41–43)
Pelvic Exam	• (19) • • • • • (21–25) •• (27) • • •• (29–31) •• (33) • •• • (35–38) •• (40) •• • •• • (41–43)
Rectal Exam	• (19) • (29) • (35) •• • • • (40–43)
*Hearing Assessment	• (40)
**Tetanus-Diphtheria Booster	• (16) • (18) • (26) • (31) • (35) • (40)
**Influenza Immunization	
Blood Pressure	• • • (16–19) • • • • • • (21–27) •• (28) • • •• (30–32) •• (34) • •••• (36–39) • (41) •• (42) •• (43)
***Pap Smear	••• • (16–19) •• • • •• • (21–26) •• (27) • •••• (29–32) •• (33) • •• • (35–38) •• (40) •• • •• (41–43)
Cholesterol	• (19) • (22) • (25) • (29) • (31) • (33) • • (36–37) • (41)
Stool for Occult Blood	•• (40) •• (42)
Sigmoidoscopy	
Mammography	• (40)

Source: Taken from four major studies by Frame and Carlson; Breslow and Somers; American Cancer Society; Canadian Task Force on the Periodic Health Examination.
Note: The more dots against any one screening technique, the more of these authorities recommend them.

sure just how valuable many screening procedures are. What looks like commonsense preventive medicine is often not so on deeper analysis.

The danger with the coming of cheaper and easier screening methods is that society might ask *fewer* questions, not more.

48 49 50 51 52 53 54 55 56 57 58 59 60 61 62 63 64 65 66 67 68 69 70 71 72 73 74 75 +

Procedure
History & Physical
Breast Exam by doctor
Pelvic Exam
Rectal Exam
*Hearing Assessment
**Tetanus-Diphtheria Booster
**Influenza Immunization
Blood Pressure
***Pap Smear
Cholesterol
Stool for Occult Blood
Sigmoidoscopy
Mammography

Notes: Summary of recommendations of the four major studies. *=Canadian Task Force recommends that this be done on the basis of clinical judgement. **=At first visit physician should check past immunization history per Centers for Disease Control recommendations for rubella, mumps, poliomyelitis, diphtheria/tetanus toxoids, pertussis. ***=If sexually active.

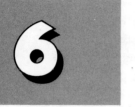

WHO SAYS PREVENTION PAYS?

If one judges investments by their returns, western medicine as currently practised is becoming progressively less cost-effective. In 1950 in the US 4.6 per cent of the Gross National Product was spent on health care. This percentage had doubled by 1975 and is now half as large again. Medicine and all its ancillary industries and back-up services employs 9 per cent of all Americans, which makes it the country's biggest industry. On the whole this service is a disease-centred one and lacks what economists would call effective market controls. The same tendencies apply to most westernised systems of medicine.

Evidence over many years shows that whatever financial and other resources are put at the disposal of western medicine will be swallowed up. In fact one researcher has calculated that by doubling the current expenditure longevity would not be altered significantly. Half of the increased expenditure since the 1950s has gone in higher prices. The other half has gone largely on more hospital beds, more technology, more hospital admissions, more health employees and more in-patient days in hospital. But in spite of all of this the major killers – heart disease, strokes and cancer – have declined little. The exception to this is the decline in heart disease deaths in the US that has occurred over the last fifteen years. This has almost certainly come about as the result of lifestyle changes and not increased expenditure on curative medicine.

Although it is difficult to make accurate estimates it is generally agreed that about 2 per cent of health-care expenditure goes on preventive medicine in most western countries, yet we are told from the cradle that prevention pays and that a stitch in time saves nine. Just how true are these claims?

Trying to assess the value of a preventive programme is a complex task. It is not too difficult to work out the cost-effectiveness of a simple curative procedure because the end-point is often fairly clear and you know what the starting point (an ill person) is. But when it comes to spending money on prevention there are many problems, some of which arise because the person involved is healthy and the benefit conferred on him or her, or on society, may not be easily quantifiable in terms of money and may occur many years after the original expenditure on the preventive measure.

When trying to work out how financially worth while a preventive health programme is we have to consider four main points: (1) The positive and negative effects of the programme; (2) how many of these effects can be clearly related to a preventive programme; (3) what value can be put on the results and (4) the balance of the advantages and disadvantages of the programme.

As an example let's look at screening for breast cancer. The effects of the programme will include: the cost of convincing women they should be screened; the cost of their time off work or other duties to go to be screened; the cost of actually getting there; the cost of the screening itself (both in people and equipment); the cost of following up the abnormal findings; the cost of treating those who have abnormalities but who would have otherwise gone untreated; the cost of any doctor-induced problems (i.e. other problems which the screening programme itself brings into being) and their follow-up treatment; and the savings resulting from the reduced use of medical and other facilities by the women who have a cancer detected early and so do not need more expensive treatment.

The next step involves putting values on the programme. There are several questions that need to be answered. Obviously the cost of convincing women to be screened has to be related to the numbers who actually come forward. If it costs £100 per woman simply to persuade her to be screened this alters the whole

balance of worth of such a screening to the community. What about the increase in doctor-induced diseases? Is it possible that by having too many false negatives we give women false confidence, causing them to ignore lumps in the future? Or that by giving too many false positives we worry people so that they end up having unnecessary and worrying operations?

The last thing we really have to be sure about is what good the screening actually does and which part of it is most worth while. Obviously doing a total physical examination and an X-ray every six months would be *a* way of detecting breast cancer early but the side-effects of the X-rays, and the costs, would be enormous.

Lastly, a price has to be put on the whole thing and this can be difficult. The actual cost of delivering the medical side of such a programme is, of course, easily worked out but the benefits (peace of mind, improvement in life expectancy and so on) are much more difficult to evaluate financially.

Can prevention be judged like any other investment?

Most economists, when asked to express a view on the value of prevention, understandably try to analyse the whole process as if it were an investment. People need and want a certain level of health, after all, not medical and nursing care. This is one useful way to look at preventive services – by spending a penny today we might be able to save a pound (spent on cure) tomorrow. Either because of this future saving or because it raises the individual's level of health today prevention at first appears to be an attractive investment.

If we really want to know what prevention costs we need to know what ill health costs so that we can see if in financial terms it is worth practising prevention. But working out what illness costs is not easy. The direct costs of ill health are relatively easy to quantify because they are the costs of delivering a medical care system and this can be worked out. In 1984 the National Health Service cost Great Britain £16 billion. But just looking at direct medical costs is not enough. Indirect economic costs include loss of productivity because of days off work, or premature death. These have to be added to the overall figure and more than double it. In the US the total cost of illness as judged in this way comes to about 20 per cent of the Gross National Product. One recent estimate suggests that about half of all these costs are for conditions that could be prevented. So money spent on prevention *could* reduce the costs both of the delivery of health care and of the number of days lost and working lives cut short.

None of these calculations take into account the suffering of the individual (on which it is impossible to put a price) or the cost to the individual of the loss of work, or other illnesses that occur in his or her

family as a result of the original (costed) illness. These things are very difficult, if not impossible, to quantify but are none the less real for that. All of this means that any pure cost-benefit analysis undervalues the real cost of illnesses to society.

Another problem in trying to put a cost on prevention is the difficulty of evaluating a human life in monetary terms. From the economic point of view the value of a person is that contribution he or she makes to the Gross National Product. This clearly falls short because it says nothing of the person's value to society in other ways and indeed says nothing about his or her value to him or herself. Judging people's worth by their wages automatically undervalues the unemployed, women and racial minority groups – who on average earn less. If wages were the sole measure of economic value in such cost-benefit analyses then these groups would be allocated very few medical services. Also, non-wage-earning jobs such as being a mother and housewife would not be included at all and special allowances would have to be made.

Another problem in using cost-benefit analysis is that the relationship between benefits and costs is highly dependent on the discount rate. A discount rate is used in calculating costs and benefits to reflect the fact that the value of future benefits is worth less than a similar quantity of benefits today. In other words a pound today is worth more than a pound tomorrow. The choice of discount rate therefore profoundly affects the value given to benefits and costs. The higher the discount rate the less important the benefits that will accrue far into the future become in the cost-benefit calculation. If the discount rate is high, benefits to future generations will be devalued in relation to the more immediate returns provided by other programmes.

Another problem with cost-benefit analysis is that very often in health care the demands for services vary enormously from one group to another. Quite often those who most benefit from a preventive programme are not those who bear the costs. This is especially true in the US where insurance companies pay such a large proportion of medical costs. Unfortunately, a sickness-orientated system such as this encourages people to wait until they are ill (when they know that the claim will be paid) rather than seek to prevent the condition in the first place (for which the insurance companies will not pay). Private medical insurance also tends to encourage the use of health screening systems which in turn produce a number of false-positive results and lead to the consumption of even more medical services quite unnecessarily.

Let's look now at the economic evidence on the three main preventive methods: changes in lifestyle; public health measures; and screening.

Lifestyle changes

These include things such as stop-ping smoking, wearing seat-belts, reducing alcohol consumption and so on. They are often extremely cheap to implement. A cost-benefit analysis on smoking and alcohol produces dramatic results. The cost of alcohol abuse and smoking accounts for one fifth of all health expenditure. When indirect costs are added the cost of smoking and alcohol abuse accounts for one quarter of all the economic costs of illness. These figures would increase even more if the costs of fire losses, car accidents and crime due to smoking and alcohol were added.

According to Dr John H. Knowles, late President of the Rockefeller Foundation:

Over 99 per cent of us are born healthy and suffer premature death and disability only as a result of personal misbehaviour and environmental conditions. . . . the individual has the power, indeed the moral responsibility to maintain his own health by observance of simple prudent rules of behaviour . . . life is meant to be enjoyed . . . but the cost of individual responsibility in health care now becomes prohibitive. The choice is individual responsibility or social failure. Responsibility and duty must gain some degree of parity with right and freedom.

So much for the *costs* of alcohol and smoking. The *benefits* are harder to quantify. The benefit *could* be the amount people are prepared to pay to indulge in these activities but this is probably an underestimate because presumably people prevented from smoking and drinking would need to do other things to answer the needs they have in the first place. Perhaps the cost of the drug bill would rise proportionately. A prevention plan to reduce smoking and alcohol use would, of course, cost money and there would be transitional costs as the two industries lost profits and put people out of work. Governments could, of course, compensate these industries temporarily in the interests of the nation's health.

Even allowing for all these costs economists still think the financial advantages could be considerable. To see just how cost-effective a reduction in tobacco and alcohol use would be one need look no further than the Mormons and Seventh Day Adventists in the US who live without these drugs and have provably lower death rates and longer lives. Their healthy eating habits also give them a cancer mortality of between 50 and 65 per cent that of other Americans.

Public health measures

These are more difficult to cost out. Immunisation against the infectious diseases such as polio, rubella, measles, diphtheria, mumps, whooping cough and smallpox has been of interest to governments all over the western world because these diseases are highly contagious, cause a provable disruption to society and are relatively easily prevented. Although any one of these diseases causes very little risk of serious life-long impairment or fatality to any *single* individual, an epidemic affecting perhaps hundreds of thousands of people really does cost society a lot of money. The costs for society of preventing these illnesses are small yet the benefits are great. However, the

benefits to society in the case of certain immunisable diseases, unless a very large proportion of the population is immunised, can be small. This applies especially to diseases in which there is considerable 'herd immunity'. After this crucial point is reached there is really not much point spending yet more money immunising the last 10 per cent of the population.

A good example of how to work out what is worth doing in the public health arena was the different ways in which German measles vaccine was used in the US and the UK, when it was first licensed in 1969. In the US children between 1 and 12 were innoculated whilst in the UK only girls between 11 and 14 were offered the vaccine. The benefits of the programme were defined to include the saving of the costs that would have been incurred in the treatment of the disease and its complications had it not been prevented. Work loss was also taken into account. The direct costs were the expenditure on the vaccine, its administration and the treatment of vaccine complications. By 1972 it was obvious that giving the vaccine had economic advantages at any age but that the most cost-effective way of using it was to offer it at the age of 12 to girls only, rather than to all children at age 6 or younger, as had been done in the US.

This raises an interesting general point in that it would be ideal to be able to prevent many diseases – whether they are communicable or not – yet as a society that already spends so much on health we have to be highly selective about what we spend money on. However rich a society its resources are not endless, and starting a preventive programme means shifting priority from other preventive programmes, acute care or even from non-health activities. This puts a considerable burden on those who are planning to introduce preventive programmes because they have to be able to justify what they do in terms of value for money. Unfortunately, the crisis-intervention sort of medicine we are all used to has rarely been subjected to such rigorous scrutiny–often with dire results.

Another example of the value of public health measures in the preventive field is the fluoridation of water to prevent tooth decay. Governments, whether local or national, tend to support water fluoridation because it is by far the cheapest way of ensuring that vulnerable people get enough fluoride. Cost-benefit analyses have shown that the fluoridation of water saves up to twenty to forty times its cost by dramatically reducing the incidence of tooth decay.

Environmental control of air and water pollution is the nearest we come in this century to the environmental problems faced in the last. A great deal of evidence has been accumulated to show that a reduction in air pollution would lead to a significant reduction in illness and death rates in urban areas. Using current costs for reducing air pollution there is no doubt that the benefits would outweigh them.

Screening programmes

These are often said to be an essential part of any preventive medical system in so far as they pick up disease early and enable it to be treated more quickly and presumably more cheaply. When calculating the cost-effectiveness of a screening programme, though, many things have to be taken into account including: the cost of the screening itself; the cost of any treatments that are thought to be necessary as a result of the screening; and the various costs of false-negative and false-positive results. This latter–the chasing of red herrings–can be very costly. On the benefit side there will be some value in catching things early and there may well be an increase in wellness of the screened population because they don't walk around worrying whether or not they have the condition.

Perhaps the most widely used and accepted screening programme is for phenylketonuria. If an affected baby is not detected and treated very soon after birth irreversible mental retardation results. The test is simple. A pinprick in the child's heel very soon after birth allows a drop of blood to be analysed. Several studies have shown that this simple, effective screening test is cost-effective even though the condition itself is very rare. Screening for other metabolic diseases has not been found to be cost-effective.

Screening for high blood pressure is cheap but because so many people do not take their medicines properly the benefits that accrue are not nearly as great as they could be and the cost-benefit analysis looks rather poor. Selective screening of high-risk populations almost certainly *is* worthwhile, but even this is not as simple as it might appear in the light of the Canadian study mentioned earlier which found that newly diagnosed hypertensives who did not bring their blood pressure under control had an 80 per cent increase in work absenteeism due to illness – attributed largely to an awareness of their condition. Here the cost of the screening was low but the accompanying costs of the drugs (a large proportion of which are not taken by blood-pressure patients) and the work days lost were high. This illustrates just how difficult it is to put a value on preventive measures.

A wide range of estimates has been published concerning the benefits of screening for cervical cancer. Evidence on the efficacy of this screening is complicated by the fact that death rates have been falling in unscreened as well as in screened populations and by uncertainty about the natural course of the disease. Those women who are most likely to be examined regularly (middle- and upper-income women) normally have a lower rate of cervical cancer than do lower-income women. Recent Canadian studies show that cervical cancer screening *is* cost-effective. The frequency at which it should take place, however, is still open to debate.

The evidence for the cost-effectiveness of screening for breast cancer is better than that for cervical cancer. A New York study found that the screening did not affect the survival rate of women aged 40–44 but it did lead to a significant reduction in mortality in women aged 50–59. It also seemed to be beneficial to women aged 60–64. The cost-benefit ratio of mammography appears to be very favourable. The US National Cancer Institute estimated that 20 per cent of breast cancers were discovered at the localised stage as a result of mammography. At a cost of $40 per mammogram the minimum cost per life prolonged is $240,000 ($24,000 per year of life saved) for women aged 55-64.

Quite recently then, and prompted by the vast and escalating cost of modern sickness intervention (as compared with *health* care), governments the world over have started to question the sense and economic viability of continuing down the 'more-is-better' path. The primary prevention of chronic disease looks like being the most cost-effective area in which to start off, if only because the after-the-fact treatments of many chronic diseases range from the expensive and basically unsuccessful to the almost endlessly expensive maintenance of a generally lower quality of life for many of the sufferers. Lifespans are getting longer, and a person with an untreated chronic disease today will probably be around with his or her condition for many years. This need not be the case, however, because the control of high blood pressure, for example, can postpone or prevent about a third of all strokes at a hundredth of the cost of living with a stroke.

But it is not just in chronic diseases that prevention definitely pays. An educational programme for surgical patients in a Massachusetts hospital explained the risk, the pain, and the post-operative effects the patients could expect. Doing these simple things reduced the need for painkilling drugs by 50 per cent and hospital stays by 2.7 days. In another study the education of asthmatics who used an emergency room produced a cost saving of $6 for every dollar spend educating the patient to care for him or herself. Even more drama-

tic results have been obtained with haemophiliacs. Education on care, prevention of injury and simple treatment reduced hospital stays from 432 to 42 days!

Quite clearly prevention *can* pay but does not necessarily do so. Every new programme has to be looked at very carefully before it is implemented on any large scale, if only to make sure that it does not fall into the trap that so much western medicine has historically—that of doing something simply because it could be done and then worrying about the cost of it all afterwards.

PART TWO
A Preventive Health Plan for Everyday Living

7 CHANGING YOUR LIFESTYLE

It would be quite wrong to suggest that all illness could be abolished by 'right living', but there is no doubt that changing one's lifestyle and behaviour even a little can result in a greater resistance to illness and quicker recovery from disease.

Most of us have become sloppy about the way we run our lives and often have only ourselves to blame when things go wrong. We flagrantly abuse our minds and bodies and then wonder why they let us down. I put 'minds' first because as many as three-quarters of all symptoms are caused by emotional and psychological dis-ease. Don't forget that the largest group of prescriptions written in most western countries is for mind-altering drugs. We also try to cope with the stresses and strains of modern life by the frequent consumption of cigarettes, alcohol and caffeine- and cola-containing drinks –all of which have provable harmful effects, at least in some people.

Obviously the list of things one could do to lead a generally better life is lengthy, so I have selected seven major ones to concentrate on. If these are right in your life the effects of everything else will at least be greatly diminished, if not totally reversed. I can guarantee that by adopting the kind of lifestyle and habits outlined in this section of the book you will feel better and enjoy life more. A useful book that takes the whole subject further is *Your Complete Stress-Proofing Programme* by Leon Chaitow.

What you eat

It is an old truism that 'you are what you eat' and it is certainly a fact that you can only get the nutrients essential for the healthy working of your body by eating them.

We are all brought up to believe in the 'balanced diet' but the adequacy of the sort of protein-and-two-veg regime generally designated by this phrase is almost certainly a myth. A 1980 study (and there have been many over the years throughout the western world) found that only 15 per cent of the UK residents interviewed were consuming a diet that could provide even the minimum dietary requirements as laid down by the Department of Health and Social Security and these are themselves reckoned to be too low by many experts. In the USA two workers did a detailed study of 860 dental patients and found that almost half had frank vitamin and mineral deficiency states and that 6 per cent had no vitamin C in their blood at all. Another US study found that 88 per cent of 120 randomly selected people had a significant deficiency of at least one vitamin and that 63 per cent were deficient in more than one. As we learn more about minerals it is becoming apparent that most people are short of these too.

Unfortunately, most people think that if they eat a little of a wide variety of foods their body will somehow balance out the goodies and end up healthy. Modern research has proved otherwise. Evidence now suggests that modern farming practices, which deplete the levels of essential nutrients in the soil by intensive cropping, mean that even the starting point–plants and animals from agricultural sources–are poor in all kinds of essential substances. Intensive farming methods, drugs used to fatten animals and so on, have provable negative effects on our health and nutrition. A further loss of vitamins and minerals occurs between the picking and the eating as modern food processing removes much of what is left. Few people realise the grave deficiencies of their modern diet, yet government departments repeatedly assure us that all is well.

All the above assumes that the consumer is really trying to eat healthily–and I am saying that this is very difficult to do, however well motivated one is. But the vast majority of

the population don't try. They consume large amounts of sugar, white-flour products, fat and alcohol, and suffer considerable nutritional deficiencies as a result.

Because most of us have enough to eat in the West we imagine we are well nourished. The truth is that we are mal-nourished because we eat too much of the wrong foods. Here is a list of things that can appear if, for example, the vitamin and mineral balance of the body is not just right. When did you last have one, or more, of these?

- Cracks at the corners of your mouth
- A bright red tongue
- Ridged, brittle nails with white flakes
- Gums that recede and bleed easily on brushing
- Dry skin
- Dull, lifeless hair
- Poor dream recall
- Skin stretch marks
- Slow healing of wounds and grazes
- Apathy
- Easy bruising

In the UK and the US various concerned authorities are now looking much more closely into western diets and the NACNE Report (named after the UK Advisory Council on Nutrition Education) caught the public interest, probably for the first time on this subject. This authoritative report, based on other learned reports and vast amounts of clinical and scientific data, came out with several recommendations for healthy eating. These, put into lay language, are:

- *Energy intake should be appropriate for maintaining optimal body weight for height and sex, with adequate exercise.* This basically means that if you tend to put on weight you should reduce your food consumption so that your weight falls and stays within the 'desirable' levels given on height and weight charts. You can do this by taking more exercise *and* reducing your caloric intake.

- *Fat intake should be an average of 30 per cent of total energy.* This means that if you add up all your calorie intake for a day fat should never make up more than 30 per cent of it. At the moment fat makes up nearly 40 per cent of daily calories. Remember when working out fat consumption that there is a lot of hidden fat in meat especially, so it is best to aim for less than 30 per cent to take this into account. Overall, most of us need to cut fat intake by a quarter.

- *Saturated fatty acid intake should be an average of 10 per cent of total energy intake.* This means that saturated fatty acids (dairy produce, meat and certain plant oils) should provide no more than 10 per cent of all your daily calories. At the moment most people's diet contains 18 per cent saturated fatty acids. So you will have to cut this intake by nearly half.

- *Average sucrose intake should be reduced by 20 kg per head a year.* This in practice means cutting sugar intake by half—from an average of 8 teaspoons a day to 4. The ideal, of course, would be to cut out added sugar altogether over a period of weeks by slowly reducing the amount you take. There is so much hidden sugar in so many processed foods that you will still be eating more than you need however hard you try to exclude it.

- *Average salt intake should fall by 3 g per head per day.* Many people eat as much as 12 g salt per day. Again there is a lot of salt 'hidden' in processed foods of all kinds so the ideal is to end up by adding no salt at all to food or during cooking. This is quite easily achieved over a few weeks or months.

- *Fibre intake should increase on average from 20 g to 30 g per head per day.* This probably means eating half as much again of fibre-rich foods as you do now. These are wholemeal flour and its products, bran-containing breakfast cereals, pulses, fruit, and vegetables.

Other main NACNE recommendations:

- Don't worry about how much cholesterol you eat

- Don't change the amount of protein you eat

- Reduce alcohol intake to 4 per cent of total calories at most. (This means in practice a maximum of one pint of beer or two glasses of wine a day.)

- On vitamins and minerals NACNE think that anyone eating along the lines they suggest will inevitably eat more of these nutrients, which is true. I, and many others involved in nutrition, see this as being totally inadequate because of the poverty of vitamins and minerals in modern foods as they actually reach the table. This is a subject of considerable debate, with government food experts maintaining that we all get enough of these things if we eat a NACNE-type diet. Certainly it is true that if we do we won't be *grossly* deficient but I maintain that much ill health is caused by marginal (as yet unrecognised by the medical profession) dietary deficiencies.

In addition to NACNE's recommendations, which I heartily endorse, I would add:

- *Avoid or cut down on foods that contain additives, preservatives, colourings, etc*. The effects of these chemicals are only just beginning to be understood. Get into the habit of reading labels and don't buy anything with any of these substances in it unless you have no alternative.

- *Greatly reduce your intake of tea, coffee, chocolate and cola drinks*. In the case of the first three dilute them and have them very weak.

- *Supplement your daily diet with a multi-mineral, multi-vitamin supplement.*

Vitamin A	500–1200 IU
Vitamin D3	20–100 IU
Vitamin B1	2–10mg
Vitamin B2	2–10mg
Vitamin B6	2–15mg
Vitamin B12	10–25mcg
Vitamin C	25–150mg
Vitamin E d-Alpha Toc.Succinate	10–50 IU
Biotin	20–50mcg
Calcium Pantothenate (Vitamin B5)	30–60mg
Choline	5–15mg
Bioflavonoids	5–25mg
Folic Acid	50–100mcg
Nicotinic Acid or	5–10mg
Nicotinamide (Vitamin B3)	10–20mg
Inositol	5–15mg
P.A.B.A.	5–10mg
Beta Carotene	2–5mg
Iodine (from Kelp)	10–25mcg
Calcium (element)	50–150mg
Chromium	20–30mcg
Iron (element)	2–3mg
Magnesium (element)	20–60mg
Selenium (element)	10–25mcg
Zinc (element)	2–4mg

Such a supplement should be free from yeast, wheat, gluten, milk, corn, sugar, and artificial colourants and preservatives. The doses given are the minimum. It is safe to take up to four times these doses daily.

Take them all with food, spread throughout the day.

- *Eat as much of your foods raw as you can*. This mainly involves fruit, seeds and nuts and vegetables, of course. Recent research suggests that raw foods not only have better nutritional qualities (which has been known for a long time) but that they have intrinsic energies which are helpful in keeping the body healthy and curing disease.

If you eat in this way and supplement your diet with vitamins and minerals you will undoubtedly feel better, and specific results can include:

- No more constipation (fibre ↑)

- A slow weight-loss (fibre ↑ fat ↓ sugar ↓)

- Reduced blood pressure (salt ↓)

- Fewer signs of vitamin/mineral deficiency

- More energy

- Less tooth decay and gum disease (sugar ↓ fibre ↑)

- Reduced chances of becoming diabetic in middle age (because you are slimmer)

- Less chance of producing gallstones (because you are slimmer)

- A reduced chance of having a heart attack (because you are eating fewer saturated fatty acids that clog up the heart's arteries and because you are slimmer and have a reduced blood pressure)

- Less chance of developing diverticular disease of the colon (fibre ↑)

- Reduced chance of bowel cancer (fibre ↑ meat ↓ fat ↓)

- You'll feel pleasantly full after a meal (fibre ↑)

- Reduced problems with (or complete cure of) your piles (fibre ↑)

- An increased ability to withstand stress.

Exercise

For many years it was thought that deliberate physical exercise was unnecessary for health, but recent research has proved how *positively* valuable it is. We all know that exercise makes us *feel* better but until recently it was not known why. It appears that naturally occurring pain-killers in the body called endorphins are released during exercise. These have the effect (like morphine and its synthetic derivatives) of making the person feel 'high'. Adrenaline (epinephrine) is also produced in larger than normal amounts during exercise and this too causes a 'high' feeling. This well-being clearly spills over into the individual's life and improves its quality. It also appears that he or she will eat less (most people eat too much as a sort of comforter when they feel low – which is not good for their weight). Also, recent research has found that a person's metabolic rate remains raised for several days after taking serious exercise, so this too is good news for slimmers because meaningful exercise two or three times a week can keep their metabolism burning up fat all the time.

Most people who don't take regular exercise fail to realise just how unfit and unhealthy they are. When faced with a broken lift and a moderate run of stairs they are puffing and panting by the second floor, and a modest run for a bus exhausts them and gives them aches and pains.

Regular, controlled exercise is best and symmetrical exercises are probably ideal for 'the non-professional'. These include walking, running, swimming, skipping, cycling and rowing. Such exercise at least three times a week, will tone up the muscles, the heart and the breathing system and improve your sense of well-being. Stimulation of the circulatory system reduces the amount of lactic acid in the bloodstream. Lactic acid results from shallow breathing and inactivity and can induce feelings of fatigue and lethargy.

It is now known that muscular tension and poor body posture (a common sign of stress) feed back impulses via the nervous system to create a degree of central nervous system activity which prevents you from relaxing mentally. So, just as mental states can create physical tension, so a prolonged degree of physical muscle tension can cause stressed emotional and mental states. Physical activity and massage reduce tension in both the muscles and the mind.

The problem with taking exercise is that most people don't know how much they need to take for it to be beneficial. A lot of research has now been done on this and it appears that the best guide is your heart rate. Get used to feeling your own pulse and take it before and during exercise. From 220 deduct your age. Calculate three-quarters of this and this is the exercise pulse rate to aim for.

So, at age 40:
$$220 - 40 = 180$$
$$\tfrac{3}{4} \times 180 = 135$$

So 40-year-olds taking exercise should ensure that, whatever they do and however they achieve it, it puts their pulse rate up to 135. Any higher and they could be overdoing it – any lower and the exercise is not doing them much good. As you become fitter you will notice that you need to do more work to reach the goal.

The ideal is to do a form of physical exercise that maintains your pulse at your ideal exercise level for about 20 minutes three or four times a week. If you are at all worried about any medical condition you have or if there is a history of heart disease in your family, talk over your plans with the doctor first. When it comes to taking exercise the secret is to do it regularly in a controlled way and to do things you enjoy. If you exercise as I have suggested you will benefit in the following ways:

- You will feel healthier and more lively generally

- You will tend to lose weight slowly (if you don't eat more)

- Your muscular strength will build up

- Your reflexes will sharpen

- You will feel less stressed

- You will want to be more physically active generally

- Your appetite will improve

- You will look healthier

Breathing

Breathing is an activity to which most of us give little thought yet we are aware that when we are tense we breathe shallowly or sigh a lot. When a person is relaxed and happy his or her breathing is slow and rhythmic and healthy breathing involves the whole ribcage. When we are tense breathing becomes rigid, shallow and only the uppermost part of the chest will move. Many relaxation and meditation programmes involve breathing manoeuvres, mainly because thousands of years of experience have shown that breathing control can alter a person's state of mind and vice versa. Learning to breathe properly can be a valuable part of stress control. This works because stretch receptors in the lungs feed back information to the brain and alter central functioning in a way which tunes up the rest of the brain. Teachers of the Alexander Technique claim to be able to abolish all kinds of physical and even some emotional complaints solely by altering body postures and improving breathing techniques.

Breathing is one vital function of the body over which we have conscious control, and because it can be so easily mastered to our benefit it is worth learning how to breathe more healthily. The main purpose of learning breathing exercises is to be able to use them in stressful and painful situations. You can also use them to help you to get to sleep. If you doubt that breathing exercises can be of help in tense and stressful situations just watch tense people and see how they sigh a lot, catch their breath, gasp or show laboured breathing. Panicky people overbreathe and can get tingling in their fingers and toes as a result.

There are many good breathing exercises and the reader should refer to a specialised book on the subject, but here I will just outline one – three-stage breathing.

- Start by lying down on your back with your lower back touching the floor. You may have to bend your knees to achieve this.

- Rest the palms of your hands on the upper part of your chest and breathe gently. Breathe out slowly and completely and repeat this cycle ten times. Your hands are simply registering the movement of this part of your chest.

- Place your hands on your lower ribs on either side of the breast bone so that the fingertips almost touch when you breathe out. Watch and feel your fingertips being parted – one hand from the other – as you breathe in. Breathe in and try to separate your fingertips as far as you can. Breathe out and try to get them to touch in the midline. Close your eyes, relax and repeat this ten times.

- Place your hands on your tummy at the level of the navel. Repeat the slow breathing and see if you can make your tummy expand as you breathe in. This shows that the diaphragm is working fully. Your fingertips will move back and forth as they did on your chest but probably more so. Repeat this ten times.

- With your hands on the floor breathe out completely, then expand your abdomen with your breathing. Then fill your lower chest – then your upper chest until all three areas seem 'full of air' (of course there is really no air in your tummy but it expands because of the diaphragm pushing down from the expanded lungs). Carry on until your whole respiratory system is full of air. This should take about 10–15 seconds.

- Reverse the process to exhale. Expel air first from your upper chest, then your lower chest, then your abdomen. Expel the last of the air by contracting your abdominal muscles slightly. Pause for 2–3 seconds and then restart the whole cycle.

- Repeat the cycle ten times.

The benefits of learning to breathe more deeply and fully include:

- You will feel more relaxed while you do the exercises

- You will be able to call on them at times of stress and tension

- You can use them to get to sleep

- You can use them as a prelude to meditation or other relaxation exercises.

Sleep

Rather like breathing sleep is something we all tend to take for granted. As long as we are managing to sleep we don't think too much about it. But depression and stress affect sleep profoundly, and both are affected by inadequate sleep, so it makes sense to try to get the best possible sleep to combat these two common ailments of everyday life. Many people have difficulty getting off to sleep, wake after an hour or two, wake up feeling unrefreshed, sleep fitfully, and so on. This kind of disordered sleep is the norm for millions of people who then wonder why they feel so unwell during the daytime. Unfortunately, it becomes a vicious circle because the stressed person sleeps badly, lies awake and worries more; lack of sleep then leads to poor performance during the day; which brings more stress, and still more difficulty in sleeping, and so on. A lack of sleep has many provable ill-effects including: poor energy; a reduced ability to do fine tasks; an increased sensitivity to pain; memory lapses; poor judgement; reduced motivation; decreased sex drive; a feeling of negativity; poor reaction times and general irritability. We look in more detail at how to prevent insomnia and how to enjoy more relaxed sleep on page 266.

Benefits you can expect if you get more and better-quality sleep include:

- You will feel more relaxed and happier

- You will have faster reflexes (especially valuable and even life-saving when driving)

- You will be more mentally agile

- You will be better tempered

- You will feel more positive

- Your memory will improve

Other aspects of your lifestyle

We all live in a way which does little to help us and the list of changes that would help prevent disease is almost endless. However, there are some things which are notably worth changing and which the motivated individual *can* change.

- *Reduce the crutches you think you need to 'cope' with life.* This means cutting down or cutting out prescribed tranquillisers, tobacco, alcohol, soft drugs and caffeine-containing drinks (tea, coffee, chocolate and colas). All of these have provable ill-effects that produce illness and disease.

Another coping mechanism that does harm is the between-meals sugary snack. This, like the aids already mentioned, stimulates the person back to life, if only for a while. Blood sugar rises as a result of this consumption, and the pancreas has to work overtime to produce insulin to counteract the glucose peaks. If the pancreas fails to produce enough insulin the person will become diabetic, and if it over-produces the individual's sugar level falls and he or she suffers a hypoglycaemic attack (see page 248). Either way the situation is not healthy and produces many symptoms that baffle doctors. Such people know they don't feel well yet neither they nor their doctors can put a finger on what is happening. The answer is to cut right down on all of these stimulants – preferably cut them out altogether.

When it comes to smoking, if you can't stop – it is probably the most difficult prop of all to give up – try to make up for at least some of the damage you are doing by continuing to smoke by taking the following:

Vitamin B complex – 1 tablet daily
Vitamin C – 1-3g daily
Vitamin E 200-600 IUs daily.
All these should be taken with food and spread throughout the day.

- *Look at the way you live and change*

things for the better. Here are some suggestions.

1. Exercise for 10–20 minutes every day, or at least three or four times per week.
2. Relax or meditate at least once a day for 10 minutes. Mornings and evenings are best, *not* after a meal or you could fall asleep.
3. Don't work more than ten hours a day.
4. Take holidays to suit you. Some people prefer several short breaks to one long annual holiday.
5. Eat and drink healthily, as outlined on pages 70-74.
6. Make a real effort to be more relaxed about things.
7. Do all you can to promote an active sex life. Seek help if you have any problems.
8. Don't let worries niggle away at you. Sort them out before they sort you out!
9. Take positive steps to reduce stress-inducing factors that are within your control. You may need, for example, to move house to something smaller or nearer your job, or to work out your finances better (perhaps with professional help). (See below.)
10. Take up a creative and non-competitive hobby such as DIY, gardening, collecting something, etc. Make sure your hobby doesn't just continue into your spare time the stresses and strains of your working life.
11. Don't create unnecessary deadlines in your work or social life.
12. If in doubt, cut down on the amount you do when not at work so as to make time to communicate with your partner and family. This will increase the quality of your life a lot more than you think.
13. Take up some kind of interest or do something that helps others less fortunate than yourself. This makes most people feel a lot better about themselves.
14. Face the fact that you are, to a considerable extent, responsible for your health and that of your children, and that they have every right to look to you for guidance so that they too will live long and happy lives. Older family members have a responsibility to the next generation and this involves helping the children avoid some of the hazards the older members have negotiated.
15. Explore the value a spiritual dimension could have in your life, and share what you enjoy with your family.

Many of these changes in lifestyle depend to a great extent on altering the way you think about health and indeed about life generally.

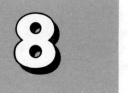

STRESS

As we saw in Part One the way we think and the attitudes and beliefs we subscribe to have a great influence on our health and the way we look at prevention.

In a stressful world which is full of change most of us have to cope with the problems of growing up, going to school, leaving school, forming relationships, having children, making a home, holding down a job, bereavement, problems with children, illness, and much more besides. Many of these problems are in no way 'our fault', yet they can have a profound effect on our health, often reducing our ability to withstand infections and even making us susceptible to killer diseases such as cancer. Several studies have confirmed that stress impairs the functioning of the immune system. We shall look at methods of stress reduction on page 87.

The typical responses of individuals to bad luck and stress vary enormously. A few people seem to thrive by overcoming obstacles, but it is probably true to say that more 'illness' and 'dis-ease' is caused by stressful events in people's lives than is caused by 'real' disease. But as well as these 'external' sources of stress and emotional upheaval there are many more 'internal' – or self-gener-ated – causes and some people are much more likely to be troubled with these than are others.

Some people hold beliefs that are almost bound to make them suffer more than necessary in the hurly-burly of everyday life, and others have personality types that make them exceptionally vulnerable. Both of these can be modified – at least to some extent – and increasingly people are realising that their personalities have an enormous influence on their health and illness patterns.

Uncertainty is a potent cause of stress in many people's lives but rational, clear thinking can overcome or reduce many of the stresses associated with uncertainty. For example, if you think you are about to be made redundant you can explore all the possible alternatives ahead of time, perhaps even starting to look into retraining. This positive action will make you feel a lot better and you will be less uncertain about your future because you will at least have explored, and probably sorted out, some alternatives ahead of the crisis point.

Uncertainty over a physical symptom is a major source of stress to many people who, often quite wrongly, imagine they have a serious disease. The answer here is to seek a professional opinion, and get the necessary tests done, so that your suspicion is either confirmed or proved wrong, and you can deal with the resultant situation appropriately. We all seem to have difficulty coping with problems which don't have definite boundaries, yet can do so much better once the problem is defined clearly. Fear of the unknown is a disease-producer, yet so much information is available today that there is no need to fret unnecessarily over all kinds of imagined horrors.

Another source of stress is the inability many people have to make decisions at all. This in itself tears them apart because the very act of choosing one direction in life by definition rules out certain others and such people cannot bear to have any doors closed – they want all their options open all the time and so decide on nothing. In such circumstances it helps to write down the problem in logical steps and then to work out on paper all the possible answers you can see. This is best done with the help of a partner or a friend, but for some people in certain circumstances a professional counsellor may be the answer. Often an outsider can see a way through an apparently insuperable problem, partly because he or she is outside the problem that looms so large in the troubled person's life, and partly because he or she can bring experi-

ence from dealing with other similar problems to bear on this particular one. Often an outsider sees a totally new way out of the dilemma that is entirely invisible to the individual involved because of his or her upbringing, education, way of thinking, emotional state, or whatever.

One of the things that makes many people 'ill' is coming to terms with the fact that in modern life many problems simply don't have an answer. Things are so complicated today that the simple answers of our grandparents often can't be made to apply. Coping with the unchangeable is a sign of emotional maturity and again professional help may be necessary.

A large number of people harbour negative feelings such as hate, distrust and resentment, sometimes holding on to grievances for years. These feelings work away inside them to make them ill even though the source of the problem is often someone else. Whilst serious grudges and really intransigent problems may need professional insights and expertise, many such negative emotions can be overcome by individuals themselves once they realise that they are doing themselves more harm than anyone else. The starting point is to realise that the past is done and gone and that nothing can undo what we have done. The aim should be to come to terms with what has happened and then try to make amends for it in some way. Often simply having the strength to say 'sorry' after many years can lift a burden off your shoulders. Sometimes such feelings are best put down in writing rather than discussed face to face, or it may be better to open the door in writing and then meet to talk it out. Very few people can throw a heart-felt apology back in someone's face and if time has healed the emotional wounds even a little then things can go very well from there. It was a wise man who said, 'He who cannot forgive breaks the bridge over which he himself must pass.'

The secret of all attitudes, beliefs and behaviour is to know yourself and to have insights into these facets of yourself. This can be very difficult but there are excellent books that can help. Perhaps one of the best is *'I'm OK – You're OK'* by Dr Thomas Harris. A few sessions with an insight-trained counsellor of some kind can also be invaluable in opening doors for you which then alter the whole way you think in the future. It pays to listen to what good friends say too. There are few people who will be really honest with you in life and, ironically, your partner may not be the best person.

So many emotions, types of behaviour and beliefs are destructive and harmful to us that it is a shame that so little is said about all this in health education of all kinds. It should really be a major strand of preventive medicine – the benefits would be enormous. The burden on doctors would fall dramatically if they were trained to deal with their patients in this way – giving insights into their personalities as an explanation for their ill health. Alas, few doctors are capable of doing this and those that are have too little time to

exploit their skills. Hopefully there will soon be a shift away from dealing with the obvious complaints to dealing with the underlying personality problems that produced them in the first place.

If you doubt the importance of the personality in illness and health, think of all the major diseases that we are heir to. Smoking, for example, has an enormous psychological component to it and most smokers won't or can't give up until they understand the underlying psychological mechanisms that make them do it. The problem with overeating is much the same. Both are oral pleasures for people who are arrested at the oral stage of their psychosexual development. Most VD is caused by promiscuous behaviour which could be prevented if the individuals concerned had insights into themselves and their actions. The majority of car crashes are in no way 'accidental' and neither are the thousands of unwanted pregnancies that occur each year. And so I could go on. And I haven't even mentioned the obvious emotionally-based problems within marriages, families and working groups – all of which produce disease. The greatest tool of preventive medicine, then, is self-knowledge, and until our medical-care system comes to grips with this people will continue to injure and kill themselves quite unnecessarily.

An increasing number of people in the West are finding that a spiritual dimension to their lives is invaluable to their physical and mental well-being. Since antiquity humans have felt the need to commune with super-natural beings, and almost every culture has a concept of God. To many, Christians included, an essential part of their God is his ability to heal sickness and even to prevent illness. Examples of miracles abound in historical and religious literature and there is little doubt, given the enormous power of the mind over the body, that such phenomena can be real enough. Current research into parapsychological phenomena makes it all much easier for us to believe in today than it would have been for those living in biblical times, but even so there are still sceptics.

There is little doubt that we are learning in the West that humans are far more remarkable than we previously thought. Telepathy, clairvoyance, clairaudience, psychokinesis and the ability to heal are so well documented that it is difficult to be sceptical about them any longer. What is interesting is the idea that we all possess such gifts as a part of being human beings but that most of us have lost them. Research in Russia, for example, has found that most people can be taught to dowse and to develop all kinds of parapsychological abilities they never knew they had. Susceptible people can learn such skills in as short a time as a weekend.

It appears that western thinking and behaviour inhibits these intrinsic – or some would say God-given – abilities. A doctor working in a very primitive area of Africa was astonished at how the local people regularly and quite naturally com-municated with each other over long distances without speaking. They quickly lost this telepathic ability once they came into regular contact with westerners because, they said, they felt so much in awe of the cars, watches, explosives and so on. These things, they said, seemed to dwarf their 'simple powers'.

Much of the maintenance of good health and even the curing of ill health resides, I believe, in these realms of the mind that are currently called parapsychological. Some, in different parts of the world, attribute them to God or Gods, others to the wondrous nature of mankind. Needless to say I am in no position to say which is correct but I do recognise a higher force of health and ill health than man and his personal behaviour. The healing power of one person upon another is a skill that has been all but lost in many westernised cultures although it is being revived among certain Christian groups, especially in the charismatic wing of the church. Of course for many so-called primitive people the laying on of hands and absent healing are a long-established part of their culture. With the increasing interest in the mystical and the supernatural and with a growth of 'natural' medicine in the West I feel sure that all of this side of healing and maintaining health will be of greater importance in the future.

The causes of stress

We hear a lot about stress today, and

it is often claimed that stress-induced illnesses have now replaced the infectious illnesses as the epidemic diseases of modern life. Whether this is true or not is difficult to say but there is little doubt that certain modern diseases appear to be more common in those who are stressed or who have certain personality types.

Stress is a natural part of life and it is perfectly reasonable in some situations–if, for example, a car is coming towards you too fast when you are on a pedestrian crossing. The problems occur when a person finds totally inappropriate things stressful. This brings us to the core of the whole problem of discussing stress – the fact that different people find different things stressful. Each of us, with our unique personality, defines certain very different things in life as stressful. One's personal beliefs and perceptions greatly influence just how stressful any one life event is.

Almost anything in life is capable of causing stress but a number of 'life events' that are generally found stressful have been identified in the work of T. A. Holmes and R. H. Rahe. They are the authors of the key study on life's stressful events (1967). Holmes and Rahe graded forty-three life events using major changes such as the death of a spouse as an arbitary 100 on the scale and marriage as 50. It was found that four out of five people who were experiencing many dramatic changes in life all at the same time could expect a major illness within the next two years. Here is a selection from Dr Rahe's list:

Death of a spouse	100
Divorce	73
Personal injury or illness	53
Fired from work	47
Retirement	45
Sex problems	39
Gain of a new family member	39
Change in responsibilities at work	29
Outstanding personal achievement	29
Leaving school	26
Change in living conditions	25
Change in working hours or conditions	20
Change in sleeping habits	16
Change in eating habits	15
Holiday	13
Christmas	12
Minor violations of the law	11

It was found that when the score (using the full forty-three items identified in the study) came to 300 or more there was likely to be a serious illness, and a score of over 100 indicated that remedial measures should be taken to limit the reaction to change. Fewer than 30 per cent of individuals with scores of under 150 became significantly ill.

Because we are all made so differently things stress us for different reasons. Some people are stressed by 'internal' events such as guilt, fear of the future, remorse, failure, anticipation of failure, self-pity, brooding over past events and so on, whilst others find these no problem yet find the 'external' world a mass of stressful triggers. It is interesting that many comparatively pleasant things can also be very stressful. Getting married is a happy event for most of us yet it is half-way up the stressful events list. Holidays and Christmas too add stress to our lives.

A lot of stress is quite unnecessary and comes about because of an individual's inability to accept the world the way it is. 'Wouldn't it be nice if . . .' 'If only . . . .' and similar statements (usually said with a sigh) are the hallmark of this kind of person. Such people are always longing for better things, are never satisfied with their life the way it is, always find fault, and so on. The best advice to such people is to 'live for the present'. Many people behave as if life were a sort of rehearsal for something! Tied to this feeling of disappointment about life is an inability to express feelings clearly without getting upset. Feelings bottled up or expressed inappropriately are very stressful. Wishing secretly that things were other than they are is usually stressful.

Unfulfilled expectations are another very potent source of stress. We all grow up with expectations, most of which are gained quite unconsciously from our parents and other authority figures around us. When we come face to face with the real world our expectations are often too high and we blame the situations, ourselves or those around us. Perhaps the biggest single example is marriage. Most people have unrealistic expectations of a lifelong marriage and can only be disappointed with the realities as they unfold. How much better it would be to educate children to be realistic about major life events during their teens, and even earlier if they could cope with it.

The physical effects of stress

These are many and profound. When an individual, whether with justification or not, finds a situation stressful, his or her body undergoes a 'fight or flight' reaction. This is a primitive response seen in all animals but most animals don't meet life-or-death situations that trigger off this response very often. The problem with human beings is that their way of life has set them up to perceive many things as stressful and they react biologically to stimuli that do not affect the animal world generally. This occurs partly, of course, because humans are so complex emotionally and psychologically.

The body's reactions to stress are:

- The hypothalamus (a part of the brain) initiates a number of hormonal changes.

- The pituitary gland is activated by the hypothalamus and in turn activates the adrenal glands to produce more adrenaline and noradrenaline. These powerful hormones do many things but the main ones are:

- The heart beats more powerfully and faster

- The pupils of the eyes dilate

- The blood pressure rises

- The muscles tense

- The breathing rate increases

- Blood is directed from the digestive system and the skin to other more vital functions

- Blood flow to the kidneys is reduced so as to reduce urine output

- Saliva dries up

- The liver releases stored glucose for energy

- The immune system (which fights infection) shuts down temporarily

In the average stressful situation these changes are temporary and normality resumes after the stress-inducing situation is past. However, for many of us in the West today many or all of these changes become an almost permanent feature of the way our bodies work, as one stressful event follows another. This produces symptoms such as:

Headaches

Dizziness

Sweating

Coiled legs

Hair twisting

Finger drumming

Clenched fists

Nail biting

High blood pressure

Allergies

Ulcers

Skin rashes

Depression

Unreasonable fears

Breathlessness

Sighing

Little interest in life

Poor appetite

Nervous tics and twitches

A fear of becoming ill

Poor self-esteem

Difficulty in relaxing

Difficulty with concentration

Hunched shoulders

A worried frown

A gripped thumb

Clenched teeth

Insomnia

Blurred vision

Swallowing difficulties

Sex problems

Heartbeat irregularities

Indigestion

Backache

Colitis

Irritability

Disturbed sleep

Fatigue and tiredness much of the time

A tendency to cry

Aching shoulders and neck muscles

Food cravings between meals

Smoking or drinking to calm yourself

Feeling neglected or let down

Feeling a failure towards others

Rarely laughing

Feeling uncomfortable touching or being touched

None of these conditions is a 'disease' in itself but a combination of several reduces the quality of life and many of them together can reduce a person almost to the point where he or she is unable to cope with everyday life. Many of these conditions will be dealt with more fully in the body of the book and even though there are other reasons for many, if not most, of them stress is probably the commonest.

How to combat stress

The first thing to do when trying to combat stress is to read the preceding parts of this section of the book. Start by improving what you eat, by taking more exercise, by breathing better, by getting more and better-quality sleep and by changing your lifestyle and attitudes. Even if you do nothing else and your life continues to have just as many potentially stressful events as before you'll feel a new person and many of the above list of symptoms will disappear over a few weeks.

There are other steps, though, that you may find helpful. They include three activities with proven value in reducing stress both at the stressful time itself and in between.

Relaxation exercises

There are so many types of relaxation exercises that a book such as this cannot even give an overview of them. Here, however, is one example of an exercise sequence that is simple and effective:

- Take the phone off the hook

- Make sure the room is warm and quiet and that you won't be interrupted

- Choose a time of day that is free from stress (morning or evening is best)

- Avoid doing the exercises after a meal

- Try to do them twice a day

- Put a blanket on the floor or sit directly on the carpet

- Wear loose clothing–nothing constricting

- Remove shoes, ties; undo bra or belt

- Sit up in a supported position

- Clear your mind of intrusive thoughts and let things happen

- Breathe deeply and regularly (see page 76 for details)

- Once the breathing is established try to introduce thoughts such as of a wave of warmth or happiness coming over you. All this relaxes tense muscles and the action of the sympathetic nervous system and prepares you for the relaxation exercises you want to do. For example:

- Systematically and consciously relax all the areas of the body in sequence

- Start with the feet–deliberately tighten the foot muscles and then relax them after 10 seconds of holding them in tension. Feel them release as you let go. Try consciously to register how good this feels

- Work up to the top of the body, tightening and relaxing area by area

- Do this for ten minutes and then spend a further ten minutes returning to normal. Just sit or lie there feeling relaxed and carry on with the deep breathing. Get up slowly and gently to resume your normal activities.

Biofeedback

This is a useful tool for learning how to relax. A biofeedback system uses the 'feedback' to the individual of biological information that is otherwise unavailable to him or her so that he or she can exert some control over a particular body system. Using such techniques people have been able to control the temperature of a particular part of their body, their pulse rate, their blood pressure, their perspiration rate, the relaxation of various specific muscles, and so on. Although there is no guarantee that learning to reduce *certain* of the effects of stress will reduce them all, biofeedback is definitely a valuable tool and shows the stressed and tense person what can be done with the power of the mind alone.

The simplest piece of biofeedback equipment (it can be bought from good chemist shops and specialist health and sports stores) is a simple skin resistance meter. Pads attached to the fingers detect the level of sweat production–which relates fairly closely to the level of activity of the flight-or-fight stress system of the body. The machine produces a noise, and the idea is to use your mind to silence the noise produced by the machine. How you do this is up to you. Some people think of pleasant, calming scenes. Others imagine a favourite pursuit. Others just gaze at a beautiful picture or object. As sweat production falls, the skin resistance falls and the machine stops making a noise. Such equipment is available for under £50, but there is also much more sophisticated and expensive biofeedback equipment on the market. Perhaps the most complex device is the 'mind mirror', a type of electro-encephalograph which displays twelve printouts of brain waves.

Whichever method is used, the idea–just as with relaxation exercises–is that one recalls the method when the situation gets stressful. Many thousands of people have used relaxation exercises or biofeedback to relieve themselves of stage fright, nerves before exams or a job interview, etc. What you learn at home is put into use whenever you need it.

Meditation

This is the final type of stress-reduction method to be described briefly here. There are many forms and there is no room in this book to describe them in detail. Most are best learned in some kind of formal setting–many local authorities have evening classes on the subject, and there are also private groups, church groups, and many other places one can go to to learn.

Before doing any meditation spend a few minutes doing relaxation exercises and deep breathing, which will make you more receptive to your chosen method of meditation. There are many techniques of meditation but they all have in common the conscious attempt to focus the mind on one subject. Concentrating on your breathing as described on page 76 is a simple form of meditation. Concentrating on breathing is relatively easy compared with concentrating on an abstract thought or image. The crux of meditation is the clearing from the mind of everyday clutter. Some claim that meditation, if taught well and done properly, will lead to a raised spiritual awareness as well as relaxation but this may not be what you want.

The device or 'distracting object' which you concentrate on can be a mental picture, an image, a sound, a word, an idea, an activity, etc. Various forms of meditation have used repetitive chanting or even the repetition of a simple single-syllable such as 'Om'.

Postures and positions for meditation vary greatly but the most important thing is to stay immobile. Whatever position is adopted it is important to incorporate the meditation into one's daily routine and so look upon it as an oasis of calm and peace.

As the weeks go by many, if not all, of the signs of stress should disappear and you should feel a lot healthier generally. Also, the positive benefits of any of the activities described in this section will boost your natural immunity to disease and the ability of your body to heal itself when others around you are falling ill.

This is the essence of preventive health–boosting the body's natural defences so that it can withstand the stresses, infections and cancers that are being continuously produced in all of us, as well as emotional strife, environmental onslaughts and so on. Many people experience many or all of these yet never get ill. If more of us lived along the lines detailed in this section we could join them.

For more on stress, see page 335

DISEASE AND THE WESTERN LIFESTYLE

To many, if not most, of us living in the West, the notion that some of the diseases we all take for granted as the major killers are preventable is indeed hard to accept. Strokes, heart disease and cancers between them kill most westerners yet they are relatively uncommon in the non-westernised world. Why should this be, and is it possible that by altering the way we live we could reduce or even abolish these conditions?

At first, the suggestion that it is our western lifestyle that causes many of our major diseases seems quite ridiculous, but the pioneering work of a group of doctors who spent decades in non-westernised parts of the world must make us think again. They noticed that certain non-infective diseases were very much less common in traditional societies than they were in the West. They wondered at first what to call these diseases. 'Diseases of civilisation' (meaning modern, western civilisation) is not quite right because evidence suggests that some of them were around but uncommon in the ancient civilisations of Egypt, Greece, Rome, India and China. Given that the conditions they found to be so common were now mainly seen in communities that had adopted our western, technological way of life, they decided to call them 'western diseases'.

The first two criticisms that are immediately thrown at such a suggestion are, first, that people in the Third World tend not to live to be old enough to get 'our' diseases, and second that their medical systems are so poor that they simply do not diagnose the conditions even when they *are* present. Neither of these criticisms stands up when examined in depth, and studies which show that migrant populations (originally without western diseases) adopt the diseases of their westernised brothers in their new country, prove without doubt that it is not simply that whole populations in the non-industrialised world are somehow immune to westernised diseases. It is also impressive (if depressing) to watch peoples with traditional lifestyles take on our disease pattern as they adopt our way of life.

So what could possibly be causing these western diseases? Obviously motor-car accidents can only occur where there are motor cars, and pollution from industrial effluent or cigarette smoke is only found where these two abound, but these are not the diseases I mean when I refer to western diseases. The conditions in question are such disorders as: high blood pressure, obesity, diabetes, heart disease, appendicitis, piles, varicose veins, gall-stones, kidney stones and cancer.

Of course, any of many changes in western lifestyle in recent years could account for the frequency of all these conditions today and their virtual absence until the last century in the West and in most of the world today, but because many of them seem to affect the digestive system it makes sense to start looking for clues in the food we eat. Modern technology has radically altered the production and preparation of food and it now seems that food changes are at the heart of many of these 'new' western diseases. Let us look in turn at each of the diseases listed above to see why it should be that they are so common in the West and yet so uncommon elsewhere.

High blood pressure (hypertension)

Blood pressure goes up with age in most people in most populations that have been studied, but one study reports thirteen small populations where this does not occur and a major study in Kenya in the 1930s found that high blood pressure was hardly ever seen. A study of 1,000 post-mortems in Kenya in 1936 found that only 36 of the deaths were the result of heart disease and there were no cases of high blood pressure. In the early 1940s one doctor found 23 cases of high blood pressure over four years – most of those were salaried and prosperous. At this time strokes and angina were still considered to be very rare and serious hypertension was not seen in East Africa until 1953.

Today, hypertension has become a very common disease in East Africa and a review of deaths in hospitals there found that hypertension was responsible for 'something like 40 to 60 per cent of the heart disease hospital diagnoses'. By 1978 it was the second commonest cause of death among the urbanised Bantu. Research has implicated many factors in this dramatic story but apart from the stresses of urbanisation (which are difficult fo quantify and are arguably not much greater than the stresses of tribal life), the amount of salt a population eats seems to be crucial. An analysis of the Kikuyu diet in 1930 found that salt was never added to food. The vast majority of the diet was unrefined starch in the form of carbohydrate (72 per cent of calories consumed); the rest was made up of fat (9 per cent) and protein (19 per cent). Salt intake started to rise in the 1920s and 1930s, first in urban areas. In places where diets were supervised by Europeans salt use was common.

Western man consumes 6–18 g of sodium (as common salt) daily. Primitive hunter-gatherer man consumes about 0.6 g daily. A recent study of such peoples found that their blood pressure does not rise with age.

Ethnic groups who do not add common salt to their food have lifelong low blood pressure and no exceptions have been found to this rule. A part of this might be explained by different sensitivity to dietary salt. Genetically controlled salt sensitivity varies considerably both in animals and in man. It is now suggested that most people can tolerate a daily intake of up to about 4 g of salt but that above this level an increasing proportion of salt-sensitive subjects develop blood pressure with age. Above 6–8 g almost all salt-sensitive people will develop blood pressure with age. It is interesting that although fat people so often have hypertension in the West, obesity itself is not the cause – it is the high salt intake that so often goes with the obesity.

This knowledge has led to many trials of low-salt diets to alleviate hypertension. One major study found that reducing salt intake to 3 g daily was as effective in lowering blood pressure as drugs prescribed to another group for the same purpose. Many centres now claim to achieve normal blood pressure in their patients within a few weeks of putting them on a low-salt diet (4 g a day or less) and many people can then stop taking drugs entirely.

Obesity

It is impossible to be sure what proportion of the western world is obese but current estimates suggest that about 30 per cent are 'clinically'

overweight. That obesity increases one's chances of suffering from diabetes, heart attacks, gall-stones, hiatus hernia, cancers of all kinds, painful feet, arthritis of the hips and knees and several other conditions is now beyond dispute. It shortens life and reduces the quality of life for countless millions of people. Obviously obesity is a terrible health and social problem.

In the 1920s obesity was rare in African rural peoples and a 1960 study suggested that low body weights were lifelong in rural Zulu men. There is now overwhelming evidence that in certain ways the control mechanism of body weight somehow breaks down in an affluent society. Individuals in primitive societies have a kind of automatic regulator which controls the amount of effort they spend searching for food and the amount of food they consume. According to one world expert, 'Supermarket Man has no such automatic facility.'

An adult man, wherever he lives and however he eats, who eats 1 per cent more energy every day than he expends accumulates 1 kg of fat per year. At 30 such a man would weigh 30 kg (66 lb) more than someone who had been in good energy balance for a lifetime. Obesity is a real hazard to hunter-gatherers because it slows them down, affecting their ability to catch prey and to escape animal predators. So in survival terms it pays the hunter-gatherer to keep slim. Such peoples get their food mainly from plants, and individuals spend 2–3 hours a day gathering food, three-quarters of which is supplied by women and children gathering and one quarter by men hunting. Many hunter-gatherers live long enough to become obese but they do not do so. In one study of such a group 7 per cent of the men were over 65 but they were all slim.

The first agricultural revolution, in about 10,000 BC, changed things radically for most of the world's population as man began to farm cereals and to store food. The diet of today's peasant agriculturalist has changed little since this time. Although food shortages occur in developing rural peasant communities, resulting mainly from population density and poor soil fertility, competent scientific observers say that even where the population is not dense, the soil is fertile and there are two harvests a year, body weight remains low throughout adult life.

Pastoral peoples plant no crops but raise animals and eat meat, blood and milk. Studies show that their blood cholesterol levels remain low despite the high intakes of animal fat and cholesterol, and that obesity is rare.

The second agricultural revolution started in Europe towards the end of the eighteenth century and crop rotation and fertilisers, together with better machinery and animal husbandry, changed western eating habits totally. The upper classes became wealthy; meat, butter and milk could be consumed throughout the year; and sugar intake went up, as did that of alcoholic drinks. Obesity suddenly became extremely common in the upper social classes, towards the end of the seventeenth century and even more so in the eighteenth century. Portraits of even quite young people of the time show double chins.

With the coming of the Industrial Revolution in the nineteenth century the production of goods and wealth really took off. This enabled radical changes in the production, storage and transport of food. Dietary fibre began to be milled out of bread–the staple diet of the masses. Salt, sugar and fat intakes rose and the consumption of starchy foods fell. Fruit and vegetable intakes rose steadily. People got less exercise, as machines began to do the work. Slowly food became so plentiful, even for the masses, that people began to eat snacks between meals as well as regular meals–themselves a luxury for many until 200 years before.

So why is obesity so common in the West and hardly ever seen in non-westernised peoples? The main answer is that our food has radically changed *in character*–it is not simply that we eat too much of it, as was previously thought. Over half the energy in the food of a hunter-gatherer or peasant agriculturalist comes from high-starch foods. Such a diet eaten even 'to excess' does not cause obesity, partly because it is almost impossible to eat an excess, so bulky and filling is it. At least two-thirds of the energy in a western diet comes from fibre-free fats and sugars and low-fibre cereal products. Undoubtedly, there are other factors in the production of obesity but, looking at populations overall, food is undoubtedly at the heart of the problem. That westernised people can slim by adopting a high-fibre (rich in unrefined carbohydrate) diet is no longer in doubt; and the observation that slim, rural dwellers in non-westernised countries can be made obese very quickly on a western diet is not easy to refute.

It seems that food intake stops when we feel we have had enough and that we feel satisfied sooner on foods rich in dietary fibre – i.e. unrefined carbohydrate foods. It is simply so easy to over-consume refined foods that have no appetite-controlling capacity that we in the West eat ourselves to obesity.

Diabetes

Studies in East Africa in the 1930s found that diabetes was rare. Nowadays there are diabetic clinics in all town hospitals.

Diabetes is undoubtedly an ancient disease and Galen, who lived in the second century and was the greatest medical authority in the Roman Empire, certainly described it. What most people do not realise is that he only saw two cases! The condition was further described in the seventeenth century in Europe, but it was rare until the eighteenth century, when it became a common disease among the English aristocracy. Obesity and diabetes emerged together as societies became affluent and ate more fat, oil, sugar, meat, wine and

beer, together with refined cereals. In 1971 one researcher reviewing diabetes in the tropics wrote that, 'The incidence of diabetes is likely to increase with urbanisation or as the complexity of civilisation takes hold of any racial group.'

Diabetes is not one simple condition, but a family of conditions. There are, however, two common types. The first (now called Type I diabetes) most commonly first occurs in children but can affect people of any age. Such people need insulin by injection – usually for life. This is a very rare condition among the children of many tropical communities and is also rare in Japanese children. Type II diabetes is the adult-onset type that usually, but not always, occurs in the obese (usually women). In both types genetic and environmental factors are important.

The cause of diabetes is as yet unknown but it has recently been suggested that a high intake of foods rich in high-fibre starch is protective and might even be a good treatment for diabetes. Trials have now shown that slimming on a high-fibre diet can 'cure' many cases of adult-onset diabetes completely. Other studies have shown that eating a high-fibre diet can reduce the need for insulin in Type 1 diabetes, and in certain trials patients have been able to stop taking insulin completely when eating the correct diet rich in unrefined starches. Obviously this all has to be done under the watchful eye of a doctor who is expert in diabetes – it is not a do-it-yourself treatment for diabetics.

Heart disease

Now the biggest single killer in the western world, cardio-vascular disease emerges last of all the western diseases as a population becomes westernised. Even today rural peoples around the world have very little coronary heart disease. Among the rural Bantu in southern Africa coronary heart disease occurs at a level of only 1 or 2 per cent of that seen in white South Africans of similar age and sex. As obesity rises in a community, usually along with blood pressure, death rates from heart disease also rise.

Appendicitis

Most of us think of appendicitis – the emergency operation most often performed in the western world – as inevitable but this again is a relatively recent western disease. In fact it is the first of these diseases to appear once a population changes its eating habits and lifestyle.

Studies of appendicitis in pre-1920 Africa show that it was a rare disease among the indigenous population but relatively common in the Europeans and Indians. It is still possible to find hospitals in Africa where the surgeons have not seen a case of appendicitis for ten years. In contrast, British hospitals remove 56,000 appendixes every year. During the past twenty-five years the number of people with acute appendicitis admitted annually to large western hospitals throughout sub-Saharan Africa has risen from less than 5 to over 50 per year. When appendicitis emerges in a community it appears first in the adults. Two dramatic examples of a western diet as the cause of appendicitis come from China and Africa. In China a flour mill was installed in a town in which appendicitis was almost unknown. Within a few months of the mill opening cases of appendicitis began to appear in the wealthier middle class, who had taken to eating white flour. During the 1939-45 War appendicitis appeared for the first time amongst African troops when they were supplied with British army rations during their attachment to British regiments.

It is not known for certain what causes appendicitis but the initial problem is likely to be an obstruction to the hollow cavity within the appendix; pressure builds up and deprives the lining of the appendix of its blood supply. This paves the way for infection to enter and the organ becomes inflamed. The original obstruction probably comes about as a result of the passage of sluggish, thick, tarry stools along the large bowel off which the appendix branches. It is known that low-fibre diets, high in refined carbohydrates, are the biggest culprits in this story.

Piles

It is hard to tell how common piles are in any community because the term is a relative one and most people with the condition do not seek medical help. A study of seventy-seven rural hospitals in Africa found that fewer than 3 people a year were diagnosed as having severe piles. This is dramatically less than in the West where the condition is said to affect half of the entire population over the age of 50!

Piles used to be thought to be a kind of varicose vein of the back passage, but recent research shows that this is not so. They should now be thought of as a prolapse of special anal cushions which, when of normal size and in their normal position, help maintain faecal continence. These cushions are now known to prolapse when hard, sticky stools pass over them and shear them away from their underlying tetherings. This can be entirely put down to a diet too low in dietary fibre. Many early cases of piles can be cured by putting the affected person on to a high-fibre diet.

Varicose veins

It is much easier to estimate how common these are than is the case with piles. In North America 19 per cent of men and 44 per cent of women over the age of 30, and 42 per cent of men and 65 per cent of women over the age of 50 have varicose veins. In Third World countries the figure is nearer 10 per cent of people over the age of 30.

The erect posture of humans, constrictive clothing, repeated pregnancies and heredity are no longer acceptable causes in view of the differences in worldwide distribution of the disease. It is now thought that the main problem is the increased pressure in the leg veins that is produced while straining at stool. We in the West strain to pass our hard stools and do so in a sitting position. Peoples who don't get varicose veins squat to open their bowels (so shutting off the leg veins at the groin) and pass their motions easily because these are very soft (like toothpaste) as a result of their high-fibre diet.

Gall-stones

The most common type of gall-stone is made of cholesterol and is the result of altered bile metabolism produced by dietary changes in the West. It is difficult to be sure exactly how common gall-stones are because many produce no symptoms at all and are discovered by chance on X-ray or at autopsy. However, accurate enough figures enable us to say that the proneness to gall-stones of westernised countries varies between 30 and 60 per cent—the highest figures being from Chile, Sweden and Czechoslovakia. Third World countries have much lower figures, for example: Uganda 3 per cent; Thailand 4.4 per cent; and Ghana 0 per cent. A survey of hospitals in Africa, India, Arabia and New Guinea confirmed that gall-stones are extremely rare in the rural parts of these countries. On the other hand, in the urbanised black population of Johannesburg, gall-stones are quite common (12 per cent in elderly women).

Since World War II there has been a worldwide increase in the number of people undergoing surgery for gall-stones. The increase has been between 2.5 and 6 times, depending on the country. There has been an increase not just among older women –the most susceptible section of the population–but also among young people and in men. This suggests that whatever is causing gall-stones has increased its influence since the last war.

All this evidence suggests that gall-stones are directly related to a western way of life. It is also interesting that people with one of four other western diseases are much more likely to have gall-stones. These other conditions are obesity, diabetes, diverticular disease and hiatus hernia. A woman with gall-stones has on average put on more weight since maturity than one without, even if she is not seriously overweight.

The common factor between all these conditions is the over-consumption of refined foods and of high-energy foods. A reduced calorie intake is the best treatment for maturity onset (Type II) diabetes as we have seen; it also reduces harmful blood fats and is slimming. But–more to the point when it comes to gall-stones–it results in a lowered concentration of cholesterol in the bile and so in fewer gall-stones. Wild animals rarely have gall-stones but they can be made to have them by being fed artificial diets such as our western diet. Of all the dietary factors that have been studied in the laboratory and clinical trials the lack of dietary fibre and too much sugar and white flour are the main culprits. Increasing the intake of these reduces the likelihood of an individual forming gall-stones.

Kidney stones

The incidence of kidney stones has gone up considerably this century. It used to be mainly an adult disease but now it occurs in children too. The occurrence rate is between 3 and 13 per cent in westernised countries, with the rate in the USA about 12 per cent, yet kidney stones are rare in people living in poor or primitive conditions.

What could have caused such a change? The greatest difference between the poor and the affluent countries of today is their diets. In the richer countries, the fat and animal protein content of the diet is five times greater than in the typical diet of the poorer countries. Most kidney stones are made of calcium and it is known that both protein and glucose can increase the amount of calcium the body puts out in the urine. One researcher has found that the glucose effect is exaggerated in stone-formers. Sugar can be shown to increase the amount of calcium put out by the kidneys in normal people and to produce damage to the tubular cells of the kidneys of animals.

It has been found that people who repeatedly form kidney stones eat more animal protein than do other people. The stone-formers in one study consumed more meat, fish and poultry and less grain and starch than did non-stone-formers. A high-fibre diet might well be of value in this condition in so far as it reduces blood-glucose swings–which are known to be critical in producing a urine rich in calcium, which then crystallises out to form kidney stones. Lastly, there is evidence that a western diet reduces the production of normal stone-inhibiting substances in the urine.

Cancer

The most recent collection of cancer incidence figures from around the world shows that the highest of all is in black African males in Bulawayo, Zimbabwe, while the next highest level is in the black population of the San Francisco Bay area of the USA. These men have a 19 per cent chance of developing cancer by the age of 61 if they don't die of something else first. The lowest levels of cancer incidence occur among men in Nigeria, who have a 6 per cent chance of developing cancer by the same age. In women the highest cancer rate in the world is among the better off (i.e. white) groups in the US but women from less affluent areas (i.e. mostly racial minorities) still have quite high levels.

It is interesting to look at the different types of cancer prevalent in different areas, especially if they are occurring in the same country. While the total rates of cancer in black males in Zimbabwe and the USA and in females in North and South America are all similar, the organs in which they occur are quite different. Cancers of the liver and gullet are more often seen amongst black men in Zimbabwe where they are fifteen and three and a half times more common respectively than in the USA. Cancer of the cervix is five times more common in Colombian women than in women in the USA, and cancer of the breast is three times more common in the USA than in Colombia. In both sexes cancer of the colon and rectum occur between four and six times more frequently in the USA than in either Zimbabwe or Colombia.

Undoubtedly cancers were known in antiquity but evidence suggests that they were rare until this century and things have changed dramatically in the West in recent years. Three National Cancer Surveys in the US span thirty-two years and give a very accurate picture of what is happening to cancer incidence. The occurrence of cancer has gone up for some types and down for others but the overall trend is upwards. Colorectal (large bowel) cancer, and that of the prostate and bladder, and of course lung cancer, have all gone up whereas cancers of the mouth, pharynx, gullet, stomach, liver and biliary tract have all become less common. Over this period women have fared relatively well compared with men because they have not shared in the rise in lung cancer and have experienced a sharp drop in cancer of the cervix. Interestingly, in a country like Japan, cancer incidence figures were much like the Third World until 1930 but have now changed to a westernised pattern. The incidence of cancer of the stomach, gullet and liver is falling in Japan, and that of lung, pancreas, bowel and rectum is rising. Cancer of the breast is also on the increase in Japan.

All of these findings suggest that westernisation does something to a population to induce not only *more* cancer overall but rather different sorts of cancer. Let's look at what these factors could be in a westernised life.

Reproductive and sexual behaviour

These both influence the incidence of certain cancers, and change with westernisation. Early first childbirth and having large numbers of children both reduce the incidence of breast cancer. In the West we delay the birth of the first child and women have few children. Both of these things have produced substantially higher levels of breast cancer in the West. Cancer of the ovary is also seen more in populations with reduced fertility.

Cancer of the cervix, in contrast, increases in incidence with greater fertility. This relationship may be related to the proven link between early promiscuous sexual activity and cervical cancer. No one knows why this should be but the current theories are that smegma (the white

matter that can collect under an uncircumcised man's foreskin) or even semen itself might be carcinogenic. A more recent suggestion is that cancer of the cervix is caused by a venereally transmitted virus such as herpes. Genital hygiene and the use of a condom (sheath) reduce these risks.

Occupational exposure to chemicals

This is an unfortunate side-effect of moving off the land and into factories. It has led to increasing numbers, of men especially, being exposed to carcinogenic chemicals, for much of their working lives in certain industries. It has definitely caused an increase in tumours of the bladder and the skin. A particular type of lung tumour is seen commonly in those who work with asbestos dust.

No one knows how great a problem industrial exposure to carcinogens is and today many known hazards have been reduced or totally removed, but westernised peoples are still exposed to food additives, washing-up liquid residues, air pollutants, water pollution from industry and agriculture and frank chemical hazards at work in varying amounts. The harm done by some of these agents is well known and provable, yet we continue to bombard ourselves, often quite unnecessarily, with chemicals of a dubious nature.

Improved hygiene

Better sanitary conditions are a reason for falling levels of certain sorts of cancer as populations become westernised. Cancer of the liver is the best example here. There is increasing evidence that hepatitis B is an important factor in the production of liver cancer and this infection falls with improved personal and community hygiene. Greater personal hygiene in the West has also led to a reduced number of cancers of the penis.

Tobacco and alcohol

Consumption of these substances plays a substantial part in the rise of cancer levels as a community becomes westernised. Tobacco consumption is directly linked to cancer of the lung and bladder and probably to that of the pancreas. Cigarette consumption was low until 1973 in developing countries but as the public in the westernised world became aware of the dangers and tobacco consumption fell, the companies switched their sales to Third World countries. We can expect to see far more cancers in these countries as a result.

Alcohol interacts with tobacco as a causative agent in cancers of the gullet and larynx and independently of tobacco raises the level of cancer of the liver by producing cirrhosis. In contrast to the situation regarding tobacco consumption there is no direct and consistent relationship between alcohol consumption and economic development. Alcohol consumption is going up everywhere and there is evidence that cancer of the gullet is rising along with it.

Diet

Eating habits have always been a prime suspect as a cause of cancers but are difficult to convict conclusively. In general, westernised countries consume a diet high in energy, fat, protein and sugar and low in unrefined starch, dietary fibre, vitamins and minerals. Western diets make people fat and obesity has now been linked with an increased susceptibility to cancer. Several studies have found that tall, fat women are the most likely to develop breast cancer. Studies of Japanese women have linked the consumption of meat, eggs, butter and cheese to breast-cancer incidence. Breast cancer rates in rats can be greatly increased by feeding them diets high in fat. This raises their levels of prolactin (a hormone that acts on the breast).

Cancer of the body of the uterus (not the cervix) is more strongly linked with obesity than is breast cancer. Fat women seem to produce more oestrogens and these in turn may have a carcinogenic action on both breasts and uterus.

When we look at cancer of the colon the link seems to be with the increased consumption of meat and animal protein more than with fat. A study of Japanese migrants to Hawaii found that sufferers from cancer of the large bowel were more likely than control patients to have adopted a western style of diet and were about two and a half times more likely to have regularly eaten meat, particularly beef. Further support for this finding comes from the many studies done on the Seventh Day Adventists and other vegetarian groups in the US. They all have lower than expected colon-cancer rates. The Mormons, who are big beef consumers, also have low colon-cancer rates, so clearly beef is not the only answer. The worldwide level of cancer of the colon is related to the consumption of unrefined cereals and several experts have suggested that dietary fibre is protective in some way. This may be the result of its bulking action (which dilutes any carcinogens present in the food residue), or of its ability to increase the speed at which food residues pass through the colon (so reducing the amount of time a carcinogen is in contact with the bowel wall). Nobody knows for sure. Certainly studies have found that people with bulky stools have less colon cancer than those with hard, tarry stools. Fibre lack may well not be the only factor here though, and the answer will probably be found to be a combination of fat, meat and fibre – each of which causes has its champions in the scientific world of cancer research.

But we don't learn about diet and cancer by looking only at the negatives. Stomach cancer has *fallen* dramatically this century and always falls when a country becomes westernised. No one knows why this should be but in Japan this decline in mortality is paralleled by an increasing consumption of meat, milk, eggs, oil and fruit. Studies of individual Japanese have found that two glasses of milk a day seem to be protective. The daily consumption of green or yellow vegetables appears to be protective too. Perhaps this decline is due to the increased consumption of vitamins A and C. Vitamin A has been shown to reduce the risk of experimentally-induced cancers in laboratory animals and there are several studies that suggest that it reduces the incidence of lung cancers in humans.

This brief survey of the major diseases of the western world shows clearly how they are linked to a western lifestyle, a fact that can be established both historically and by making comparisons with non-westernised peoples around the world today. Perhaps we should round off this section by looking at the effect of particular aspects of our western lifestyle on health. We shall look at how to combat the negatives of this lifestyle in Part Three of the book.

Personal lifestyle and disease

Although we all live against the backcloth of western civilisation we are able now, at least to some extent, to manipulate our environment so as to reduce some of the hazards. There are three reasons for linking health and lifestyle.

1. The major causes of death, serious illness and disability in the West today are the chronic diseases and violence. Chronic disease accounts for about 80 per cent of all deaths, and violence in the form of accidents,

suicide and homicide for about 8 per cent.

2. Behind most of these deaths are behavioural and environmental factors, many of which can be prevented. About 80 per cent of all cancers in men, and 75 per cent in women, for example, are attributable to environmental or behavioural factors or a combination of both.

3. A few individual and societal lifestyle changes could make an enormous difference to rates of death and disease and levels of suffering in any westernised society. The most blatant examples of harmful behaviour are tobacco and alcohol abuse, over-eating, lack of physical activity, drug abuse, sexual promiscuity, the irresponsible use of motor cars, and carelessness about contraception.

Smoking

Of the eight risk factors listed above smoking has been the most widely studied. Nearly 20 per cent of all western mortality is smoking related. Lethal diseases associated with smoking are: heart disease, lung cancer; chronic bronchitis and emphysema; and cancer of the kidney, stomach and pancreas. It also plays a part in the forming of peptic ulcers and has adverse effects on the fetus. In spite of this being well known and widely publicised 36 per cent of the UK population and 41 per cent of adults in the US, still smoke.

Alcohol

The extent to which alcohol contributes to disease, disability and premature death is not always appreciated. Many authorities agree that 'alcoholism' is the most devastating socio-medical problem faced by human society apart from war and malnutrition. It plays a major part in liver disease, peptic ulcer, many digestive disorders, nervous system damage, nutritional disorders, and metabolic changes. It contributes to half of all deaths in car accidents, half of all murders, and a quarter of all suicides. The true alcoholic's lifespan is shortened by 10–12 years and even that of the heavy social drinker is shortened.

Drug abuse

This is now increasingly common in the form both of legal and illegal drugs. People living in the industrialised world are increasingly dependent upon readily available drugs as aids to coping with the stresses of modern life. These range from prescribed tranquillisers such as Valium and Librium to alcohol, tobacco, caffeine, cannabis, cocaine and heroin. Six out of ten of all prescriptions in the US are for mood-altering drugs. Legally prescribed drugs in the form of tranquillisers and sleeping tablets are used in suicide attempts – successful and otherwise – and the number of narcotic addicts is rising all over the western world. Narcotic drugs are now the second biggest killer under the age of 40 in

New York (violence and accidents are the main cause). The withdrawal of both legal and illegal drugs can cause real suffering (as millions of tranquilliser patients know to their cost).

Overnutrition

We saw on page 92 how obesity caused by eating too much of the wrong things can result in all kinds of diseases and disabilities secondary to obesity, and the link between cancer and obesity is now too well proven to ignore. It is estimated that one in three Americans are clinically overweight; juvenile obesity is a growing cause for concern (with post-mortem studies on young teenagers finding serious deposits of atheroma in their arteries); too much fat and too much energy have provable ill-effects and produce cancers, diabetes and gall-stones (see pages 94–100); the over-consumption of salt produces high blood pressure, and the decrease in dietary fibre produces many ill-effects. We have seen what constitutes a healthy eating pattern to prevent disease on pages 70–74.

Lack of physical activity

Ninety-three per cent of UK homes have a TV set and the average family watches more than three hours a day. The average western person now spends more time watching TV than doing anything else other than sleep or work! The modernisation of industry and the universal use of cars and labour-saving devices in the home makes us all unused to strenuous muscular effort.

There is now good evidence that regular and fairly strenuous exercise is positively valuable to health, helps keep us slim, helps control food intake, improves our sense of well-being and keeps old people fitter and happier.

Motor-vehicle accidents

Road accidents kill about 50,000 US citizens and injure another 5 million each year. Speeding, failure to use seat-belts or motorcycle helmets, and alcohol and soft or hard drugs are frequently involved. We saw on page 37 the effect on the death and injury rate in the US of the imposition of the 55 mph speed limit after the Arab oil embargo of 1973.

Violence

All western countries are becoming more violent. Between 1960 and 1975 the rate of violent crime in the US (murder, rape, assault and robbery) tripled. The US has one of the highest murder rates in the world (about five times that of the average European country). Violence and vandalism are now an increasing reality in inner-city schools throughout the western world and even within the family violence is on the increase, with battered children and spouses an increasing problem. The suicide rate in the western world is rising. Many quite sober and responsible experts now see violence as a culturally sanctioned way of problem-solving in American life!

Failing family relationships and marriages

There is a provable link between divorce and poor health and early death, and more than a third of all western marriages now end in divorce. The married have a significantly longer lifespan and in England and Wales the married have less chronic illness (especially mental illness) than the formerly married and make fewer demands on the health-care system. Divorced people have more days off work, more mental illness, and are more likely to be admitted to mental hospital and to have minor ailments than are the married. Recent US research has found that *all* illness – including cancer – is more common in the formerly married than in the married.

Children raised in single-parent families have more illness and make more demands on the health-care system than do those with two parents. A lack of physical and psychological support is probably largely to blame but many single-parent families also become poor (if they are not already so) and poverty brings its own health hazards.

Sexual promiscuity and contraceptive carelessness

The role of women in society is changing very quickly and sexual attitudes have changed in parallel with this over the last thirty years. Earlier sexual experience results in more babies born to young girls which in turn increases the statistics for still-birth, prematurity and 'poor quality' births. Low-birth-weight babies are two to three times more likely to be born to such youngsters. The results of sexual promiscuity, with more than half of all married people *admitting* to having had an extramarital affair, and the considerable rise in premarital sexual activity have resulted in more VD, more cervical cancer and more unwanted pregnancies. At the most dramatic end of the scale AIDS kills hundreds of people a year in the West and genital herpes causes substantial sexual disability among millions.

About a third of all pregnancies in the UK have been calculated to be 'unwanted' – at least at the time of conception. We look at this complex question more on page 44 but in addition to all the factors mentioned there is contraceptive carelessness, especially among the young. Young girls who get pregnant have a 20–50 per cent increased chance of having a low-birth-weight baby, which in turn can be associated with an increased mortality rate among the babies.

Depressing though all this appears to be at first sight it is quite clear that many, if not most, of these conditions can be modified given enough understanding, motivation and behavioural skills. In a highly fluid society such as we now have in the West nothing stays still for long and change *is* possible. Twenty years ago hardly anyone of influence was talking or writing about lifestyle, but today specialist health magazines, articles in other magazines and news-papers, health food stores, books and self-help groups attract the serious attention of millions of people every year. People are at last starting to realise that they can't go on abusing themselves and that simple changes can make a real difference to their life-expectancy in the future and their general well-being in the here-and-now.

Things are already changing for the better, especially in the US where change, both for good and evil, happens quickly. Both in the US and in the UK the consumption of to-bacco, eggs, butter and cream is down and recreational exercise is greatly in fashion. Non-smokers have been vociferous to assert their right to breathe clean air, and no-smoking areas in public places are now the norm rather than the exception. There is an increasing awareness of the family's role in promoting health and more effort is being put into the support of families in troubled situa-tions. Of course, it is still a drop in the ocean compared with what *could* be done but it is a start.

Public views are changing on sexual promiscuity and the 'anything goes' attitudes of the sixties and early seventies are now gone. AIDS and genital herpes have made both the homosexual and the heterosexual communities less promiscuous and, given the current falling family size throughout most western countries, the problem for the future in the West looks like being *under*-population not the reverse. Public criticism of vio-lence on TV and sex and violence on

videos for home consumption has had some effect on programming, and even the rise in violent street crimes associated with drug abuse, prostitution and pornography has slowed, if not reversed, in the US.

These valuable and positive changes have come about mainly for the following reasons. First, there has been a growing disenchantment with the ultra-permissive society which so obviously produced so much disease and *dis*-ease, and second there has been a slow but steady realisation that even a rich country like the US can no longer afford to pick up the pieces of such self-destructive ac-tivities as those listed on pages 99–104. Expenditure on personal and community health care now repre-sents so large a proportion of the total national expenditure that even the ordinary person in the street is get-ting the message loud and clear. The total ill-health cost of smoking and alcohol abuse alone in the US runs at over $100 billion a year. Such mind-blowing figures impress even the most sceptical. A new develop-ment in the US is a refusal by some managements to increase their com-pany's risk of having to pay out under workmen's compensation or employer liability laws by declining to employ individuals who have unhealthy lifestyles.

Even among the general public concern is growing along these lines. Non-smoking life-insurance policy-holders, for example, are starting to ask why they should pay increased life-insurance premiums to cover the other policy-holders who choose to smoke. Forward-thinking insurance companies are now offering reduced premiums to non-smoking and non-drinking individuals to take into account their reduced health risks and car-crash potentials.

With a growing realisation that we have finite resources; with the slowly dawning truth that fossil fuels will run out in our grandchildren's lifetime; and with a greater reluctance to generate wealth simply to squander it on insatiable 'health-care' systems, people all over the westernised world are beginning to question the old notions of absolute freedom and are starting to think more about social responsibility. Just as a heart-attack patient reaches his or her 'teachable moment' in the coronary care unit (the realisation dawns that he or she has just missed knocking on the pearly gates), so too society is starting to realise that its 'teachable moment' is close. In a sense, this is what this book is about. If I had written it ten years ago it would have been ignored or laughed at.

Part Three looks at individual diseases or ailments and gives practical tips on what to do to prevent them.

PART THREE
A Guide to Self-Help Prevention

SELF-HELP PREVENTION FOR VARIOUS CONDITIONS

In Parts One and Two we have looked at some of the background to prevention – in this Part we see what we can do as individuals to help ourselves. I have focused on self-help simply because it is an area of life over which we all have at least some degree of control. A few of us would like to conduct public campaigns for and against various pursuits that promote or harm health but, being realistic, the vast majority of people are not very politically minded and want to get on with living their lives in a way which produces benefits for them and their family.

Large-scale progress is usually made by a minority of activists who doggedly pursue a particular idea; such campaigners will always be vital. This part of the book does not address itself to such people, rightly or wrongly. Arguably such individuals will continue to campaign for what they believe in whatever the rest of society does or does not do – and much of the time they will be right.

When using this part of the book please be wary about combining prevention with treatment. If you are under your doctor for a particular condition that involves the use of drugs, don't stop taking them because you are following a particular preventive regime. Continue with the drugs and next time you see your doctor for a check-up tell him or her what you are doing and discuss whether it is possible to reduce or even stop the medication altogether. Be prepared for at least some hostility to many of the ideas in this book. Most doctors don't read the literature from which I have drawn many of the preventive measures and are naturally sceptical or even hostile. None of the ideas I outline here can do any harm and many can be proved to do a lot of good, so stick to your beliefs and if you find a particular thing works, tell your doctor, or other health-care professionals you come across, because it will help increase their confidence in such unfamiliar approaches.

ACCIDENTS

To most people an accident is an 'act of God', a random occurrence or the result of carelessness or thoughtlessness. But just because accidents occur quickly, often instantaneously, doesn't mean that they are not preventable – many are. Studies show that even the most apparently random of 'incidents' occur according to recognisable patterns and are in fact often quite predictable. So in preventive terms many accidents are not random happenings at all.

The size of the problem

To many readers the inclusion of accidents in a book about preventing disease and illness might come as something of a surprise but it should not do so. Unintentional injury is the fourth leading cause of death in most westernised countries and in the US caused 104,000 fatalities in 1977. Homicides and suicides are not included in this figure!

Accidental injury is *the leading cause* of death under the age of 40 in westernised countries and among the young contributes more deaths than *all other causes combined*.

Approximately one in three of the US population has a non-fatal injury sufficient to make them have a day away from their usual activities *every year*, and about half of these injuries need medical attention. Accidental injury accounts for about a quarter of all permanent disability in most western countries. For example, it is estimated that more than 20,000 people in the US alone suffer from on-going epilepsy as a result of a car accident.

Obviously this is a vast subject which could fill a book in itself. What I have done therefore is to summarise a few useful hints on the prevention of 'accidents' of all kinds, on the provable basis that many, if not most, can be prevented with some thought and planning.

Even with the best planning in the world some people will still suffer

'accidental' injuries because of psychological and emotional factors. People will continue to have rows and marital problems, to be depressed, to feel ill and so on, all of which can make them drive badly, drink too much and fall down the stairs, cut themselves and so on. In addition, certain personality types 'need' to indulge in dangerous or potentially dangerous pastimes which expose them to injury and even death. We cannot possibly abolish all accidents, but we can definitely reduce them. Here are just a few tips as to how to achieve this in day-to-day life. Most accidents occur at home so let's start there.

Safety in the home

Although many learned researchers talk about the 'psychodynamics' (i.e. the interplay between physiological and other factors) of accidents, especially accidents in the home, there is little doubt that most accidents are caused through carelessness and thoughtlessness. Over 2 million people are involved in accidents in their homes every year in the UK, a figure which considerably exceeds (in numbers if not severity) the far more widely publicised figure for road accidents. In Britain, accidents at home account for one in 112 of all deaths, and 37 per cent of all accidental deaths. This represents over 6,000 deaths in any one year. The very old and the very young are especially at risk from domestic hazards.

Most accidents at home occur in the kitchen (12 per cent) or living room (12 per cent), with the seemingly more dangerous garden next (9 per cent). In very young children, falls, burns and scalds, fires, suffocation and poisoning head the list of dangers, whereas older children suffer cuts, bruises and broken bones. Old people may accidentally take too many drugs. They may also fall more as their senses dull and this leads to an increase in cuts and burns. Seventy-five per cent of all injuries needing hospital treatment are cuts and bruises, sprains, fractures, dislocations, burns or scalds. Prevention often simply involves careful planning of your environment and daily life to reduce the risk of accidents.

There are special hazards encountered with fire, electricity, gas and water. Fire can often be prevented. The Home Office booklet *Dangers from Fire* is free to every household and is well worth reading. It is aimed at prevention and is available from local authorities, local fire prevention departments and county fire brigade headquarters. Electricity and gas in the home should be treated with respect. Always consult experts if in doubt. Many domestic fires start because of unsafe wiring, plugs and appliances. The Electricity Council has produced a booklet, *Safety in the Home,* which is available from electricity showrooms or the Council itself. Another very good booklet is *Electricity for Everyday Living.* This is available from EAW (Publications Dept Ltd), 25 Foubert's Place, London W1V 2AL, price 75p. The British Gas Corporation publishes the useful

booklet *Help Yourself to Gas Safety,* available from your gas showroom.

For more information about safety at home, write to RoSPA and ask for the information you require. *Safe as Houses* is a particularly useful booklet and may be obtained (price 55p) from the Royal Society for the Prevention of Accidents (RoSPA), Cannon House, The Priory, Queensway, Birmingham B4 6BS.

It is never too early to start thinking about safety. If you have small children you have moral and certain legal responsibilities to protect them from danger. Remember too that a child under the age of 16 cannot be held responsible for his or her own safety and well-being, or for that of another child under 16 – you as the adult are responsible. Get your children to respect danger, especially in connection with fire, gas, electricity and water and encourage them to think of the safety of others as soon as they are old enough.

Make today the day you get started – go around the house, check off the points on the next few pages and *do something* about them if necessary. That ten minutes could be the most profitable you spend for some time.

Kitchen

- Have cupboards that can be reached easily without having to stand on chairs or steps.

- Turn saucepans on cookers so that the handles don't stick out.

- Keep poisons, cleaning fluids and disinfectants high up and preferably locked away.

- Don't prise open cans with fingers.

- Never leave fat heating in a pan on the cooker unattended.

- Wipe up spills at once.

- Don't polish floors highly.

- Put all sharp things in drawers.

- Check the safety of plugs and wiring on domestic equipment.

- Don't overload electric sockets.

- Use a brush and dustpan to sweep up broken glass or china.

- Have a fire extinguisher or fire blanket handy and know how to use it.

- Never put water on a fat fire – put a lid on the pan or cover it with a fire blanket.

- Teach children to respect kitchen machinery.

- Have a first-aid kit handy

- Never leave a flex from an electric kettle overhanging the edge of a work surface.

Bathroom

- Keep all drugs and medicines out of children's reach, preferably in a special cupboard that locks. Place the medicine cupboard high on the wall so that children can't reach it.

- Flush all old medicines and those without labels down the lavatory.

- Ask the Gas Board to service the water heater yearly.

- Choose non-slip flooring.

- Have a non-slip backing to the bathroom mat.

- Use a non-slip mat in the bath for the young and old.

- Run cold water before hot when filling the bath.

- Ban portable, mains-operated electrical appliances from the bathroom.

- The heater should be high up on the wall or ceiling but not over the bath.

- Have a pull cord for the light switch.

- Have a proper razor socket only – no other power outlets.

- Keep razors well out of children's reach.

- Never block ventilation holes if you have a gas water heater in the bathroom.

- Never leave children alone in the bath.

Shed, garage and workshop

- Use the right tool – don't make do.

- Use ramps for cars, not piles of bricks.

- Keep garden tools hanging safely on walls.

- Keep weedkiller and other chemicals high up and out of reach. *Never* use domestic containers (e.g. lemonade bottles) for weedkiller etc.

- Check children's bikes for safety at least twice a year.

- Wear safety goggles or glasses when sanding or grinding.

- Wear a mask when spraying and ventilate the area.

- Work in a good light.

- Petrol must be kept in metal cans only (plastic degenerates and leaks). No more than 4 gallons may be stored at home.

- Keep children away when you are doing something dangerous – in one third of DIY accidents it is the watching child who is hurt.

- Never run an engine in a closed garage.

Gardens

- Make sure ladders have a firm footing.

- Don't be overprotective to older children.

- Supervise small children all the time on swings.

- Keep ponds fenced or covered if you have young children.

- Make water butts safe.

- Make sure paths and steps are even, especially for the elderly.

- Teach children to recognise poisonous trees and shrubs.

- Teach everybody to respect swimming pools.

- Put out fires before going to bed.

- Never throw inflammable liquids or aerosol cans on to fires.

- Wear stout shoes or boots when mowing.

- Clear lawns of stones and toys before mowing.

- Never leave a mower unattended when the engine is running or, in the case of an electric mower, still plugged in.

- When using power hedge clippers, keep the flex over your shoulder out of your way.

- Don't leave garden tools lying around – they are a danger to everyone.

- Keep septic tanks properly covered.

- Check deckchairs and garden furniture for safety after the winter.

- Never adjust your mower or hedge trimmer while it is running.

General

- Keep fires guarded. It is illegal to leave a child under 12 in a room with an unguarded fire.

- Keep pins, needles and scissors away from young children.

- Make sure bookshelves can't be pulled over.

- Put electric flexes where people won't trip over them but not under carpets.

- Replace flexes immediately if they are at all chafed or worn.

- Stand on something safe when dusting.

- Unplug the TV when going to bed or leaving the house.

- Never take the back off the TV or obstruct the ventilation slots.

- Keep all plastic bags away from children. This includes the inner sleeves of records.

- If you have young children, fit safety catches to all windows above ground level. Never leave open without a safety catch a window in a room where a young child is playing.

- Never put mirrors over the mantelpiece. Clothes could catch fire while the wearer is looking in the mirror.

- Don't leave small objects lying around with small children about–they may swallow them or put them in their ears or noses.

- Beware of catching fingers under sash windows and in doors.

- Never move an oil heater when it is alight. Position it where it cannot be knocked over.

- Electric convector heaters are safest for children's bedrooms.

- When using paraffin heaters ensure that there is adequate ventilation.

- Close medicine containers and return them to the medicine cupboard at once after use.

- Don't smoke in bed.

- Disconnect electric underblankets before going to bed.

- Return electric underblankets to the manufacturer for regular servicing. Never use one for the very young or the old who wet the bed. They can, however, use electric overblankets.

- Don't leave sleeping pills by the bed–repeated doses can be taken accidentally.

- Loose mats should have non-slip backing strips.

- Never carry too heavy or too big a load up or down stairs. Keep a hand free to hold the rail or banister.

- Use safety gates on the stairs with very young children about.

- Good lighting is essential–no dark corners.

- Don't store rubbish or anything inflammable under the stairs.

- Never leave things lying on the stairs, and make sure the stair carpet is well fixed and has no holes.

- Never meddle with gas or electrical installations. Call in an expert.

Dangers of fire

- Always keep a special watch on children and elderly people when fires and heaters are in use. (Remember, it is illegal to leave a child under the age of 12 in a room with an open fire.)

- Keep portable heaters away from furniture and curtains and in a safe place where they can't be knocked over. Keep oil heaters out of draughts. Never dry clothes over or near a fire or on the cooker.

- Keep all fires and heaters well guarded. A good guard covers the whole fireplace area, not just the actual fire itself.

- Use a sparkguard in front of real fires whenever you leave the room and overnight.

- Never leave lighted cigarettes or matches on upholstered furniture. When buying furniture look for the 'Resistant' label. This means that the furniture's covering is less likely than other coverings to catch fire but it is *not* fireproof.

- Never smoke in bed.

- Never overload power sockets with too many plugs.

- Use only the recommended fuse wire in your fuse box – never use thicker metal of any kind or you could start a fire elsewhere in the house. Electrical fires are still a major cause of domestic fires.

- Replace worn cables or flex at once.

- When deep-frying always watch the pan carefully to ensure that it doesn't overheat. Never fill the pan so that it is more than a third full with the food in.

- If there are children around keep matches and lighters where they can't find them.

  Store inflammable fluids such as petrol, paraffin and oil out of the sunlight and where they can't come into contact with heat or flame. Keep them in recommended containers with tops that fit.

- Plan your escape from your home so that if your home catches fire you will know exactly what to do. Find out where your nearest outside phone is (perhaps with a neighbour) to call the fire brigade.

- Always call the fire brigade for any fire, however small.

Firework safety

- Keep fireworks in a closed box. Take them out one at a time and put the lid back on at once.

- Follow the instructions on each firework carefully. Read them by torchlight – never a naked flame.

- Light fireworks at arm's length – preferably with a safety firework lighter or fuse wick.

- Stand well back.

- Never return to a firework once lit even if you think the flame has gone out–it may go off in your face.

- Never throw fireworks.

- Never put fireworks in your pockets.

- Keep pets indoors.

- Never fool with fireworks.

- Watch that bonfire too:

  –Site the bonfire away from the house, garage or shed.

  –Light with firelighters–not paraffin or petrol.

  –Keep a bucket or two of water handy, just in case.

  –Pour water on the bonfire embers before going indoors.

Having taken all these precautions enjoy your firework party. Ten million people do every year–safely.

Safety at work

- Be sure to use protective equipment, guards etc., where they are provided. If a particular situation seems to you to be dangerous and to need protective clothing or equipment, tell your manager or employer, or your union representative.

- Help newcomers to be aware of any dangers in your place of work.

- Ensure that people are properly trained to do their job with safety in mind.

- If you are in charge of people, be prepared to explain to them what the dangers are in any particular situation–once they understand they will probably be more willing to comply with the safety regulations.

- Keep accident records so that you can be more aware of what is actually going on.

- Keep all your tools and equipment in a safe condition.

- See that wounds and injuries are looked at straight away–even a small wound can make it more likely that you will have a serious accident.

- Remember that a low accident rate helps improve productivity and keeps costs down.

Safety in the office

Every year at least 5,000 office workers sustain injuries serious enough to keep them off work for three days or more. Almost all office accidents are caused by falls–next comes the handling and lifting of goods, materials and equipment. Here are a few useful tips for safety:

- Try to avoid cramped conditions. The law governs very strictly how much space there should be for any given number of people. Currently this is set at 40 sq ft per person (with his or her essential equipment–such as a desk and other furniture).

- Keep the temperature sensible. The law says that the temperature must not be less than 16°C (61°F).

- Be careful about furniture and fittings. Probably the most dangerous are filing cabinets that can topple over when top drawers are pulled out. Spread the load over the drawers and open only one drawer at a time. Metal furniture, particularly shelves and drawers, can cause nasty injuries.

- Badly placed telephones with trailing cables are a serious hazard, causing people to trip and fall. Put all cables under special cable covers if they cross the floor where people walk.

- Keep the office tidy. Keep floors, passages and stairs clear of goods, litter and so on. Place litter bins where no one can fall over them. Do not put broken glass into litter bins–dispose of it direct into the dustbins.

- Most accidents in offices are caused by falls over cables and objects lying about. Spilt liquids on shiny surfaces, rugs with holes in them, and worn carpets and rugs are also common causes of accidents. As you walk about, look where you are going. Walk, don't run.

- Learn to lift properly so as not to hurt your back (see page 152).

- Ensure that you are properly trained to operate the equipment you are supposed to be using. Never dabble with electronic or electrical equipment unless you are trained to do so. Be careful of chemicals used for copiers and other equipment.

- Be aware of the fire regulations for your office.

- Don't play around in the office– horseplay results in accidents, and the office is no place for practical jokes.

- Know who is in charge of first aid in your office.

- Be thoughtful about your actions and how they could make life unsafe for your colleagues.

Driving safety

Most families now have a car and many have two. Of all our everyday activities, driving is one of the most dangerous, killing 5,599 people in 1984 in Great Britain and injuring a further 319,000. The cost to the nation of all these accidents is £2,650 million. The fact is that by adopting some fairly commonsense preventive measures much of this illness, suffering and financial cost could be avoided. Here are the top twenty guidelines for safe driving drawn up in the UK by the Royal Society for the Prevention of Accidents.

- Plan journeys in advance and ensure that rest periods are allowed for on long trips.

- Keep your vehicle in good condition with frequent inspection and regular servicing.

- Ensure that you are fit and alert before driving. Do not drive after drinking and be sure that medicines will not affect your ability to drive.

- Maintain your observation well ahead and plan your approach to hazards. Use mirrors frequently.

- Handle your vehicle with positive precision and aim for the smoothest possible drive.

- Give clear and early signals for all manoeuvres. Help other road users to understand your intentions.

- Always think ahead and exercise caution. If in doubt – don't.

- Assess speed carefully to take account of all conditions. Avoid sudden changes of speed or direction on slippery surfaces.

- Never drive so fast that you cannot stop safely in the distance you can see to be clear.

- Remember the additional hazards of driving at night. Adjust your speed accordingly.

- Know the problems which a truck driver faces and make due allowance when such vehicles are manoeuvring.

- Traffic legislation has been developed to improve safety for all. Do not break the law.

- Be considerate of the comfort and safety of your passengers. Ensure that children are properly restrained and drive as you would wish to be driven. Remember that the law says you as the driver, and your front-seat passengers, must wear seat-belts at all times.

- Know and understand signs, signals and road markings – they all have valuable information for the driver.

- Remember that 95 per cent of accidents are caused by human error. Always maintain maximum concentration on the task in hand.

- Always drive within the limits of your capability and within the limits of your vehicle.

- Park in such a way as to cause minimum inconvenience and danger to other road users.

- Learn some basic first aid so that you know what to do if you see an accident.

- Maintain courtesy on the road. Be considerate towards the needs and problems of other road users.

- Take a pride in your driving, but remember that all drivers have room for improvement.

Safety for the elderly

Growing old is a growing business, with an ever increasing proportion of the population being over 65. People over 65 are at much greater risk than other age groups of having a fatal accident. The problem gets worse as the person becomes older, and women are more likely to be hurt than men.

Suffocating and choking

These accidents are chiefly associated with food. The problems may be exacerbated by arthritic hands which have difficulty cutting up food, ill-fitting dentures, or a total lack of teeth with which to chew the food. There is little that can be done positively to prevent such hazards.

Falls

Falls are the most common type of accident amongst elderly people. More than half of them occur when the elderly person is moving about on the same level but a substantial proportion also take place on the stairs.

Environmental hazards such as poor lighting and worn carpets play a part in this type of accident but physical factors are a more potent factor. These could include physical impairment, drugs or alcohol, inactivity and the reduced ability to retain one's balance.

Cuts

This type of accident is rarely fatal, with only about twenty-five deaths a year across all age groups. Although the younger groups suffer most there is still a substantial number of acci-

dents in the older range too. There can be medical consequences too as wounds may heal more slowly in the elderly.

Among the younger retired group lawn-mowers and garden tools are major offenders. Handling difficulties among the older group may lead to hitherto unlikely accidents with kitchen knives and can openers.

Fire

Fire and flames are the second major hazard for the older age groups. Nearly 10 per cent of cases are fatal in the 65-74 age group, and 13 per cent in the over 75 age group. Non-fatal accidents are likely to be serious.

Many accidents occur because of physical problems in elderly people. Dizziness, blackouts, strokes and heart conditions are often involved in a fall on to a radiant or open fire.

Blows

Once again there are few fatal cases of a person being struck by another person or an object but there are a significant number of such incidents causing injury to elderly people. The younger age group of elderly people are typically hurt trying to retrieve an object from the top of a wardrobe or cupboard while the older age group bump into furniture while moving about.

The general lowering of shelves and improvement of low-level storage is a task for pre-retirement days with a view to making life easier later.

Poisoning

Over half the fatal poisoning cases amongst elderly people involve drugs and medications. This is not surprising as people receiving a variety of treatments may become confused as to which medicines to take, when, and in what quantities.

Gases and vapours are responsible for a third of the deaths by poison amongst the elderly. This usually takes the form of gas poisoning – from faulty gas appliances or as a result of failing to have flues cleaned regularly.

Where accidents to the elderly occur

As people grow older they tend to concentrate their activities in the living-room and bedroom. This is clear from the marked difference in percentages of domestic accidents shown between the age groups in these two rooms:

	64-74 years	75+ years
Living/dining room	15	21
Kitchen	20	15.5
Garden/grassed area	16	9
Inside stairs	11	10
Bedroom	8	18.5
Yard/drive/path	10	6

The dangers of water

Whether you are walking near a pool, boating on a lake, cruising down a canal or sailing on the sea, water is a real hazard that demands great respect.

When at the seaside:

- Don't bathe when a red or other warning flag is up. It is not clever and could endanger the life of someone else who tries to save you.

- Keep a close eye on children – never let them play at the water's edge unattended. Babies and small children can drown in a few centimetres of water before you even know they are in trouble.

- Ensure that non-swimmers and all children wear approved and properly constructed life jackets if they are on the water.

- Look before you dive – many people suffer serious illness because they have hit their heads on rocks or dived into inches of water.

- If you are on the water either in a boat, water skiing or windsurfing, watch out for bathers. Keep well out of the way or fun can turn to tragedy within a few seconds.

- Beware of poisonous jellyfish. Most jellyfish are harmless but the Portuguese man-of-war (distinguished by its air-filled bladder that stands up like a sail) is poisonous. Never swim behind a Portuguese man-of-war because the tentacles can stretch up to 45 metres (50 yds) and bear poisonous capsules.

- Listen to the locals when swimming anywhere unfamiliar. With holidays taking people into tropical and sub-tropical waters today some are getting bitten by poisonous fish. Some of these bites can be dangerous so ask if it is safe first.

For details on the prevention of drowning, see page 200.

ACHING FEET

What is it?

A family of conditions around the foot that cause pain and aching.

What causes it?

Aching feet are hardly a subject for high-tech medicine and more often than not elicit a laugh rather than sympathy. After all, no one ever died of them. However, when your feet hurt you hurt all over and aching feet can make the most easy-going person irritable and tense. Painful feet in turn can cause back pain, knee problems and even stress and fatigue because of the abnormal postures your body takes up. All of this will make you less likely to want to play games and to take exercise and the cycle continues.

Almost eight out of ten people have aching feet at one time or another, according to surveys – in fact it is the third most common medical complaint. But why is the foot so vulnerable to aches and injuries? For a start it is a very complex structure of 26 bones, 56 ligaments and 38 muscles. This means there is a lot to go wrong – and the heavy punishment our feet take can accentuate problems that in other parts of the body might go unnoticed. By the age of 35 the average person will have walked 45,000 miles and the ball of the foot may be subjected to a force of 200 lb all the time and far more on running and jumping. Being furthest from the heart the feet have the poorest circulation of the body and this reduces with age as the arteries supplying the lower limbs narrow. Most of us wear shoes which immobilise the feet to a great extent and as a result the foot's muscles are in a pretty poor state a lot of the time.

The greatest single cause of aching feet is poor footwear. Under constant pressure from tight or ill-fitting shoes, the skin of the foot becomes hardened and forms corns. Shoes which are too tight can cause ingrowing toenails or a painful thickening of the nail of the big toe.

Women have by far the greatest number of foot problems (about 85 per cent, according to several experts), mainly because of the style of women's shoes. High heels make the body slide forwards, and to re-balance it a woman has to alter her whole posture. This takes the form of sticking her buttocks and her stomach out. The higher the heel the more the weight of the body is thrown on to the ball of the foot and a woman with a wide forefoot will end up with corns, bunions and hammer toes when her foot is jammed into a pointed shoe. High heels, if worn all the time, can also shorten the Achilles tendon at the back of the heel and leave the wearer open to injuries.

Platform shoes can cause painful bleeding under the big toenail and tight boots can actually cut off the circulation. Bunions (an inflammation of the joint where the toes meet the foot) are often caused by shoes that force the big toe into an unnatural angle.

The way people walk reflects the way they feel. Depressed people walk sloppily with a shuffling gait, and the stresses that this can put on the feet can cause problems. Though plantar warts (verrucas) are caused by a virus, there is a school of thought that says that they only occur when the individual is emotionally run down or stressed.

With the current vogue for walking and jogging an increasing number of individuals are suffering from a condition called plantar fasciitis. In this the thick band of fibrous tissue that runs the length of the sole linking the heel to the ball of the foot becomes inflamed. Sometimes the insertion of the fascia pulls away from the heel bone and a bony spur forms. These heel spurs are themselves very painful but the increased pulling of the tissue away from the bone that often accompanies fasciitis is the most common source of foot pain among adults who exercise. The earliest signs of fasciitis are a bruised sensation in the heel which won't go away or pain in the sole as you get out of bed in the morning.

Prevention

- The key to preventing foot problems is buying sensible shoes. The shoes should be at least ¼in longer than your longest toe, and high and wide enough not to squash your feet at all. Ideally, the heel should be no more than 2 in, and the sole should be flexible enough to bend with your foot and thick enough to absorb some of the forces when jumping on to hard surfaces.

- Buy shoes made of natural material if at all possible, because man-made materials promote sweaty feet and increase the likelihood of athlete's foot (see page 148).

- If you suffer from aching feet, use specially made shoes, or inserts such as heel cushions or arch supports, but see a specialist if these don't quickly relieve the aches and pains. There are several kinds of inexpensive cushion insoles to absorb the shock of running and walking.

- If you are overweight, go on a diet. This helps take the weight off your feet and can work wonders in itself.

- When starting to increase your activity level do so gently and get good advice from a sports shop or health professional about what footwear to choose. Remember that when you run the force carried by your feet is 3–4 times the weight of your body, so treat them carefully.

- Do foot-muscle exercises to strengthen the muscles and so reduce the chances of aches and pains. Here's what to do:

  Sit down on a chair with your feet off the floor and your shoes off. Vigorously point your toes up and then in, down and then out so that you make circles with your toes. At the same time flex and extend your toes.

  While standing with your feet apart and pointing in, roll on to the outside of your feet several times and curl your toes slightly. Practise walking on your toes. Deliberately walk with a spring in your step.

  Stand a few feet away from a wall. Place one foot ahead of the other and pretend to push the wall as if it were a broken-down car. Keep the rear leg straight and the foot flat on the floor. Bend the forward leg and raise that foot. Switch legs and do it again. This exercise is especially good for heel pain.

ACNE

What is it?

Spots, usually a mixture of blackheads, red or purplish spots of various sizes, pustules, scars and pits on the skin. They are mainly found on the face, the back of the neck, the back and the chest, but can be found in the armpits and on the buttocks. The complexion is often greasy and muddy and the individual usually has lank, greasy hair.

Acne is most common during adolescence and most people grow out of it in their twenties.

What causes it?

During adolescence profound hormonal changes are occurring and the oil-producing glands in the skin begin to over-produce their secretions. These secretions often become dammed up in the sebaceous glands and the topmost part of the duct blocks up with oxidised sebum to produce a blackhead. If this is squeezed a worm of sebum appears.

Some women have acne or similar types of spots every month premenstrually and others have them when they are pregnant but these are easily explained and usually disappear quickly.

Of the specific things thought to cause acne here are just a few:

- Refined foods, especially sweets and chocolates. Having said this, most acne researchers dismiss the effect of diet.

- Cosmetics and oil-based make-up and thick, greasy skin creams can contribute to a mild form of acne called 'acne cosmetica'.

- Caffeine-containing drinks such as tea, coffee and cola.

- Stress. Some people definitely

have more spots at times of stress. This may well come about as a result of the increased levels of androgens (male hormones) produced by the adrenal glands during stress.

- Woolly clothing next to the skin.

- Environmental factors are not uncommon in acne. Mechanics, fast-food workers and anyone who works in a greasy atmosphere can develop acne because the atmospheric grease blocks the pores in the skin. Those who work with chlorinated hydrocarbons found in paints, varnishes, mineral oils, pesticides and roofing materials may develop a type of acne called chloracne.

- Iodine and bromide-containing medicines. Iodised table salt contains too little iodine to worry about but some asthma medications and multivitamins contain a lot. Other drugs that cause pimples are steroids, male hormones, lithium and certain anticonvulsants.

- Tar and oil products.

- Infrequent washing. Ordinary oily skin has very little to do with pimples. The oil that reaches the skin is usually *not* the problem – it is the oil trapped in the hair follicle that produces acne. Antibacterial soaps have been found to be of little value compared with normal soaps.

Prevention

Avoidance of any or all of the above offending substances is a good start to preventing acne. The following are probably useful:

- Wash several times a day with a bland soap and water. Don't scrub, wash gently. Dry well with a rough towel.

- Use non-greasy, water-based cosmetics.

- Get into the sunlight as much as possible. Ultraviolet light not only cures but prevents acne. Some people's acne gets worse in hot weather. This is probably a combination of perspiration, humidity, and suntan lotions.

- Eat a healthy diet rich in vegetables and fruit and keep away from refined foods and sweets if you find that they worsen your problem.

- Vitamin A has been used by itself to treat acne but without much success. However, 100,000 IU vitamin A *and* 800 IU vitamin E daily do seem to help. The doses of the vitamins can be reduced as the condition improves over several months.

- Keep away from soft drinks – they may contain brominated vegetable oils or stabilisers and bromides are known to irritate acne. Drink fresh fruit juice instead.

When the Food and Drugs Administration in the United States looked at the myriad of acne preparations available over the counter it found that only three active ingredients were worth bothering with. These were sulphur, sulphur/resorcinol mixtures and benzoyl peroxide.

Of these three only the last actually prevents (rather than treats) acne. This has led several distinguished experts in the field to promote the use of benzoyl peroxide as a preventive for acne. The chemical is a powerful bactericide that comes in various strengths. One study showed that two weeks of application to the skin had the same effect as four weeks of treatment with oral antibiotics.

When starting with this substance go gently and use the lowest possible concentration. One study found that the lowest concentration had just as much effect as did the more powerful concentrations but that the former caused less skin irritation. Benzoyl peroxide can cause the skin to peel, flake and burn. Apply it on alternate days until your skin 'hardens' and then begin daily or twice-daily treatments. People with fair skin, freckles and/or red hair tend to be most sensitive to it. Also, be sure to treat the entire face and not just the existing pimples. Gels are more effective than creams or lotions. This preparation should not be used if the skin is inflamed—antibiotics are best in such cases. For successful prevention of acne antibiotics must *not* be taken with food.

AFTERNOON SLUMP

What is it?

Many individuals are familiar with this phenomenon but it is one that the medical profession discusses very little. It takes the form of restlessness, lethargy, depression or dullness, or a mixture of them all, after lunch. About an hour after having had lunch is the most common time but it hits some people as late as 4 p.m.

To most sufferers afternoon slump is simply a time each day when they feel at a low ebb—they can't concentrate, drive poorly, shout at the kids or whatever. Doctors call it the post-prandial dip and it is characterised by low body temperature, low blood sugar, fluid retention, a reduced work efficiency and a depression of mood. For some people it is a blight on the whole afternoon.

What causes it?

- Too much stodgy, refined carbohydrate for lunch. One study found that people who had eaten a heavy lunch were less able to detect signals and couldn't differentiate as well between varying sizes and intensities of light.

- We all operate on a 12-hour cycle superimposed on a 24-hour day. Many scientists think that our bodies are crying out for a rest at about this time of the day. In Mediterranean and Latin countries the siesta is the rule rather than the exception–people go home at lunchtime to sleep and then return to work later in the afternoon and work into the evening. People who enjoy a siesta need less sleep at night, so it is not a waste of time sleeping during the day as is often thought.

- Skimping on breakfast. A research study found that 79 per cent of the subjects studied who complained of fatigue, fluid retention, or both, had skimped on breakfast. After being placed on a high-protein breakfast, forty-nine out of fifty-eight patients reported obvious, in some instances dramatic, reductions in fatigue and fluid retention.

Prevention

- Eat a 100 per cent raw lunch. Avoid all refined stodge.

- If you can't eat 100 per cent raw then remove sugar, honey, refined carbohydrate foods and very sweet fruits such as dates, figs and bananas.

- Have a glass of orange juice with brewer's yeast stirred in.

- Take some light exercise straight after lunch.

- Eat a sensible breakfast.

AGEING

What is it?

Ageing is a normal process that starts in our mid-twenties. It is characterised by a decline in cardiovascular and respiratory fitness, a loss of muscle and bone, a thinning and wrinkling of the skin, a stiffening of the joints, a fall in sexual potency (especially in men) and many other more subtle changes. Many, if not most, of these changes appear simply to *accompany* the advancing years– there is no solid evidence that they are *caused* by growing old. For this reason it is at least theoretically possible that they can be slowed down, halted or even, on occasions, reversed.

The elderly and the very young are the greatest consumers of health services and the elderly are becoming very numerous. It is estimated that one third of all the people who have reached the age of 65 in the last 2,000 years are alive today! By the turn of the century one person in three will be over 75 and one in thirteen over 85.

The consequences of survival of the elderly on such a scale are so great that as yet few people have grasped them, but it is certain that the physical, mental and social demands of such a vast number of old people will be great and could even be beyond the ability of a decreasing working-age population to sustain.

All of this makes preventive strategies for the elderly vital for the community at large – not just to make life more pleasant for older people themselves (valuable though this undoubtedly is).

There is evidence that although people's life expectancy is rising actual lifespan is not. On average people are already remaining fitter for longer and have a shorter period of terminal dependency as a result of medical, social and economic changes that have taken place over the last century. The aim of prevention in old age is to prevent illness rather than postpone mortality. As one old lady put it, 'I want to die old, and healthy.'

But preventing the problems of old age does not just involve preventing illness in the commonly accepted sense of the word, because in the elderly, perhaps more than at any other age, social and other less well-defined factors come into play.

What causes it?

No one knows what causes the degeneration that currently goes hand in hand with advancing age, but we are only too aware of the results and it is these that need to be tackled in any preventive regime for the elderly. The most common specific problems are: iatrogenic disease; depression/anxiety; alcoholism; hypothermia; 'flu; constipation; tetanus; malnutrition; and high blood pressure. These are brought about not just by the degeneration process itself, but also by a general loss of fitness, and the social consequences of old age in our society.

Prevention

Of diseases generally

- By far the commonest type of illness in old age is iatrogenic– doctor induced. Many old people are on medication that greatly handicaps them in all kinds of physical and psychological ways.

- All the conditions listed above can be found in other parts of the book and so are not discussed further here, but remember that many of them may have started well before old age. This puts the onus on all of us both within and outside the medical profession to recognise these conditions early and to treat them so that people do not already have them as they embark on old age.

- Stop smoking cigarettes. However late you stop it reduces your chances of getting lung cancer and improves your breathing, your senses of taste and smell, and your appetite.

- Control your weight. Eat sensibly to prevent obesity. (See page 290).

- Keep active and involved with other people.

- Keep physically fit.

Screening measures that are definitely worth taking.

- Have your blood pressure taken

at least once every two years.

- If you are a woman, have a mammogram done every year in your fifties.

- If you are a woman, have a cervical smear done at age 50, 55 and 60.

- Have a tetanus immunisation every ten years and 'flu immunisation every year.

Screening measures that are probably worth taking.

- Have a stool sample examined yearly for blood so that any colon cancer is picked up early.

- Have your hearing and eyesight tested yearly.

- Look after your feet.

- Visit your dentist once a year.

- Treat pressure sores and eczema.

- Have your blood tested for anaemia every two years.

Screening measures that can be useful but are not of first importance

- Have your eyes tested for glaucoma.

- Have a rectal examination once a year for rectal cancer.

- Undergo screening for depression.

- Undergo screening for mental functioning generally.

- Have blood tests for reduced thyroid function every five years.

Screening measures of no proven value

- Routine electrocardiograms.

- Routine blood tests.

- Routine barium enemas or meals.

- Routine urine analysis.

Of unfitness

All four aspects of fitness–stamina, strength, suppleness and skill–can be improved with advantage in old age. As well as actually *being* fitter many old people *feel* so much better when carrying out such a fitness programme. Here are some useful hints.

- Check with your doctor that you have no physical illness or disability that would make a fitness programme unsuitable or dangerous.

- Bear in mind that the dictum 'use it or lose it' applies at any age but especially in old age.

- Continue with a sport or activity that used to give you pleasure when younger, or take up a new activity. Swimming, yoga, keep-fit, music and movement, and gentle aerobics are all good, as are walking and gardening.

- Find out about your local leisure centres, adult education classes, and so on.

- If you get ill or have to go into hospital remember that fitness takes longer to return the older you are. A few days' inactivity can take several weeks to overcome.

Of social problems

We all have social problems but the elderly are worse off than most for three reasons. First, they are often pessimistic and hold negative beliefs and attitudes, many of which are totally false. Many old people, for example, see old age as an inescapable downhill slide to illness and death whereas the former of these two is in fact no longer inevitable. Some are too depressed or too tired to summon up the energy to do anything much.

Second, many young people tend to write off the aged and are pessimistic about the scope for prevention in old age. Some are overprotective or guilty and so don't give the help they could.

Third, there are very real practical problems, including poverty, and poor heating, housing and mobility. Also, many old people are very lonely and isolated socially. They often know little of the social and other amenities and benefits that are available and are often too proud to seek them out or even to accept them when they are specifically offered.

All of these problems can only be prevented, in our culture, by a team approach–the family, the elderly ·person's doctor, the health visitor, the local authority, and any others involved, all have to pull together to reduce the social burdens that are almost inevitable in a society that pushes its old people out of family homes to live alone for many years.

Finally, here are a few facts that should encourage the elderly in their preventive-health-care programme:

- A study of 200 men and women aged between 56 and 87 who participated in a programme including walking, jogging and stretching 3–5 times a week found that 'dramatic changes' began as early as six weeks into the programme. Regular exercise turned back the clock for the volunteers, and men and women of 60 and 70 became as fit as people twenty or thirty years their junior. Over a forty-two week training period the amount of oxygen carried per heartbeat went up on average by 29 per cent.

- At the Pritikin Longevity Center in California the effects of exercise and diet have been tested over many years. After twenty-six days serum cholesterol dropped from 222 to 179mg/100ml; blood triglycerides (fats) fell from 156 to 141mg/100ml, and nine out of eighteen subjects studied had falls in blood pressure sufficient to allow them to stop taking their drugs. The calibre of certain arteries increased, thus improving blood flow dramatically.

- The most critical measurement of cardiovascular and respiratory fitness is the 'VO2 max'. It declines at the rate of 1 per cent a year after age 30. Using controlled exercise programmes 70-year-olds can improve their VO2 max by 15 years. Again, physical exercise is the best way of keeping young and fit.

- The more you exercise the more energy you have. For millions of people getting old means slowing down and being almost constantly tired. The problem for such people is that they tire at the slightest exertion. In one study of old people the volunteers became *less* tired after each work-out and claimed to have more energy than before to carry them through the day.

- Wrinkled skin is a normal part of ageing as the connective tissue weakens and fat is lost. However, studies show that this process is worsened by spending long periods in the sun, by smoking and by the use of alkaline soaps. The remedy? Stay out of strong sun; stop smoking; use sunscreen creams when you go into the sun; and nourish your skin by taking vitamins A, C and E.

- Physical exercise also has beneficial effects on the skin. In one study, twenty older women who exercised regularly on a trampoline were compared with twenty who did not take exercise. The exercisers looked younger, and had fewer wrinkles and better skin colour than the sedentary group. They also had less pronounced bags under the eyes.

- Blood pressure creeps up with age in almost all westernised societies. The fact that this is not inevitable is shown by its absence in many traditional-living countries. Reducing salt intake and using relaxation exercises have been found to halt the gradual increase in blood pressure and even to reverse it. Taking plenty of calcium has also been found to help reduce blood pressure.

- As we age (after the age of 25) we lose 3–5 per cent of our muscles, glands, connective tissue and internal organs every ten years. The breakdown products are passed out in the urine, and fat takes the place of the once active tissues. So unless you lose this 3–5 per cent of your body weight each ten years you will get more fatty and less muscular. But this is not an irreversible part of ageing. A study of two champion runners aged 70 and 71 found that they had the same amount of body fat as university students. Just dieting, however, is not enough – you have to exercise to build up lean muscle and other tissues.

- Exercise can also be an excellent treatment for varicose veins in old age. The author of a leading book on the subject claims that old people with the condition should run, jump, jog and 'do anything but sit still'. The pumping action of the calf muscles helps improve leg circulation, and it also helps to keep your legs elevated when rested (above heart level if possible).

- Many elderly people have lost a lot or even all of their teeth and see this as inevitable. It isn't. Tooth loss in middle and old age is mainly the result of gum disease. This can be totally prevented by regular brushing (from gum to tooth), the use of dental floss and regular visits to the dentist. Vitamins A and C are vital too. Calcium and vitamin D are now known to help prevent the loss of bone from tooth sockets. One researcher supplemented, for a year, the diet of women with very low bone density with 750 mg calcium daily plus vitamins D and C. Within a year he found the rate of bone growth around their teeth roots had roughly doubled.

- The brain also lives by the principle 'Use it or lose it'. There is no doubt that you *can* teach an old dog new tricks. Experiments with rats have shown that those raised in 'enriched environments' – roomy cages, with other rats and a variety of playthings, had heavier, more chemically active brains than did rats raised alone in 'impoverished' environments.

Physical exercise can also help. In one study reaction times, short-term memory and reasoning power were all improved in a group of elderly, out-of-shape people when they were put on a four-month walking programme. The walking group improved in six out of eight areas of mental functioning; a group who did weight lifting and push-ups in one; and an idle group in none.

There are various 'cures' and 'preventives' for old age for which claims have been made over the years but none has yet withstood scientific scrutiny – even ginseng with its well-known pharmacology and the vast scientific literature on its success in other areas. At the moment all such rejuvenation and old age-preventing techniques should be regarded with suspicion.

AIDS

What is it?

A potentially lethal venereal disease that affects mainly the homosexual community and those who have received infected blood by transfusions. The letters of the name stand for Auto-Immune Deficiency Syndrome – the condition is so named because it produces a breakdown in the body's ability to combat infections.

AIDS appears to be a new disease and at the time of writing the total number of cases reported worldwide is less than 12,000. Just why some people who develop AIDS die and others seem to be able to cope with the infection is not known but most people who contract the disease probably do not realise they have it. Only about one in ten of those with the AIDS virus go on to develop a more serious form of the disease.

There is no treatment for AIDS and this makes prevention all the more vital. Gamma interferon, Interleukin and bone-marrow transplants have all been tried unsuccessfully.

The first signs of AIDS are night sweats, fevers, rapid weight loss, lethargy and general malaise. Sometimes these symptoms are clear-cut and then disappear. Swelling of the lymph glands and the appearance of skin blotches are signs that the full AIDS condition has developed. Symptoms can take from six months to four years to appear after the initial contact with someone with the virus.

People who have AIDS usually die from pneumonia or skin cancer as a result of the breakdown of the immune system.

What causes it?

AIDS is caused by a virus that was only identified in May 1984. Since then the entire genetic structure of the virus has been discovered but vaccines may take a long time to develop because the AIDS virus, unlike that of certain other viral diseases, appears to be able to live alongside the antibody to it in the blood. The virus is also very changeable (rather like the 'flu viruses) and this again makes for problems in combating it.

Infection with the virus does not necessarily mean death as was thought until very recently. Having said this, once someone has the disease itself (as opposed to being infected with the virus) at the current state of knowledge death is certain.

The disease has only been around for six years or so and it is clear that the incubation period can be this long. There is now concern that carriers of the virus might remain symptom-free for perhaps much longer and then finally develop the disease – all the time passing it on to others unwittingly.

Prevention

If you are not in a high-risk group the chances of contracting AIDS are negligible. The virus has been found in saliva, which gave rise to scares about catching it from poorly washed cups and glasses, but so far there is no evidence that people in close non-sexual contact with AIDS sufferers have contracted the disease. Those most at risk are:

- Homosexual males.

- Drug addicts who 'main-line' (inject themselves).

- Those who receive several or repeated blood transfusions, such as haeomophiliacs.

- Those who have intercourse with someone of the opposite sex with the disease.

- Those who share a razor or a syringe with an AIDS sufferer.

As a result of this knowledge preventing AIDS is relatively straightforward, at least in theory.

- If you are homosexual cut down or cut out altogether your promiscuous sexual activities. There is good evidence that both homosexual and heterosexual promiscuity has fallen since the AIDS scare began and the level of all venereal disease is falling as a result. If you are homosexual, stick to one partner.

- If you are a woman, be aware of the possibility that a sex partner may be bisexual and a carrier of the disease. Although AIDS is very uncommon in women in the West it is estimated that about 100 women in the US have contracted AIDS from a bisexual partner.

- Haemophiliacs have repeated blood transfusions for their condition and often use pooled blood products which may have been contributed to by hundreds or even thousands of donors' blood. According to a US study virtually all haemophiliacs have been exposed to the virus yet only a tiny percentage go on to develop AIDS. The only preventive measure possible here is to reduce the situations in which haemophiliac children hurt themselves and so require blood or clotting factors, thus reducing their chances of exposure to the AIDS virus. Various countries around the world are enacting laws to forbid homosexuals and drug addicts to give blood or to donate organs for transplant. In the UK all blood products are now screened for the AIDS virus and the special substances given to haemophiliacs are heat treated.

- Don't share a razor, or needles for administering drugs, with anyone who could be in a risk group.

- Don't have anal sex with anyone who could be infected. The delicate anal tissues are more easily torn than those of the vagina and thus let the virus in.

ALCOHOLISM

What is it?

A complex and ill-defined condition in which a person is addicted to alcohol either physically, psychologically or socially. It is almost impossible to know exactly how many people are affected by alcoholism, if only because the boundary between heavy social drinking and true alcoholism is so difficult to define. Alcohol certainly affects the lives of millions of people in one way or another, whether financially, medically, socially or legally.

Over the past twenty years the consumption of alcohol has gone up throughout the western world and it is estimated that between 4 and 9 per cent of the total dietary energy of the British population comes from alcohol. A figure of £1.6 billion per year has been put on the consequences of this level of consumption in terms of costs to industry, to the National Health Service, and arising as a result of drink-related offences. It does *not* include any valuation of family stress or the extra burden put on services such as the probation and social services.

That alcohol in all but the smallest of amounts is bad for you is beyond doubt. It causes: cirrhosis of the liver (which kills far more people a year than do illicit drugs such as cocaine and heroin); gastric troubles; heart disease; acute and chronic muscle disorders; nervous-system problems; nerve disease; metabolic disorders; blood disturbances; altered drug metabolism; and an increased susceptibility to infections. People who drink have more accidents at home, at work and on the road; alcohol is often involved in suicide; it makes people fat; it makes them aggressive, anti-social, more likely to indulge in domestic violence and less efficient at work; heavy drinkers are more likely to be sexually impotent; and so on – the list is almost endless.

Despite all this, alcohol is the most widely used social drug. It is used as a sedative, a stimulant, a medicine, a social lubricant, a religious symbol and an indicator of the transition from work to play. It will undoubtedly continue to be used widely, but given the vast costs to society and to individuals some sort of preventive strategy is essential if the situation is not to go from bad to worse.

Prevention can be divided into three different levels. The first would be a primary preventive programme aimed at youngsters who have not yet started drinking seriously. Preventive measures would help them to realise the many pressures that influence their choice, and enable them to make a sensible decision about whether to drink. For those who do choose to drink education would help them to drink safely and moderately without harming themselves or others. Such a programme would be a major nationwide task because it would have to take into account very complex factors, such as the different personality, social skills, social environment and so on of different individuals. A self-confident, well-balanced person is less likely to come to harm in the hands of alcohol but we do not have, and cannot realistically expect, a nation of such individuals.

Secondary prevention is aimed at those who have already started drinking but who have, as yet, no obvious problems as a result. Preventive action here would encourage such people to see that they are likely to be drinking too much and would help them to cut down to a safer level. It could also tackle the considerable social and financial pressures on people to drink more. Such secondary prevention would promote light drinking and discourage excessive drinking.

Tertiary prevention would be aimed at true alcoholics to enable them to recognise their condition and to get help to prevent further deterioration and early death.

This kind of strategy generally has to be formulated and carried out by health authorities on behalf of the individual, but here are some things that the individual can do to prevent alcoholism or simply cut down on his or her drinking.

Some practical tips on prevention

Anyone who drinks alcohol is affected by it–at least to some extent. In general, the more you drink and the more regularly you drink, the higher the risks.

The problem with controlling drinking has always been that it is so difficult to set safe limits. One aspect of this is the inability of most of us to compare one type of alcoholic drink with another. If you think of it in this way though you won't go far wrong:
1 standard drink = 1 single measure of spirits *or* 1 pint of ordinary beer *or* lager *or* 1 glass of wine *or* 1 small sherry.

There are some surprises. For example, a half a pint of beer has the same amount of alcohol as a double whisky. Extra-strength lagers are very powerful and can contain as much as three times the alcohol of a normal beer. A glass of wine is as strong as a single whisky.

The first stage in prevention is to work out what you really drink. Don't guess. Don't cheat–it's your life and your family's future we are talking about. Start off by recalling, day by day, all the drinks you had last week. If this is too difficult start a diary today and enter at the end of each day what you drank, where and with whom. In another column put down how many standard drinks this added up to each day. Do this for a whole week. Bear in mind that if you pour yourself a 'short' at home it will probably amount to at least two or three standard drinks. Then total up the number of standard drinks.

If you are a man drinking up to 20 standard drinks a week (or a woman up to 13) you are probably safe. Try to keep your drinking at or below this level.

Men taking between 21 and 36 (14 and 24 for women) are probably unlikely to come to any great harm if the alcohol intake is spread throughout the week. But if you have binges and get drunk you risk having an accident. On average it takes the body an hour to get rid of the alcohol from one standard drink and you are much more likely to have an accident at work, at home or on the road if you have been drinking. One in five men admitted to hospital are there with an alcohol-related problem. One in three drivers killed in traffic accidents in the UK is over the legal limit (2½ pints of beer or the equivalent).

If you score between 37 and 50 (25 and 35 for women) you are getting close to the danger level and you could start to be a danger on the road and a misery to live with at home. It makes sense to cut down on your heavier drinking days and to reduce a little right the way through the week.

Between 51 and 95 (36 and 63 for women) you are already harming yourself. Your liver and stomach are being damaged, perhaps permanently, and the drink will now be affecting your life seriously. You will be dull at work and play and may be drifting into sexual, marital, legal and social problems. You will probably be getting into debt and may have been involved in drinking-and-driving offences. You must take serious steps, probably with professional help, to get your drinking down.

- So, in summary, a sensible limit for men is 2 or 3 pints (or their equivalent) two or three times a week, and for women 2 or 3 standard drinks two or three times a week. Women are more affected by a specific amount of alcohol than men because a smaller percentage of their body weight is made up of water. Alcohol is distributed throughout all the body's fluid and so is more 'dilute' in men than women. Also, women's livers seem to have a smaller capacity for detoxifying alcohol than do men's. Recent research shows that the effect of even very moderate drinking in pregnancy is harmful to the baby so the rule should be–if you're pregnant, don't drink.

    If you are drinking the equivalent of 4 pints of beer or 8 whiskies a day (for men) or 2½ pints of beer or 3 glasses of wine and 2 glasses of sherry (for women) you are almost certainly in for serious trouble with alcohol.

- Look back over your drinking diary and see if there are particular times or occasions (or even people) which encourage you to drink. Try to cast your mind back to how you felt at the times when you drank. Were you, for example, frustrated, angry, sad, depressed or tense? Could it be that by

getting professional help from a doctor or counsellor you could re-order your life to avoid the situations that make you drink in these particular moods? Sorting out the underlying problems, be they a failing marriage, a disappointing sex life, a poor job, or whatever, could be the real cure for your drinking.

- Reward yourself with something nice (such as some new clothes, a visit to the cinema, or a meal out) if you succeed in cutting down on the amount you drink in situations that have previously trapped you (as judged by your drinking diary). Start saving the money you would have spent on drinks and buy something you really want or save for a holiday you otherwise could not afford.

- When out with friends who buy rounds say you would rather buy your own–that way you will drink less. Make drinks last longer (actually go by the clock if that helps) and alternate alcholic drinks with non-alcoholic ones.

- Set yourself limits for a particular occasion and stick to them. If you are going to a wedding reception, for example, tell yourself that you will have only two drinks, plus the champagne for the toast, and have soft drinks the rest of the time.

- Most of the above advice about prevention can prevent the moderate drinker from becoming a real alcoholic. But millions of individuals are already further down the road than this and sadly an estimated 85 per cent of all dried-out alcoholics eventually go back to drinking. Why this should be is not known but undoubtedly many have psychological problems that make it likely that they will always need a prop of some kind.

An increasingly vocal group of doctors believes that better results would be achieved by more radical dietary approaches to alcoholism. They suggest a switch from sugar, cigarettes and coffee to whole grains, fresh fruit and vegetables and vitamin supplements. Only a few US alcohol treatment centres use this nutritional approach but those that do claim good results. One expert in the field claims that alcoholics have a metabolic problem that makes them convert alcohol into a highly addictive morphine-like substance called tetra-hydro-isoquinoline (THIQ). Most alcoholics also develop hypoglycaemia, she claims. They crave alcohol and sugar in any form. She puts them on a six-week programme which involves analysing their mineral and vitamin status. This is often very poor in alcoholics, and even in serious drinkers, as such people tend to eat little and what they do eat is often junk food. She then gives them full doses of vitamins B and C and takes them off all refined foods, sugar, coffee and tobacco.

On this programme one US unit has 82 per cent of its patients still sober after a year. These results are,

it claims, far better than the US National Institute of Alcohol Abuse and Alcoholism can achieve. The NIAAA's figures show that only 15–20 per cent of all treated alcoholics are still dry after two years.

As long as twenty-five years ago Dr Roger Williams, the renowned US nutritional physician, used the amino-acid glutamine for the treatment of alcoholics. This reduces the terrible craving alcoholics have as they come off the alcohol. B vitamins also reduce the craving.

If you are drinking more than a few drinks it makes sense to take a good vitamin B complex supplement and to change your diet to a healthy one (see page 70) as a preventive against the proven harm the alcohol will do you in the long term.

ANAL FISSURE

What is it?

An anal fissure is a painful crack in, or ulceration of, the skin at the opening of the back passage. It starts off as a small tear, which is then reopened every time the person opens his or her bowels.

What causes it?

Constipation. As hard, difficult-to-pass stools are forced through the delicate lining of the anus, the skin tears.

Prevention

- As for constipation (see page 182).

- While the high-fibre diet is starting to act use a little lubricant on the bowel opening. Saliva will do, or you can buy some KY jelly from a chemist's. This enables the hard stools to pass more easily and reduces pain and bleeding a little.

ANAEMIA

What is it?

A condition with many causes in which the oxygen-carrying power of the blood is reduced. By far the commonest cause is iron deficiency, which is still a very common condition indeed, even in westernised countries where one would imagine almost everyone had access to healthy foods. In the Third World much of the iron consumed is in relatively unusable forms and is bound to phytic acid in cereal fibre. The best sources of usable iron are red meat and poor people eat little red meat. In the Third World millions of people have intestinal worms that cause a continuous loss of blood from the digestive system.

Although iron has been known to be an essential nutrient since ancient times there is much that is not known about it and doctors still debate what iron deficiency is and how it should best be treated.

Iron is essential in the body mainly because without it red blood cells could not carry vital oxygen to the rest of the body. About two-thirds of the body's 4 g of iron are tied up in haemoglobin, the red blood-cell pigment. Some is stored in the liver and yet more in the muscles as myoglobin. Red cells live for about 120 days and are then broken down and some of the iron is re-used. Some, however, is totally lost and so needs to be replaced if the person is not to become anaemic.

Only about 10 per cent of the iron we eat is available to the body and some foods yield less than 5 per cent of their iron.

It is easy to see how people can end up eating too little iron when we see the foods that are rich in it. Meat and fish contain the most readily absorbed form of iron. Iron absorption, even from iron-containing foods that do not readily yield up their iron, is somewhat enhanced by including meat in the diet. But even in people eating iron-rich foods (see below) blood losses may outstrip what is eaten or absorbed. Women in their childbearing years are most at risk of developing iron-deficiency anaemia because of losses during pregancy (into the baby) and in the monthly menstruation. Breast-feeding too makes heavy demands on a woman's iron stores. As if to combat these problems women are better able to absorb dietary iron than are men. (It is also interesting to note that the body of someone who is short of iron absorbs more of the element than does that of other people. A normal child or someone who is iron-deficient can absorb twice as much iron as a normal adult.)

But it is not only women who are susceptible to blood loss. Millions of people have bleeding piles, some have gastric and duodenal ulcers that bleed a little every day, and others take aspirin or anti-arthritis drugs which cause an increased loss of blood from the intestine.

Vitamin C is now known to be essential in the absorption of iron. Copper too is an important co-factor – and most food refining removes copper fairly thoroughly.

Anyone eating a low-quality diet – as people on low incomes and fanatical slimmers may be doing – is especially at risk. Vegetarians are also prime targets, unless they take care to eat enough of the non-meat sources of iron, of which there are several. The best are soya beans, yeast extract and almonds. Because vegetarians eat a lot of foods with a high vitamin C content they get more value out of the iron they do eat.

Millions of people throughout the world are mildly deficient in iron without realising it. They are more tired than they should be, have more infections than they should have and generally lack energy. As the anaemia becomes more severe the person becomes physically and mentally tired on the slightest exertion, and eventually even breathless at rest. Angina pectoris can occur as the heart finds it difficult to extract enough oxygen from the blood it receives and some iron-deficient people complain of 'poor circulation',

especially in their legs. Evidence is accumulating that suggests that voluntary activity is reduced in experimental animals with a mild iron deficiency in which severe anaemia has not yet developed. Although this is still controversial the finding has been supported by one human study. If this is confirmed it could make doctors totally review their current views on optimal iron levels. This would be of special interest to haematologists who assume that unless iron deficiency produces anaemia there is little or no adverse effect on a person's health. It is also interesting that mild iron deficiency (producing only a mild anaemia) increases the absorption of the potentially toxic elements lead and cadmium.

What causes it?

There are literally scores of causes of anaemia but the commonest are:

- Too little iron in the diet (or, at least, too little iron in the right form for absorption).

- A loss of blood. Anaemia caused in this way is also a form of iron-deficiency anaemia – the body does not have sufficient iron to make the replacement blood.

Prevention

- Look for and treat any cause of blood loss. This will need the help of your doctor.

- Increase your intake of bread, cereals, potatoes and vegetables. These supply two-thirds of our iron in the UK because although meat and fish (which supply the rest) are richer in iron, we eat much less of them. Other iron-containing foods include black pudding, sprats, liver and sardines. Green, leafy vegetables are rich in iron (but not spinach more than others!).

- Take an iron-containing preparation during vulnerable times (heavy periods, repeated pregnancies, unoperated bleeding piles, peptic ulcers, etc.).

- Take 1 g vitamin C a day as this appears to increase the absorption of iron from the intestine.

APPENDICITIS

What is it?

Inflammation of the appendix – a small, finger-like organ, the thickness of a pencil, attached to the first part of the large bowel.

What causes it?

An obstruction, possibly caused by a hard lump of food residue, that produces a blockage in the tiny canal in the centre of the appendix. Beyond the blockage pressure builds up and the appendix loses its blood supply. This, in turn, paves the way for bacterial infection and subsequent inflammation.

This is an elegant explanation for the commonest of all emergency operations in the western world (the removal of the appendix) but in nine out of ten cases a hard mass is never found once the appendix has been removed. In such cases it is thought that the obstruction is caused by an exaggerated contraction of the muscles in the wall of the appendix in response to the passage of thick, sticky food residues.

Evidence is accumulating which suggests that appendicitis is seen frequently only in populations which have hard-to-pass, sticky stools. Water is absorbed by the large bowel (a major part of the function of which is to retain water in the body) in excessive amounts because there is too little dietary fibre to hold the water within the bowel contents.

Prevention

- Eat more dietary fibre. To achieve this eat more: vegetables and fruit; wholemeal bread and wholemeal-flour products generally; wholemeal pasta and whole grains; whole-grain breakfast cereals and, if necessary, added wheat bran. At the same time reduce your consumption of refined carbohydrates (white-flour and refined-sugar products – bread, pasties, cakes, sweets, etc.).

- Drink more fluid – preferably water or water-based drinks.

ARTHRITIS AND RHEUMATISM

What are they?

Arthritis and rheumatism are woolly terms used to describe a host of painful conditions of the joints and muscles. True arthritis is either *osteo-arthritis*, in which the bone surfaces are worn away with age (a degenerative condition), or *rheumatoid arthritis* in which inflammation destroys a joint and its surrounding tissues. General aches and pains in muscles and joints that we all seem to get as we get older are often referred to as 'rheumatism' or 'arthritis' when in fact they are neither.

Arthritis is, however, just about the commonest disease in the western world, according to the World Health Organisation. Almost half the population have at least some signs of osteoarthritis and almost 1.5 million in the UK alone suffer from the effects of rheumatoid arthritis. In the USA 26 million working hours are lost each year through arthritis, which claims a million victims every year.

Only 2 people in every 100 will reach the age of 70 without experiencing some kind of rheumatism or arthritis. Lorry drivers, those who lift a lot and housewives are most affected.

Although drugs have done much to alleviate the pain of many arthritis sufferers, and joint replacement has come a long way, there is still no 'cure' for these diseases, which blight the lives of millions of people.

What causes them?

The true causes of arthritis and rheumatism are not known and there is no cure. However, there are many factors that are known to contribute to these conditions and some can be prevented. Preventable factors are:

- Too little exercise.
- Too much fat in the diet.
- Food allergies (for example to gluten-containing foods).
- Too little vitamin C.
- Too much sugar.
- Too little calcium.
- Too little zinc.
- Undernutrition in general.

Prevention

- Osteoarthritis, often thought to be caused by too much exercise, in fact benefits from the right kind of exercise, according to a study done at Albert Einstein's Medical Center in Philadelphia. The authors conclude that 'by strengthening the muscles around the joints exercise makes the joint work better'. Stronger muscles mean less wear and tear on the cartilage and bone and less chance of a deterioration of the osteoarthritis. Other researchers argue that exercise helps because it increases the blood supply to the cartilage and keeps it healthier. When Finnish researchers examined the hip joints of seventy-four former championship runners they found *less* osteoarthritis than in a control group, not more as one might have expected.

If you exercise wrongly it can hasten the advance of the disease. Avoid exercising unless you have warmed up thoroughly – when your muscles are tight the joints move unnaturally. Learn how to swim, play golf, tennis or whatever properly so that you don't make odd movements and put unnatural strains on your joints. If running is your sport, be sure to wear good quality shock-absorbing shoes and warm up well first. You should not exercise while using pain-killers or you could do damage to your joints without realising it.

- The worst thing for those with arthritis is to sit still. Swimming is the best exercise because it involves the use of so many joints. Walking through the water is also very good exercise if you can't swim. When you immerse your body in water it becomes lighter. Your limbs float and so do not have to work against muscle and bone. You can use your own bath to do simple hydrotherapy for 20 minutes a day. Slowly the exercises you do in the bath will be easier to perform outside the bath too. After a few weeks you will be able to do things that you would previously have found impossible.

- Hot-and-cold therapy is also very effective. In a study at Germantown Medical Center in Philadelphia twenty-four patients with rheumatoid arthritis applied an ice pack in a plastic bag to their sore knees three times a day for four weeks. At the end of the trial all of them reported more pain-free movements and increased muscle strength. They could stand up faster and sleep better and on average cut their medication dose by half.

The best way to carry out cold therapy is as follows. Take two packs of frozen peas (unopened) and wrap one round above the painful joint and one below. Cover them with a towel wrapped firmly round and leave everything in position for 20 minutes. At first you will feel coldness and burning, then numbness. This should last for 5 minutes or so. Carry on for another 15 minutes.

Arthritis of the hands and feet often responds to alternate baths of hot and cold. Carry out the frozen-peas treatment as above for 15–20 minutes and then plunge your painful hand or foot into a bowl of water at 110°F. Switch from hot to cold up to six times, putting the hand or foot into the hot water for 4 minutes and into the ice pack for 1 minute.

- Low-fat diets have been found to reduce the suffering of patients with rheumatoid arthritis. This was first discovered by chance in a group of obese people in a diet trial. All the rheumatoid arthritics noticed that the pain got better as long as they were on the diet. The Pritikin Diet claims to work on 90 per cent of those who have arthritis in their hands, wrists and fingers and on 50 per cent of those who have the disease in their knees and hips. The diet mainly consists of complex carbohydrates (vegetables and whole grains) with very little fat indeed.

- Some people who are allergic to foods have arthritis as their main symptom. One US expert believes that as much as 80 per cent of arthritis pain is triggered by food or chemical allergy. He uses an elimination diet (see page 218) and then slowly adds foods until the arthritis pain returns. The commonest group of culprits he has found are the nightshades, which include potatoes, tomatoes, aubergines, tobacco and peppers. According to a study done by *Prevention Magazine* in the US the arthritic symptoms of some 50 per cent of those who tried a nightshade-free diet diminished.

    Gluten is also currently under suspicion. In 1964 a paper published in *Medical World News* blamed gluten–a protein present in wheat, oats and rye–as a culprit in arthritis. People who eat a lot of cereals (especially wheat) are more likely to have rheumatoid arthritis, according to the author, than those who live mainly on maize or rice. Two-thirds of his patients became symptom-free on a gluten-free diet. If you want to give a gluten-free diet a trial, talk to your doctor, who will be able to give you a diet sheet.

- Vitamin C is essential for the formation and health of connective tissues. Arthritis and rheumatism appear to be disorders that mainly affect connective tissue, a fact which has led various researchers to look at the role of this vitamin. A leading US expert who has studied this connection believes that in those who are vitamin C-deficient there is instability and fragility of bones, cartilage, muscles and vascular tissue, mainly as a result of the breakdown of an intercellular cement substance which, in turn, causes tissues to rupture easily. Two other researchers have correlated a shortage of vitamin C with rheumatic disease. They found an impairment of the joints of animals artificially deprived of vitamin C. When the animals had any kind of infection the joint symptoms became worse. Those animals exposed to the same infection while on a diet rich in vitamin C did not have arthritic symptoms. The same two researchers then looked at vitamin C levels in arthritic patients and found them to be extremely low. One report found that rheumatoid arthritis patients who were receiving plenty of the vitamin in their diets excreted less of it than average, suggesting that perhaps the vitamin was being used faster than normal. Another researcher found that the bioflavonoids occurring naturally with vitamin C had a favourable influence on the condition of blood vessels in infections. Perhaps these flavonoids (often known as vitamin P) act along with vitamin C in a way which is more natural. After all, synthetic vitamin C is to some extent 'unnatural'.

To be sure of getting enough vitamin C, eat foods that are rich in it, stop smoking and take 1 g of synthetic vitamin C a day.

- One researcher in Florida analysed the diets of arthritics and found that they were all very similar – full of refined foods and sugar, all of which are low in trace elements, minerals and vitamins. He postulated that sugar upsets the calcium – phosphorus balance in the body, resulting in extreme swings of these two vital minerals, and claims good results from eliminating all sugars and refined foods from the diet of arthritics.

- Poor nutrition generally is now thought by some experts to be a cause of arthritis. Too little protein and a diet poor in vitamins and minerals can bring on osteoarthritis much younger than was ever previously seen. One US authority thinks that osteoarthritis can no longer be considered to be a disease of old age now that people in their thirties and forties are suffering from it. A generation ago it was rarely seen before the age of 60.

Decreasing mobility and general inactivity in old age further reduces the local blood flow to joints and their surrounding tissues, and hardening of the arteries, often caused by a poor diet, yet further reduces the blood supply.

Drugs, medications of various kinds and environmental hazards all affect the digestion and absorption of various nutrients, which in turn produces poor nutrition. Part of this poor nutritional picture includes too little calcium. This leads to a thinning of the bones generally (osteoporosis) but often produces no symptoms unless the person falls and breaks a bone. A San Francisco doctor as long ago as 1953 reported his findings that calcium shortage caused osteoarthritis. He suggested that because the bones were so weak as a result of the calcium lack local deposits of calcium occurred around joints to strengthen them. These extra bony deposits then caused pain, tenderness, stiffness and inflammation. Letters to *Prevention Magazine* in the US tell how people have taken extra calcium (in the form of bone-meal or Dolomite tablets) and been relieved of their arthritic symptoms.

At the Royal Free Hospital in London

a doctor was talking about the importance of raw fruits and vegetables for arthritis as long ago as 1936. The twelve patients in one study done by her were put on a diet consisting totally of fresh, raw fruits, vegetables, nuts, cream, salad oil, milk and raw oatmeal. After two weeks a few cooked foods were added. The diet was totally salt-free. Eight of the twelve patients started to feel better in the first few weeks on the raw diet. Two improved for 5–6 weeks and then relapsed. Two showed no improvement at all. All the patients lost weight on the diet which in itself was very helpful to the pains in the joints. Dr Hare who carried out this study and indeed many others since her have asked whether cooking foods might destroy valuable elements as yet unknown to science. All this is considered in much more detail in Leslie Kenton's book *Raw Energy* .

Zinc supplements have been found significantly to relieve the symptoms of rheumatoid arthritis in people who have not responded to any other treatment. A rheumatologist at the University of Washington, Seattle, noticed that a zinc deficiency coupled with high levels of copper was common in rheumatoid arthritis sufferers. He then took twenty-four rheumatoid sufferers who had received no relief from conventional drug therapies. For the first twelve-week period half the group were given zinc sulphate tablets (providing 50 mg zinc a day) and half were given placebos. For the second twelve weeks all received zinc. Over the first twelve-week period those taking the zinc fared better on all clinical measurements. Their joint swelling went down by 26 per cent, compared with no change in those not taking zinc. Joint tenderness also diminished. After twelve weeks morning stiffness decreased significantly in the zinc-takers. Further improvements occurred over the next twelve weeks. When the patients themselves were asked to evaluate the changes those taking zinc (and none were told what they had been taking) felt better overall than those not taking it.

Much of this evidence is scrappy and none of it amounts to a 'cure' for rheumatism and arthritis. However, arthritis and rheumatism are already recognised as being a whole family of complaints and I feel that the family is even larger than most doctors are prepared, or able, to admit.

Most of the above preventives involve eating more healthily in one way or another or taking more exercise. Don't wait until you have arthritis or rheumatism, although in many cases you will get relief. Rather the lessons learned from such studies should enable us all to model our lives in ways that discourage arthritis and rheumatism in the first place. This involves:

- Taking more exercise.
- Cutting down on the amount of fat we eat.
- Identifying and cutting out foods to which we are allergic.
- Taking more vitamin C-containing foods and, if necessary, additional vitamin C.

- Cutting down on sugar or cutting it out altogether.

- Ensuring that old people especially are well nourished.

- Ensuring that we eat plenty of calcium-containing foods.

- Eating more raw foods.

- Eating more zinc-rich foods (see page 314 for list).

ASTHMA

What is it?

A disease in which the air passages in the lungs become narrowed, producing difficulty with breathing. Asthma is a condition that is underdiagnosed and undertreated. Between 10 and 30 per cent of those asked say that they have experienced wheezing at some time in their lives, but real asthma is thought to occur in only about 5 per cent of the population in the UK and the USA. Among children, boys are affected more than girls (3:2) but in later years the sex incidence becomes equal.

In children a cough (especially at night) may be the only symptom. The problems in adults include chest tightness (which may show up like angina) and breathlessness at night – which can be confused with heart failure.

Parents of asthmatic children often ask whether they will grow out of it, and in fact most wheezing children improve in their teens. More than a half of all children with infrequent wheezing will be free of their symptoms by the age of 21. Asthma is less likely to get better in this way if there is a strong family history of asthma, eczema or hay fever.

What causes it?

- There is definitely a familial element to the condition. The chance of an individual developing asthma by the age of 50 is increased twenty times if he or she has a first-degree relative with the condition.

- Bottle-feeding with cows' milk is said to increase the likelihood of a baby suffering from asthma (especially if there is a family history of allergies) because it reduces the protective effect that is gained from the natural antibodies in breast milk and exposes the baby to the foreign proteins in cows' milk very early on in life before its immune system can cope.

- Abnormal sensitivity of the airways to irritants such as cold air and tobacco smoke.

- Exercise brings on an attack in some sufferers and some adults with the condition experience asthma on making love. Swimming in a warm, indoor pool is the best sort of exercise for asthmatics. Wearing a simple face mask may be an inexpensive (non-drug) way around exercise-induced asthma, according to one study.

- House-dust mites are a common cause of asthma. Susceptible individuals are sensitive to the faeces of the mites.

- Pollen and spores are another potent source of asthma for some. Generally, asthma occurring in June and July is usually related to grass pollens. Tree pollens cause trouble between February and May.

- Pets are a common source of trouble. Cats have allergens in their dander, saliva and urine, but in fact any domestic animal can trigger asthma.

- Occupational asthma is caused by chemicals,dusts and enzymes at a person's place of work or–less commonly–at home. The yellow food colouring tartrazine is a common offender.

- Food allergies can cause asthma. The commonest culprits are nuts, milk, eggs and wheat.

- Drugs. Aspirin and aspirin-containing drugs are the commonest of these sources but beta-blocking agents can also cause asthma.

- Emotion. This is undoubtedly a cause in those who have an underlying susceptibility to the condition. In children, the emotional reaction of a parent when the child has an asthma attack

undoubtedly often makes matters worse.

Prevention

- Feed your baby at the breast alone for at least 4–6 months, especially if there is any family history of asthma, eczema or hay fever. This protects the susceptible baby from cows' milk proteins and makes asthma less likely to occur in later life.

- If there is a history of allergy in the family it makes sense to take this one stage further and restrict the intake of eggs, milk, wheat and nuts during pregnancy. Recent research suggests that intra-uterine sensitisation can occur in highly susceptible families so an excess of any food, drug or chemical is best avoided during pregnancy.

- Avoid cold air whenever possible. Keep away from smokers and don't smoke yourself.

- Get a good air filter. The best models are high-particulate smoker's air filters and can relieve asthmatic symptoms in 10–30 minutes. A summer camp in West Virginia installed air filters in the sleeping accommodation and found that the number of asthmatic episodes among the children was significantly reduced.

- Drink plenty of fluids to keep chest mucus thin and coughable. Drink ½–1 cup of fluid every waking hour. Drink only warm (i.e. not cold) fluids or you could actually trigger an attack. Warm drinks dilate the airways and can be used as a way of preventing an attack as you feel one coming on.

- Clear your house of the dust mite if this is what troubles you. Scrupulous cleaning of a child's room helps. Vacuum the mattress thoroughly and enclose it in an impervious plastic box-type cover. Blankets made from synthetic fibres, foam pillows and vinyl floor coverings are best. Frequent, damp dusting and vacuuming will keep the mite population to a minimum. Certain children obtain relief from a series of desensitising injections to the house-dust mite.

- You may have to get rid of your pet if it is causing really troublesome asthmatic attacks but this is often not necessary with scrupulous domestic hygiene. Keep all animals out of the bedrooms.

- Avoid foods you know bring on your asthma. Similarly, avoid all drugs containing aspirin if they affect you adversely.

- If you feel an attack coming on—don't panic. Practise the following deep breathing exercise to abort the attack.

1. Think of your stomach and chest as two containers of air. Breathe slowly through your nose and fill first the bottom container. Continue until your abdomen bulges out.

2. Exhale through your mouth. The abdomen should now feel empty and your tummy should feel flat.

3. Repeat this inhaling and exhaling gently and slowly twelve times. You can also try some of the relaxation exercises outlined on page 87. The average asthmatic breathes at only 60 or 70 per cent of his or her total capacity, and during an attack this can fall to 20 per cent. By learning to breathe deeply an asthmatic can increase the amount of oxygen he or she takes in and can reduce the severity of an attack or abort it altogether.

- Reduce weight. Even being only a little overweight can be a problem for an asthmatic because carrying too much fat, especially around the diaphragm, is like wearing a tight garment—it restricts breathing.

- Take vitamin C. In one study volunteers who usually suffered from exercise-induced asthma were given 500 mg vitamin C before an exercise test. Their tolerance to exercise was doubled. In another study 1 g vitamin C a day seemed to protect against having asthmatic attacks. Those who took it had 75 per cent fewer attacks than those receiving a placebo. When they stopped the vitamin C they once more suffered from their attacks.

ATHLETE'S FOOT

What is it?

An itchy, red, peeling of the skin between the toes. Patches of soft white skin come off to leave sore, raw areas.

What causes it?

The ringworm fungus.

Prevention

- Allow air to reach the feet as often as possible. Go without socks and shoes whenever possible.

- Dry feet well after bathing or swimming.

- Use a dusting powder (preferably one with a fungicide) between the toes after drying.

- Wear roomier shoes and thinner socks.

- Shoes made of natural materials enable the feet to 'breathe' better and help to prevent sweaty feet.

BABY BATTERING

What is it?

A form of child abuse involving direct physical assault. More subtle types of abuse include mental and emotional cruelty, and neglect, such as failing to remove obvious dangers around the house so that the child hurts or poisons itself. The 'abuser' is usually a parent but can be anyone who looks after the child. Such adults are often at the end of their tether emotionally or physically and sometimes both. Some were abused themselves as children. More than half of all battering adults have had a neglectful, cruel, violent or unhappy upbringing themselves.

Physical assault on an older child can start off as a form of punishment and then get out of hand, especially when the child persists in doing something it knows is wrong. Once a child has been assaulted once it is more likely to happen again.

Almost all research on child abuse has centred on the parents but several studies have found that a substantial minority of battered children were of low birth weight. About half of all battered children have an IQ of less than 80 – which puts them well below the average. In one study, 22 per cent of such children were found to be suffering from a deviation of some kind. Another study found that children who were blind, otherwise physically handicapped or retarded seemed to suffer the worst abuse.

- This must raise the thought that certain children may be so difficult that they are much more likely to end up being abused. Even nurses have suggested that certain babies and children in their care are virtually unmanageable from birth. The majority of studies show that only one child in a family is abused so again it points to something to do with the child as much as, if not more than, the parent. Of course, not all disadvantaged children provoke abuse. There are probably four conditions that are necessary for child abuse to occur: a special child; a special parent; some kind of crisis; and a tolerance of physical punishment by the parents.

What causes it?

- Rejection of the parents by an apparently unloving baby who screams and screams in spite of all its parents do for it.

- A parent who is at the end of his or her tether emotionally and physically.

- Social disadvantage, often a combination of poor housing, poverty, 'feeling trapped' and feeling hard done by oneself. Single-parent mothers are more likely to be stressed and feel unable to cope and so lash out at their babies or young children. The very young mother and the unmarried mother are particularly vulnerable too, partly because they are often lonely.

- Stress in the parent caused by physical or psychological illness.

- The parents' bad relationship reflecting on the child.

Prevention

- Perhaps the greatest single preventive action one can take as a parent is to breastfeed a baby on demand and to be very close to it, keeping it near you all the time and showing it that it is loved and wanted. Such babies don't cry as much and are less likely to frustrate their parents. Of course, any baby, however well handled or loved, *can* still drive its parents to distraction but a baby who is comforted as soon as it needs to be, and feels secure, will give much less trouble.

- Get treatment for any medical, emotional or psychological problem you have yourself, especially depression, so that you never get to a state in which you are unable to cope with the strains of a baby because of ill health. Don't let depression creep up on you – get help as soon as you feel low.

- Talk to the social services, your health visitor or your general practitioner about your bad housing or lack of money. There are many sources of help available – you should not have to fight these problems alone.

- If you feel that being alone with your baby or young child is too stressful, get out and about. Go to a mother-and-toddler group and when your child is old enough, let him or her go a morning or two a week to a group of some kind so that you can have a few hours to yourself, if only to allow you to go shopping alone from time to time. Share child care with other parents by looking after their children sometimes and having them look after yours at others.

- If your relationship with your partner is bad and you are taking it out on the children, get professional help quickly and sort it out.

- If things are getting on top of you and you feel that in spite of all of these preventive measures you will hit your baby if it screams a moment more, just stop what you are doing; have a cigarette; have something to eat; have a bath. In short, do something that is pleasant for you and leave the baby to cry.

    If you are really desperate you can phone Parents Anonymous (their telephone number is in the directory). This organisation is run by ex-battering parents. They understand the problems, will not report you to the authorities, will give you useful advice there and then, and will help you for the future too.

- Mothers of premature or low-birth-weight children could be assessed to find out what their attitudes to their babies are. Research has found that such mothers have more negative attitudes towards pregnancy, more hostility towards their babies, and less emotional maturity than mothers of full-term babies. Unmarried mothers and those with multiple births (twins etc.) are also more overwhelmed

by the whole business of having and caring for a baby. Many of these factors could be assessed professionally and 'at risk' mothers given special help.

BACK PAIN

What is it?

Pain in the back, usually low down. According to statistics 5 per cent of the population of Europe suffer from back complaints at any one time. In the UK back troubles cause the loss of more hours' work than do strikes and eight out of ten adults will seek medical help for back pain at some time in their lives. Approximately 88,000 people in the UK are absent from work because of back pain on any one day.

Back pain can be acute, even putting the person to bed for a few days, or chronic – making life miserable for years.

What causes it?

- Psychological stress. Many people with back pain are highly stressed. Treat the stress and their back pain goes.

- Injury. This is by far the commonest physical cause of back pain. A sudden, twisting injury, a blow, a fall from a height or the strain of lifting a heavy object wrongly can all cause an injury that produces back pain at the time or later.

- Chronic trauma results from sleeping for years on a poor mattress.

- Poor posture. Humans are up-right creatures but the balance of the bones and muscles in the back is delicate – a combination of leverage, gravity and muscular contraction helps keep the system in normal balance. Also, the lower-back muscles seem to be rather weak to do anything very heavy. Sedentary occupations and a lack of physical fitness worsen this state further. A back that is continually subjected to mild strain also shows more signs of osteoarthritis later in life. Often the person displays poor posture, flat feet, a middle-aged tummy bulge and yet is free from symptoms until some, often quite minor, trauma breaks the camel's back, as it were.

- High-heeled and platform shoes are other culprits. They throw the body's centre of gravity forwards, alter the angle of the pelvis and force the spine to adjust to a totally new balance position.

- Poor lifting technique. Most people forget how vulnerable the back is and simply bend forward from the waist when lifting. This puts very considerable strains on the back.

- Slipped disc. This is the com-

monest cause of severe back pain. About one in every 200 people is affected in a year, and two-thirds of them are men. The pain comes on suddenly and the sufferer finds it almost impossible to move freely. Many people find that the only way to get relief is to lie flat on the floor or on a bed. Rest is the best cure but local heat and painkillers are also helpful. Nine out of ten people experiencing disc pain for the first time will be better after three weeks in bed. An osteopath can often help at the early extreme-pain stage. If these measures don't produce relief, or if there are complications, surgery can be the answer, but only about one in 1,000 back-pain sufferers need surgery.

- Standing in a fixed position for too long can also be a cause of back pain. This can occur at work or, for example, when ironing, cooking or washing up.

- Badly designed chairs or car seats are a hazard.

- With today's craze for running and jogging there is a real danger of back injury if you do not wear properly constructed sports shoes. These are made with highly shock-absorbent soles that take most of the punishment from the hard surface on which you are running.

- Insufficent exercise. This leads to weak back muscles and makes the back more liable to injury.

Prevention

- There is little doubt that back pain is commoner in 'sophisticated' countries. This had led many experts to see backache as a manifestation of the stressful life. This does not mean that all backache is imagined – this is, of course, not so. What it does mean is that given that so many of us are unfit and have weak backs we tend to over-emphasise or to be particularly sensitive to even quite minor back pains. Just as many headaches are undoubtedly manifestations of stress, so too are many back pains. That this is so can be proven by treating certain back pains with tender, loving care and reassurance, with tranquillisers or with hypnotherapy. We look at how to reduce stress on page 80.

- Poor posture is a preventable cause of back pain. Even sitting is bad for the back. Even if one sits correctly the pressure within the spinal discs is still twice that when standing and the pressure when standing is twice that when lying down.

  Try to preserve the natural slope of your backbone as closely as possible. Walk tall, lifting up out of the hips and keeping your head up (practise by walking with a book balanced on your head), your shoulders straight, your tummy pulled in and the lower back hollow. This will not only make your back better but will mean that you carry yourself and your clothes better. Avoid standing on one leg and don't slouch when sitting.

  Start off by strengthening your tummy muscles. These are often weak and flabby. A good exercise is to put your hands behind your neck as you lie flat on the floor and then lean forward to thrust your elbows towards your knees without the legs leaving the ground. Do this gently a few times every day until you can do it 20–30 times easily and without strain. As your tummy muscles strengthen you will find it easier to hold your tummy in. Do this consciously whenever you remember – at the bus stop, while waiting in a queue, and so on.

  Get into the habit of walking upright with your tummy held in and you will prevent backache as you never thought possible.

- Wear low-heeled shoes whenever possible and flat ones for doing any kind of long walk or physical work. Don't let fashion wreck your back.

- When lifting heavy weights bend your knees, keep your spine straight and balance the load equally in both hands. Lift things slowly and not jerkily.

- Avoid standing in one fixed position for more than a few minutes. On long plane journeys try to get an aisle seat and go for walks frequently. Stop the car on a long journey and walk about for 5–10 minutes.

- Choose firm, back-supporting chairs and car seats. The greatest pressure on the discs of the spine occurs when one is seated in a soft chair. Similarly, choose a firm mattress, ideally one that is a little too hard rather than too soft, especially as all mattresses soften with age. If your mattress is ten years old or more you should get a new one.

  Wear proper sports shoes for running and jogging and indeed for any sports. These will absorb most of the shock waves and protect your back. Try to run on grass rather than hard surfaces and run on your toes.

- Take regular exercise. Swimming is the best but all forms of exercise that use the whole of the body are good, and any exercise is better than nothing.

There are many good spinal exercises but here are just a few:

1. Lie on your back on the floor with your hands behind your neck. Roll your body from side to side keeping your shoulders flat on the floor.

2. Lie on your back on the floor and pull your legs up, one at a time so that the knee is on your chest.

3. Lie on your back on the floor and draw your knees up so that your feet are flat on the floor. Now do bent-knee sit-ups but don't strain your back.

4. Lie flat on the floor and lift each leg up in turn, keeping it straight.

5. Sit on the floor and twist your body from the waist so that you look first one way fully and then the other.

Do all of these five to ten times each, going slowly and gently for the first few sessions, until you become more confident.

- Ensure that working surfaces at home and at work are at a comfortable height. This is especially likely to be a problem if you are short or very tall.

- Go on a diet if you are overweight. This will improve your abdominal muscles and reduce the strain on your back. Extra pounds also make it almost impossible to lift properly. Being overweight is particularly a hazard to the back in pregnant women. If you tend to put on excessive weight when pregnant go on a diet to reduce your weight. Don't do any drastic slimming or you could damage the developing baby.

- When sitting ensure that your knees are slightly higher than your hips. Use a footstool if necessary. When driving, bring the front seat forward so that your knees are higher than your hips.

- When sleeping, try putting a pillow between your knees as you lie on your side, knees drawn up.

- Try not to sleep on your tummy.

- Don't lean over furniture to open or close windows.

- Before taking any exercise, even heavy work in the garden, warm up first with some gentle exercises. If your back starts to 'act up' stop at once and rest.

- When moving heavy objects *push*, don't pull.

Some people have pains in the neck. Here are a few practical tips for them:

- Sleep on a firm mattress.

- See that your car seat is at the right height so that you don't have to strain to see out of the windscreen.

- Take regular exercise.

- Don't stretch up to high shelves – get a ladder or a safe chair.

- Bring close work closer to your face rather than bending your head down all the time.

- Don't make sharp arm movements.

- Use chairs with arm-rests.

- Wash your hair in a shower or sitting in the bath rather than leaning over the bath or sink.

- Don't sleep flat on your tummy with your arms over your head.

- Avoid seats in theatres and cinemas where you have to strain to see.

- Don't sleep sitting up.

- Don't read or watch TV lying down in bed or on a couch.

- Don't do anything static for long periods.

- Don't carry heavy bags over one shoulder.

BAD BREATH (Halitosis)

What is it?

Foul-smelling breath produced by one or more of several causes.

What causes it?

- Infective conditions within the mouth, the commonest of which by far is dental decay and associated gum disease.

- Infections in the nose or sinuses.

- Infections in the throat. The average child with a sore throat has very unpleasant, smelly breath.

- Infections with pus in the lungs.

- Smoking.

- Dirty dentures.

- Eating smelly foods such as garlic, onions, alcohol or certain volatile substances that are excreted by the lungs or in the saliva.

- Severe toxic conditions including peritonitis.

- Fasting. This produces a smell of pear drops on the breath, caused by the body breaking down fat to produce energy in the absence of food.

- Certain drugs.

Prevention

The prevention of any of the above causes of bad breath starts with finding out which of the causes are active in any particular case. This may need the help of a doctor. By far the commonest causes are the dietary ones (in which case the cause is usually fairly obvious) and tooth decay or gum disease. Given that about nine out of 10 adults in the West suffer from some degree of gum disease, bad breath is understandably very common. If your gums bleed when you brush them they are inflamed and you should see a dentist for further advice (also see page 224).

- Sucking lozenges and peppermints simply masks the smell. Mouth washes reduce bacterial counts but not for long–soon there are even more bacteria in the mouth than before. Gargling too is not advisable because the tissues of the back of the throat can be damaged and become inflamed–leading to further bad breath. Heavy users of mouth washes have been found to have a higher risk of head and neck cancers. In one study of eleven people with these cancers who had never used alcohol or tobacco (the two main risk factors for this type of cancer) ten had been heavy users of mouth washes.

- Apart from preventing the preventable causes listed above (see page 356 for details of the prevention of dental caries) a useful preventive and curative procedure is tongue brushing.

  Tongue brushing is an ancient pursuit: Mohammed told his followers 'you shall clean your mouth including the tongue'; the Romans used iron tongue scrapers and other cultures made them from ivory, whalebone and wood.

  A study was conducted in Vancouver to find the most effective way of reducing bad breath. Eight volunteers used one of three methods to freshen their breath in the morning: brushing the teeth; brushing their tongue; and a combination of the two. The results showed that tooth brushing reduced mouth odour by 25 per cent but brushing the tongue reduced it by 75 per cent. When the two were combined odour was reduced by 85 per cent. Even those who had never brushed their tongue before soon got into the habit.

- Diet provides another preventive method. Bad breath can be caused by processes involved in the digestion of caffeine, refined sugar, white flour and cows' milk. According to researchers in the US these foods produce either the fermentation of carbohydrates or the putrefaction of proteins in the digestive tract. In both cases noxious chemicals enter the bloodstream and are excreted in the lungs to produce bad breath.

BED WETTING

What is it?

A condition in which a child wets the bed at night even though he or she is potty trained. It comes about because the child does not receive sufficient warning stimuli from the bladder to tell him or her that it is time to urinate.

Most children become dry at night when they are 2 or 3 years old but others, especially heavy sleepers, can take much longer. A half of all 2-year-olds are still wet at night; 20 per cent of 3-year-olds; 10 per cent of 5-year-olds and 5 per cent of 11-year-olds. All children become dry eventually unless there is an underlying medical problem.

What causes it?

- Immaturity–the child's 'bladder is full' sensations are not yet well developed and they go unrecognised.

- Deep sleep.

- Stress. This might be caused by upsets in the family–especially the arrival of a new baby, parental rows, marital break-ups, moving house, etc. There may also be anxiety over, for example, going to playgroup, or being left with someone else when both parents go out to work. Any or all of these can make a previously dry child wet the bed.

- Certain congenital abnormalities of the urinary tract. See your doctor if you suspect this is the case.

Prevention

- Keep both the child and his or her room warm. Dress him or her in nightclothes that fit well and are snug–all-in-ones are good.

- Lift the child out of bed when you go to bed and sit him or her on the lavatory or potty. Some children remain asleep through this but most wake and then go back to sleep at once. A few children obligingly walk to the lavatory when woken.

- Limit fluid intake during the late afternoon and early evening, but don't restrict fluids totally. Be guided by common sense.

- Look for any of the above causes that could be prevented and work on them.

- Certain electrical gadgets that ring or make other noises to awaken the child as soon as he or she wets a sensitive pad in the bed are available but have not been widely used as either treatment or prevention, and their success rate has not been established.

- A particular anti-depressant drug

has been used for some years but I do not favour its use for young children.

BREAST ABSCESS

What is it?

A collection of pus in the breast, almost always secondary to a blocked duct during lactation.

What causes it?

Most breast abscesses start as a blocked milk duct in lactating women. Milk dams up behind the blockage and causes a tender, often painful, lump in the breast. When the baby feeds, the 'let-down' reflex produces more milk, so building up even more pressure in the blocked area. Treatment at this stage cures the condition and the dammed-up milk does not then go on to form an abscess. If nothing is done the local tissues soon become inflamed and the overlying skin is reddened. Inflammatory products get into the bloodstream and the woman has a fever. She may also feel 'flu-like and achy. This inflammatory condition is called mastitis.

The stagnant milk in the blocked duct can easily become infected with blood-borne bacteria, so forming an abscess. The infection sometimes spreads beyond the affected duct and its gland, causing bacterial mastitis. This involves a larger area of the breast than an abscess alone.

A woman with a breast abscess has a tender lump in her breast, with some degree of inflammation around the lump. The abscess may spontaneously burst and drain its pus either down the duct to the nipple or even into breast tissue and thus to the skin of the breast.

An abscess should be treated as for a blocked duct (see below) and also with an antibiotic. It is unlikely that there will be any danger if the baby drinks the milk but some women prefer to feed only from the uninfected breast, especially if pus is draining from the nipple. The pain and other symptoms of an abscess are helped by aspirin and rest.

A condition less commonly seen nowadays is a breast abscess following infectious mastitis due to virulent bacteria entering the breast via the nipple. Modern thinking encourages less handling of babies in hospital by staff and also better hygiene precautions. These measures lower the chances of dangerous 'hospital' bacteria gaining access to the mother's breast.

Prevention

This is based on treating a blocked duct promptly. Immediate and thorough action for a blocked duct prevents almost all abscesses. One major survey found that women only got an abscess if they stopped feeding when they had a blocked duct with mastitis.

- The general lowering of tension in the breast gives you a chance to unblock the duct. If you have ever had a blocked duct or feel a lumpy area of the breast developing, make sure that your breasts are soft and empty after the baby feeds.

- If your breast feels lumpy after a feed give the baby more or express the milk by hand or pump. Try to fit in twice as many feeds even if you are already feeding on demand, and don't be afraid to let the baby suck for as long as he or she wants to. Make sure that your breasts never get over-full. If your baby is sleeping for long periods, either wake him or her to feed or else express some milk, in order to soften the breasts.

- Always offer the affected breast first to ensure efficient emptying and return to it several times during a feed as milk can be let down many times in one session.

- Most important–gently massage the lump towards the nipple to try to release the dammed-up milk. You can do this at any time–during a feed or when the baby is not at the breast. If you can, have several hot baths a day and submerge the affected breast under the water to keep it warm. Massage the lump and express the milk into the water.

- If you can't get into a bath place a hot water bottle over the area or splash the breast with hot water while leaning over a basin. Massage and heat together work well but be careful not to burn yourself.

- Unblocking a duct (or ducts) can take several days of perseverance. When the milk is finally unblocked, it may flow freely from the nipple. You will see that it is thicker and looks whiter than your usual milk.

- Check that your bra is not pressing somewhere and causing the blocked duct. Some nursing bras with a band across the top when the flap is open can exert substantial local pressure. Be careful how you pull down the cup of an ordinary bra–that too can constrict the breast. Some women sleep on their stomach at night and the pressure on their breasts can cause a duct or ducts to block.

- Change the position in which you feed your baby from feed to feed and even during a feed so that the direction of suction is varied. Babies can suck in such a way as to leave a particular segment of the breast unemptied at times.

- If, after 24 hours' intensive effort as described above, the symptoms are getting worse, see your doctor at once for antibiotics, but continue the treatment as above. *Don't stop feeding*.

- Rest as much as you can.

- Physical exercise, especially of the top half of the body, can help disperse the painful swelling caused by a blocked duct.

- Take 1 g vitamin C a day as soon as any painful lump appears, to help combat the infection. If you find you get mastitis frequently your zinc status could be low, so go on to a full dose of zinc as recommended on the container.

- Some doctors recommend lecithin as an additive to the diet for women who repeatedly get blocked ducts.

BREAST DISEASE (Non-Cancerous)

What is it?

Benign (non-cancerous) breast disease is a family of rather ill-defined conditions which show up as pain and lumpiness in the breast. The pain, tenderness and lumps fluctuate with the phases of the menstrual cycle and tend to get progressively worse until the menopause.

The vast majority of women who have painful, lumpy breasts will not go on to get cancer of the breast. However, the condition is still worrying and wearing on a month-to-month basis. If ever a normally lumpy breast begins to have a well-defined mass, a blood-stained nipple discharge, a turning-in or tethering of the nipples, abnormalities in the overlying skin or glands in the armpit, consult your doctor at once.

What causes it?

No one knows for sure but the prolactin antagonist drug, Bromocriptine, and the female sex hormone ant-

agonist, Danazol, both help cure the condition in some women, so presumably hormones play an important part in the story. Unfortunately, both these drugs are expensive and have side-effects.

Prevention

Research in many centres over the years has made it possible to piece together a preventive package which can also be curative.

- Stop smoking.

- Reduce the amount of animal fats you eat. The Japanese, who eat lots of fish and very little animal fat, have very little benign breast disease. Also, studies of women with breast disease suggest that there is a disturbance of fatty acid metabolism which can be corrected by reducing the amount of animal fat they eat and increasing the amount of polyunsaturated fats in their diets. Oily fish, such as mackerel, herring and salmon, are especially useful.

- Avoid tea, coffee, cola and other caffeine-containing substances. These all contain various biologically active substances called methylxanthines which have been found to aggravate breast disease.

- Take a dietary supplement containing the following:
  Vitamin E, 4–600 IU daily
  Vitamin B6, 50–100 mg daily
  Vitamin B complex, 25 mg daily
  Magnesium, 200 mg daily
  Zinc, 10–40 mg daily (especially

if your breasts are worse pre-menstrually)
Cold-pressed linseed oil, 1–2 tablespoons daily
Evening primrose oil, 4–8,500 mg capsules daily

BRONCHITIS AND EMPHYSEMA

What are they?

Bronchitis is an inflammation of the air passages of the lungs and emphysema is a condition in which the tiny air sacs (alveoli) at the ends of the passages become distended and weakened. They are usually thought of together because they so often occur alongside one another.

Bronchitis usually starts with a cold on the chest, often with a sense of 'rawness' behind the chestbone, a tightness in the chest or pain or irritation between the shoulder blades. There is often a dry cough and a moderate fever. Gradually the cough becomes looser and the sufferer starts to produce phlegm. This cough and phlegm can continue for weeks. This type of bronchitis is called acute but it can keep on recurring and become chronic. When it becomes chronic the lungs begin to shrink and permanent damage reduces their efficiency.

Chronic bronchitis is extremely common, especially in the UK. About one in twenty of all deaths are caused by bronchitis and emphysema. The total number of deaths is the same as that caused by lung cancer. These conditions also result in the loss of about 300 million working days each year.

What causes them?

- Cigarette smoking. There is no doubt that the largest single culprit is smoking, though it should also be borne in mind that deaths from these conditions are more common in parts of the country where air pollution is high. No one knows why all smokers do not get the disease but some studies suggest a hereditary link. This has been traced to a deficiency of alpha l-anti-trypsin in the blood of susceptible people. Such people are then especially sensitive to cigarette smoke and infection.

- Physical variations. The north of England has more bronchitis and emphysema than does the south and it appears that the wetness of the atmosphere could have something to do with it.

- Certain occupations are particularly connected with these diseases. Workers in the linen and cotton industry and those who are exposed to cadmium are especially at risk.

- Poor personal resistance to infections. This is caused by poor diet, bad breathing, poor posture, lack of exercise and smoking.

Prevention

- Stop smoking. Given that bronchitis is an inflammatory condition of the airways with an excessive production of mucus, the best preventive is to stop smoking if only because the smoke itself damages the air passages, so adding to the problem. Early bronchitic changes can be reversed by stopping smoking and, of course, other problems connected with smoking will go too. We look at how to stop smoking on page 332.

  There is plenty of evidence to show that children of parents who smoke have more chest infections than other children, and a London study of 10,500 schoolchildren found that even as early as 11 their lungs are being seriously affected. Those smoking up to six cigarettes a week suffered from colds and coughs and were more likely to be short of breath after exercise than the non-smokers. Obviously stopping children smoking is a major preventive measure against this vast problem.

  A study of British doctors was started in 1951. By 1964 it had been found that the death rate from chronic bronchitis of those smoking up to 14 cigarettes per day was seven times that of non-smokers, and of those smoking 15-24 daily, twenty times. In various studies pipe and cigar smokers come out better than cigarette smokers as regards bronchitis, and those who have only ever smoked pipes and cigars have a risk only very slightly greater than non-smokers.

- Clean up polluted air. Most western countries are now more vigilant about smoke pollution than in the past and the Clean Air Acts in the UK (1956 and 1968) have undoubtedly played their part in reducing the toll of these diseases. The small fall in deaths from bronchitis and emphysema seen in recent years can almost certainly be put down to these measures. Local authorities were given the power to create smokeless zones. Such measures have made the old British 'smogs' a thing of the past.

  Vitamin A appears to be valuable for those who live in highly polluted air zones. Ozone and other air pollutants destroy vitamin A by oxidation, so anyone living in a polluted area should take more of the vitamin as a protective, especially in the winter months. Liver, herring, eggs, milk, margarine, butter and carrots are good sources, but the easiest way of taking this vitamin is in fish-liver-oil capsules.

- Breathing exercises are probably worth trying at the first sign of bronchitis. See page 76.

- Take more exercise. One study of very severe bronchitis and emphysema patients who had only about 25 per cent of normal lung function left and were thus suffering from shortness of breath and limited activity, gave graded exercises in a training schedule on a stationary bicycle. When the tension on the bicycle was set to produce a feeling of 'work' but not 'exhaustion' at the end of the exercise, most of the patients felt better. At first the subjects were allowed only seven minutes on the bicycle but this was slowly worked up to twenty minutes. Exercise increases the rate of mucus production and makes it easier to cough up. People undergoing regular exercise like this report an improvement in their symptoms and are aware that the vicious circle of shortness of breath, no exercise, more shortness of breath, can be broken.

- All bronchitics cough and this is healthy. Don't use cough suppressants – the phlegm ought to come up, especially if it is infected (yellow or green). Any remedy that helps bring up phlegm can be used, including exercise.

- Poor posture can make breathing less efficient, as may nervous tension. Be sure to learn to walk upright, shoulders back and with your back straight. Be careful about bad posture when seated too. Learn how to relax and how to breathe properly (see pages 87 and 76 respectively).

- Cut down on refined carbohydrates. A study as long ago as 1933 found that girls in a boarding school were more likely to have upper respiratory problems if they ate lots of sugar. It was found that in the dormitory that consumed the lowest amount of sugar catarrh cases were 19 per cent less than in the dormitory with the highest sugar consumption.

- Cut down or cut out foods that you know produce mucus in you. Chocolate, milk, cocoa and sugar are all mucus-forming. Some people find that their mucus levels go up when they eat white bread, fried foods, cooked cheese and creamy dishes.

- Eat a wholefood diet (see page 72). Certain naturopaths think that the proportions of acid and alkali we consume should be changed in such a way as to produce a better balance of the two. A good suggestion in this respect is 10 per cent protein, 20 per cent unrefined carbohydrates, 5 per cent fat, and 65 per cent fruit and vegetables, but most people find that a diet this low in fat is extremely difficult to stick to. Eating as many foods as possible raw also seems to help. According to a leading naturopath who treats these conditions with diet, tea, coffee, cocoa and cola drinks (especially if sweetened with sugar or sugar substitutes) are also mucus-forming and should be avoided.

- Take mineral supplements. Iodine appears to be especially

useful in bronchial complaints. It can be found in seaweed, a fact first discovered during World War II when seaweed was used to supplement food supplies in the Channel Islands. There was a noticeable decrease in bronchial troubles and colds. It should also be pointed out, however, that this was also a time when the consumption of refined foods fell. Seaweed extracts can be bought in health-food shops.

Zinc and vitamin A are both valuable in the fight against any infection, as is vitamin C. Take all of these in full doses.

- The herb comfrey has been used for bronchial problems for centuries. The leaves and roots are used to make a tea which can be taken during the 'bronchitic' winter months.

- Spicy foods seem to help clear the respiratory passages, as do fluids taken by mouth. One expert in this field gets his bronchitic patients to eat large quantities of garlic, horseradish and mustard and to drink plenty of fluids during the winter months. Mucus becomes easier to cough up and so does less harm to the lungs.

- Lose weight. The fatter you are the more difficult it is to breathe effectively and to cough to bring up phlegm.

- Try to avoid places where you know there will be people with colds and 'flu. Bronchitics are more likely to get infections so it

makes sense to keep away from people with them if at all possible. It is probably worth having anti-'flu injections in the late autumn.

- If your job could be the cause of your chest condition, talk to your doctor or chest physician to see if you can get their help to change your job.

- Don't keep your house so hot that the dry air causes you problems. Put bowls of water in front of the main radiators or buy a commercial humidifier if you can afford one. Dry air thickens mucus and will do you no good. Ensure that your bedroom is well warmed before going to bed and warm the bed first too.

BRUISING

What is it?

A collection of blood and blood breakdown products in the skin or other superficial parts of the body.

What causes it?

- Trauma to the area.

- Certain rare blood or blood-vessel diseases.

- Leukaemia in children.

- Cushing's disease (overactivity of the adrenal glands).

- Certain drugs.

Prevention

The only one of these abnormalities that can be prevented without medical help is the first. Anyone who bruises easily should see a doctor to have the other conditions ruled out.

It is almost impossible to prevent all knocks and bumps in life but for those (children especially) who are liable to very easy bruising some of the hints under the prevention of accidents (see page 108) could be helpful. Here are a few tips to help prevent bruises from becoming worse than they otherwise would be.

- Arnica – the homoeopathic remedy – if dabbed on the area immediately after a knock will prevent the bruise coming out at all or reduce its severity. Arnica should only be used on closed skin (i.e. not if there is a wound).

- Ice constricts the tiny capillaries in the skin and prevents blood from leaking out to cause a bigger bruise. For immediate first aid put an unopened pack of frozen vegetables (peas are ideal) straight from the freezer on to the area.

- Pancreatic and pineapple enzymes help reduce bruising. Bromeleins – the active ingredient in pineapple – help reduce pain and swelling.

- Vitamin C and bioflavonoids might also help, according to a study in New York. These help to strengthen capillaries in people who are prone to easy bruising.

This is particularly likely to be of value in the elderly, who tend to be short of these vitamins.

- Keep off drugs that are known to thin the blood. Aspirin is the best known and most widely used but anti-histamines, anti-inflammatories and diuretics can all contribute to easy bleeding.

CAFFEINE POISONING

What is it?

A condition caused by drinking caffeine-containing drinks. The commonest of these are coffee, tea and cola drinks. There is also caffeine in certain cold remedies, pain-killers and stay-awake aids.

The signs of caffeine poisoning are shaky hands, buzzing in the ears, hallucinations, headaches, irritability, restlessness, frequent passing of urine (often making the person get up at night), palpitation, insomnia, indigestion and heartburn, and a general feeling of anxiety. Millions of people around the world have one or more of these symptoms almost all their lives, yet are amazed to learn that caffeine is the culprit.

There are many people in mental hospitals who are suffering only from caffeine addiction. A study reported in the *American Journal of Psychiatry* in 1976 found that of 135 patients on an acute psychiatric ward thirty-four were 'high users' of caffeine (more than 5 cups of coffee per day). The study also found that these thirty-four people had a higher incidence of psychosis than other patients. At first the researchers asked themselves why it was that such seriously ill people drank so much coffee, rather than looking at it the other way round. The team involved now believe that caffeine triggers psychoses (serious mental disorders) by its action on normal brain transmitter chemicals.

Caffeine taken in even normal doses can cause less dramatic but nonetheless troublesome symptoms. Light-headedness, headaches, irregular heartbeat and anxiety are common in some people drinking relatively few caffeine-containing drinks. One expert has found that high doses of caffeine can produce symptoms totally indistinguishable from anxiety neurosis. A dose of 250 mg or more of caffeine can produce troublesome symptoms at once in many people. The caffeine content of drinks is as follows:

Cup of strong, black coffee 150 mg
Cup of strong tea 100 mg
12oz can of Coca-Cola 64.7 mg
12 oz can of Pepsi-Cola 43.1 mg

Prevention

- Cut out or cut down on all caffeine-containing substances including coffee, tea, cola drinks, pain-killers and cold cures that contain caffeine (look at the labels). Throw away your coffee percolator.

You will notice signs of withdrawal–after all, you are coming off a potent drug. Caffeine is probably the most commonly abused drug in the world. Symptoms you can expect as you wean yourself off caffeine are headache, irritability, inability to work effectively, nervousness, restlessness and lethargy. Because you are trying to break an addiction, go slowly. Start drinking your tea and coffee weaker, and gradually reduce your joint intake of the two drinks to two or three cups per day.

If you find it easier, wean yourself off coffee on to strong tea, and then reduce the strength and the number of cups of tea. Using tea bags and a metal container cuts back on the caffeine in the tea you are making. Loose tea-leaves brewed for the same amount of time or to the same colour will have more caffeine than tea brewed in a bag.

- Substitute healthy drinks for the fluid you would have taken as tea, coffee or cola drinks. Drink fresh orange (diluted if it is too expensive to drink neat). Drink water, especially with meals. Take up drinking herbal teas– there are many to choose from and they are delicious.

CANCER
(see also page 98)

What is it?

Any consideration of cancer, be it

from a preventive or curative point of view, is extremely difficult because cancer is a family of conditions, not a single disease. At present only about a third of all cancers have identifiable causes, and opinions vary as to whether all cancers will eventually be found to have an environmental, and therefore preventable, cause.

Worldwide, the six most common cancers in men are of the: lung; stomach; colon and rectum; mouth and pharynx; prostate; and oesophagus. In women the most common cancers are of the: breast; cervix; stomach; colon; rectum; lung and mouth; and pharynx. These, together with those of the brain, bladder and lymphatic tissues, and leukaemia, account for three-quarters of all new malignancies. Stomach cancer is the most common cancer worldwide, closely followed by that of the lung.

The considerable variations seen from country to country, and the patterns of cancer emergence in migrant populations as they move to live in westernised countries, strongly suggest that many, if not most, cancers are linked to lifestyle and environment. Some experts claim that as many as 80–90 per cent of all cancers will eventually be preventable. Having said this, it would be easy to give the impression that only western countries have large burdens of cancer. They do not–they just have different cancer patterns.

What causes it?

Although the exact way in which the following are implicated in cancer causation is none too clear they have all been definitely connected with one type or another.

- Tobacco smoke.
- Alcohol and alcoholic mouth-washes.
- Obesity.
- Poor personal hygiene.
- Too much sun.
- Food additives.
- Pollution.
- Medicines and medical procedures.
- Certain infections.
- Exposure to radiation.
- Occupational chemicals.
- Lack of vitamins, especially A, C and E.
- Hot drinks and food.
- Too little dietary fibre.
- Viruses.
- Sexual behaviour.

There are, of course, many other factors involved in producing cancer but these are the main ones.

Although there are so many different types of cancer, more than 80 per cent of all cancers in men are caused by ten types. More than 75 per cent of those in women are caused by a different list of ten types. Six are common to both lists so there are only about fourteen types of cancer that are common and they cause between them four-fifths of all cancer deaths. Of these fourteen half are sufficiently well understood to be able to give at least some preventive guidelines. Here are a few thoughts on those which are *not* yet preventable.

- Stomach. The incidence of stomach cancer is falling in all westernised countries for some unknown reason. It is much more common in Japan but the incidence is falling there too, probably as a result of good screening measures. Perhaps the worldwide fall in this disease has something to do with the way food is stored. An alternative explanation is that people are eating more fresh fruit and vegetables and consuming less salt.

- Prostate. There has been a twofold increase in male deaths from cancer of the prostate gland this century in England and no cause has been found.

- Brain. There has been a steady rise in the figures for brain-cancer mortality this century – perhaps due to better diagnosis. Many cases would have been missed before.

- Ovary. There is an increased risk of cancer of the ovary in women who have early first intercourse, have their first pregnancy by age 20, have few children and have an early menopause. Thus it would appear likely that the cancer is linked to hormonal changes in some way.

- Breast. This, the biggest cancer killer in women, is still not preventable.

- Rectum and large bowel. Dietary factors are suggested but no single one is definitely the cause.

Prevention

- Stop smoking. Tobacco smoke is the biggest single cause of cancer in the world. In the US, for example, it is thought that about one in three of all cancer deaths is the result of smoking. Most people are aware that smoking produces lung cancer but it also produces cancer of the oesophagus (gullet), bladder, larynx and pancreas. Clearly much of this burden of cancer would be avoided if people stopped smoking. (For guidelines on how to do so, see page 332). Cancer of the mouth and pharynx are caused by chewing betel quid with and without tobacco in southern Asia, and by the combination of alcohol and tobacco in westernised countries.

- Alcohol has been found to be associated with cancers of the mouth, throat, tongue and oesophagus. Since liver cancer is often associated with cirrhosis it is possible that alcohol consumption plays a part in liver cancer either directly or indirectly. Other dietary factors have also been found to be causative in cancer. Aflatoxins are products of fungi that grow on peanuts, grains and other foods and produce liver cancer in fish and other animals. Nitrosamines and nitrosamides are carcinogenic in animals and these chemicals are often produced in the body as a result of eating nitrates and nitrites used as preservatives. Smoking and curing foods produces polycyclic hydrocarbons and this has led many cancer experts to suggest the avoidance of burned, charred or even heavily smoked foods.

- Obesity has been found to predispose to cancers of all kinds in many studies. This has been especially well studied in relation to breast cancer.

- The decline in primary cancer of the liver is probably due to improved personal and community hygiene. Hepatitis B infection is an important factor in producing liver cancer, and good living conditions and high levels of sanitation reduce the infection occurrence. If vaccination reduced the numbers of carriers by 90 per cent, and if newborn babies in Africa, Asia and China could be vaccinated, then nearly 200,000 cases of liver cancer could

be prevented every year. At the moment the vaccination is very expensive but it looks as though cheaper versions, produced by genetic engineering, are on the way.

Cancer of the penis too is declining as personal hygiene improves worldwide.

- Too much sun definitely increases the risk of skin cancer (see page 329).

- Clearly linked to sun exposure is the exposure to other forms of radiation. There is little doubt that X-rays and other ionising radiations produce leukaemias. Atom-bomb survivors have more thyroid, breast and lung cancers. Patients being treated for ankylosing spondylitis with X-rays have more stomach and pancreatic cancer. Radium dial painters have more bone cancers and uranium mine workers more lung cancers. If you work with radiation be sure to observe all the safety regulations.

- The exact proportion of cancers that are caused by exposure to environmental chemicals is the subject of considerable debate. Estimates vary from 1 to 3 per cent of all cases. Cancer mortality in England and Wales is 24 per cent higher in manual than in non-manual workers but it is thought that as much as 90 per cent of this larger risk is accounted for by factors like cigarette smoking rather than dangers associated with actual occupation. There are about forty chemicals and processes that are either known to cause cancer in humans or are suspected of doing so. Most of the known carcinogens have been withdrawn or controlled but many of the suspected ones have not. The most common environmental hazards are: vinyl chloride (liver, lung and brain cancers); some chemical dyes (bladder); some compounds of arsenic, chrome and nickel (skin, lung and nose); some wood dusts (nose); some types of tar and soot (skin); and radiation (many types of cancer). Your employer has, by law, to tell you of any known toxic or cancer-producing hazards, and you should tell him or her if you are worried about anything at your place of work. Your union safety representative could be helpful too.

• Vitamins A, C and E have been shown to be valuable protectors against cancer. It has long been realised that vitamin A is vital for maintaining the integrity of cells that cover the body's internal and external surfaces. Animal studies have shown that a vitamin A deficiency causes an increased risk of lung, bladder and colon cancers – all cancers of the epithelial (body lining) tissues. Researchers at the Massachusetts Institute of Technology found that rats so marginally deficient in vitamin A that there were no overt signs of the deficiency had an increased risk of suffering from colon cancer when exposed to cancer-causing chemicals.

Evidence from the Netherlands in a study of thirty-three patients with lung cancer found that those born in the winter months had twice the chance of developing the disease of those born in the summer months. Cows' milk has its lowest levels of vitamin A in the winter, so infants fed cows' milk formula could be getting less of the vitamin than they need. Scientists in Japan followed 122,261 men for ten years. Those who reported a low intake of green and yellow vegetables had death rates from prostate cancer over twice as high as those who ate plenty of these vegetables. The link between green and yellow vegetables was consistent across age, social-class and regional barriers. Recent experiments with vitamin A and its artificial derivatives have found that they block the effects of cancer-causing substances in the lung, breast, stomach, bladder, skin and reproductive system of laboratory animals.

Other research shows that vitamin A interferes with the conversion of cancer-causing chemicals into their active form. Many carcinogens are harmless in themselves but are converted into toxic forms in the body. In some instances, vitamin A prevents this conversion. Good sources of vitamin A are listed on page 178.

Vitamin C may be protective against cancers of the reproductive system. A New York study found that in women the risk of developing cervical dysplasia (a pre-cancerous condition of the cervix) goes down when the vitamin C consumption goes up. The women with positive cervical smears tended to be eating a diet low in vitamin C. They concluded that women who ate less than 30 mg a day of vitamin C had a tenfold risk of cervical dysplasia as compared with women whose intake was above that level.

The risk of breast cancer too can be lowered by using vitamin C supplements, according to studies at Yale University. Researchers compared three groups of women: one group with a breast cancer; a second with healthy breasts; and a third without breast cancer who had recently been discharged from hospital. All the women were asked about their vitamin C intake. Women who took more than 1 g vitamin C daily for at least a year were 50–80 per cent less likely to develop breast cancer than those who ate less.

A US study found that radiation, heat therapy, and certain chemotherapeutic drugs worked better if vitamin E was given too. In a group of thirteen patients with cancers of the nervous system which had not responded to any cure, six improved when given vitamin E. Some of them were totally free from pain for the first time too. Research in Australia found that mice fed extra vitamin E had only one tenth as many malignant chemical-induced breast tumours as did control mice.

- Hot drinks and food are linked to cancers of the gullet. The preventive answer in this case is obvious.

- Early first childbirth and having many children reduces the incidence of breast cancer. Whether breastfeeding does so is still open to debate, even after numerous worldwide studies. Cancer of the ovary is more common in women who have had few children. This could be a cause that continues to become more common worldwide as family size shrinks almost everywhere.

In contrast to cancers of the breasts and ovary, the figures for cancer of the cervix are higher amongst women who have had more children. This effect is almost certainly due to early, promiscuous sexual activity. No one knows what the connection is but smegma and/or sperms might be capable of being carcinogenic, as might herpes virus type 2 (see page 240). Genital cleanliness and barrier methods of contraception (especially the sheath) will help reduce this cancer, as will a smaller number of sexual partners. There is now a rather virulent 'epidemic' of cervical cancer in younger women–and this is occurring against a background of general improvement in the cervical cancer picture overall. Even a woman who has never had intercourse before can 'catch' cervical cancer from her promiscuous partner. Japanese women, traditionally virgins until marriage, have a high incidence of cervical cancer, perhaps as a result of their males having had premarital sexual experience with prostitutes. If a man's first wife dies of cervical cancer his second wife stands a greater chance of dying from it. These facts tend to suggest an infective cause. Prevention involves minimal penis-in-vagina sexual activity before the age of 20 and the use of barrier methods of contraception. Clearly neither of these is very realistic for most people so we can expect to see a rise in the number of women suffering from this particular cancer.

- Air pollution is probably not a major contributor to cancers but the prevention of cancer obviously must include the provision of clean air. Drinking water too can have carcinogens in it, according to recent studies.

- Hormones and certain other medications can cause cancer. The contraceptive Pill has now been positively incriminated in cervical cancer (women who have been on the Pill for five years or more have double the risk of getting the disease, according to a massive World Health Organisa-

tion study), and there are debates over its role in breast cancer. Oestrogens given ante-natally can produce cancers of the vagina and the uterus in the female children of such women. Oestrogens given to relieve menopausal symptoms increase the risk of endometrial cancer about four to eight times. Undoubtedly other drugs will be found to be carcinogenic as our knowledge increases. The answer must be to take only drugs that are absolutely necessary and to keep dosages to the minimum levels.

- Certain viruses seem to cause cancer and the avoidance of those with the viruses could be a sensible preventive measure. Herpes simplex type 2 virus is now thought to play a part in the production of cervical cancer–we saw above how to reduce the chances of contracting this virus.

  A herpes-type virus, the Epstein-Barr virus, is suspected of being the cause of a tumour called Burkitt's lymphoma, a cancer which occurs among children in certain areas of Africa. There are suggestions that the same virus is the cause of nasopharyngeal cancer and Hodgkin's disease.

- Too little dietary fibre has been proposed as a cause of cancer of the large bowel and rectum. The hypothesis is that carcinogens, whether produced by the body or occurring in food itself, are diluted by the bulky stools that a high-fibre diet produces, so reducing their effect. Because such a diet also makes food residues pass quicker through the bowel the hypothesis is that any carcinogens that *are* present are rushed through the bowel so quickly they do not have time to exert their carcinogenic effect. There is a considerable debate as to how feasible such a hypothesis is and many other theories exist as to how large-bowel cancers come about. None of this detracts from the provable value of a high-fibre diet for other conditions.

- Zinc deficiencies have been found in prostatic cancer patients, and recent work at the Sloane Kettering Cancer Center in New York concluded that 'zinc is intimately involved in immune function'.

  Selenium, a trace metal, has been found in many studies to reduce the likelihood of cancers. Studies in one part of the US compared cancer death rates in high- and low-selenium soil areas and found high selenium levels to be protective. To get plenty of selenium you need to eat wholegrain cereals, organ meats and seafoods. One study of seventeen countries found that cancer death rates were very clearly linked to selenium lack.

  The most reliable way of taking selenium is to take a daily dose of high-selenium yeast. This is probably best because so many dietary sources are unreliable in their selenium content and any-way may have been grown in a selenium-poor soil.

CARPAL TUNNEL SYNDROME

What is it?

Carpal tunnel syndrome is a condition which occurs mainly in women and consists of pain and tingling in the thumb, index and middle fingers of the hands. It usually comes on after carrying heavy shopping, or may wake the sufferer at night and is often bad on waking in the morning.

What causes it?

This unpleasant syndrome comes about when the median nerve that runs from the arm to the hand becomes compressed in the tight bony tunnel in the front of the wrist. There are many causes.

- Underactive thyroid gland.
- Pregnancy.
- Rheumatoid arthritis.
- Obesity.
- Injury.
- Vitamin B6 deficiency.
- Fluid retention.

Prevention

- An underactive thyroid gland

needs to be diagnosed medically and treated. There is little that can be done to prevent this.

- Problems occur in pregnancy because of fluid retention which is a normal part of pregnancy. Try cutting out salt from your cooking and at the table. This should help. Cutting down on the consumption of refined carbohydrates also helps.

- Arthritis is dealt with on page 140.

- Obesity is dealt with on page 290.

- Vitamin B6 has been found in several studies to prevent and cure carpal tunnel syndrome. As soon as you think you are getting symptoms, see your doctor and if he rules out the other causes it is sensible to try 200 mg a day of vitamin B6 for three months. If you add in the suggestions above that help prevent fluid retention, you will probably get results even faster.

CATARACT

What is it?

The word cataract is a generic term derived from the Latin word for a waterfall and used by doctors to describe any cloudy patches that invade the normally crystal-clear lens of the eye. Usually light passes through the lens to get to the back of the eye where it is registered by the retina. In an eye with a cataract, light hits the cloudy area and scatters.

Cataracts are very common indeed, affecting about 25 million Americans over the age of 60. At the most severe end of the scale cataracts cause blindness, but they are not always blinding. They *are*, however, disabling enough to force a third of a million people a year in the US to have their lenses surgically removed and replaced by artificial ones or spectacles.

What causes it?

The causes of cataracts are many:

- Old age.

- Congenital factors.

- Diabetes.

- Eye infections.

- Exposure to certain chemicals, drugs and poisons.

- A shortage of vitamin C.

Prevention

- Obviously if a particular drug, poison or chemical is known to cause cataracts it can be avoided. Steroid drugs and paradihydrobenzene are well-proven culprits.

- The careful control of blood sugar will tend to retard the onset of diabetic cataracts.

- Although most medical textbooks say that cataracts of old age are not preventable, evidence is now accumulating which seems to suggest otherwise.

One of the causes of cataracts is light itself. Sunlight fades carpets and curtains, as any householder knows. It also produces tissue changes in the eye. Superoxides or free radicals are produced by sunlight in the eye and these in turn attack the lens to produce cataracts.

Vitamins E and C act as 'scavengers' intercepting these free radicals and neutralising them. In one recent experiment two researchers at the University of Maryland Medical School took lenses from animals and bathed them in special solutions some of which were enriched with vitamin E and some of which were not. When the lenses were exposed to daylight the vitamin E-enriched ones suffered only one fifth as much damage as the others. In other experiments vitamin C was found to protect the lenses in similar ways. This would help explain the exceptionally high levels of vitamin C found in the normal eye – perhaps it is there to counteract the sunlight-produced superoxides. Another researcher, in Virginia, suggests that nutrition plays a vital role in the creation (and hence the prevention) of cataracts. The crucial nutrients, he suggests, are tryptophan, calcium, riboflavin and vitamin E. He did rat work which found that if they were fed a diet low in tryptophan and vitamin E they had a higher risk of developing cataracts.

A major US clinic uses 1–5 g vitamin C a day, and 200–400 IU vitamin E. The patients also go on a low-fat, complex-carbohydrate diet that encourages the consumption of fish, fowl and fresh produce. If the cataract patients improve, surgery is delayed and it is put off as long as improvements persist. The centre claims to be able to keep some people away from surgery altogether using this method. Those who do come to surgery heal faster, have fewer complications and go home the same day. The relationship between certain B vitamins and cataracts is also interesting. In a study of 173 cataract patients in Alabama the researcher found that vitamin B_2 (riboflavin) and cloudless lenses seemed to be linked. One in five of their cataract patients under the age of 50 were deficient in B_2 as were 34 per cent of the over-50 patients. All those they examined without cataracts over the age of 50 had high levels of B_2 in their blood. The researchers conclude that whilst vitamin B_2 probably does not prevent cataracts it probably retards their formation.

CHOLESTEROL: High blood levels

Cholesterol is thought to be important in producing heart disease. Here we look at ways of lowering blood cholesterol levels, and of preventing a high level from arising in the first place.

Prevention:

- Eat more fibre. This has an effect on cholesterol metabolism. Eating wheat bran produces bile that is less saturated with cholesterol (which is good because it tends to reduce the formation of gall-stones). In a study involving men eating rolled oats (1½ cupsful a day), their cholesterol levels fell by 8 per cent after only three weeks. In another study cholesterol falls of 11 per cent were produced in men fed about 2 cupsful of oats a day. Italian researchers took thirty-three volunteers and found that a typical meal took seven hours to pass through the small bowel, absorbing as it went 43 per cent of available cholesterol. When seven of the volunteers were given a substance that speeded up transit through the bowel (to 4½ hours) cholesterol absorption fell to 27 per cent.

  Pectin is a particularly good type of fibre for reducing transit time through the small intestine. It is found in fruit and vegetables and especially apples. Research in Maryland suggests that pectin helps lower cholesterol levels by slowing down the digestion of cholesterol-rich fatty foods. Also, there is a suggestion that pectin converts cholesterol into a form that is poorly absorbed by the body.

- Aubergines (eggplants) also reduce the amount of cholesterol absorbed from foods. An Aust-rian scientist fed a high-choles-terol diet to laboratory animals. If they also received aubergines they were protected from the build-up of fatty plaques in their blood vessels. The results were best when the aubergine was eaten *with* the fatty meal.

- Garlic has a long history of being useful in heart disease. An Indian research team looked at blood cholesterol levels in ten people who ate garlic along with a meal of bread and butter. Those who ate the bread and butter alone had a 20 per cent rise in choles-terol but those who ate it with garlic had no such rise. Another Indian research group found that garlic prevented coronary artery disease in rabbits fed on a high-cholesterol diet. The rabbits' cholesterol rose, but only the 'helpful' HDL fraction which might even be protective against atherosclerosis (narrowing of the arteries) and heart disease.

- Beans lower the dangerous LDL portion of cholesterol. A study of eight men with high blood choles-terol found that half a cupful of beans a day for three weeks reduced their cholesterol by 20 per cent. The dangerous LDL fraction went down by 24 per cent yet the protective HDL fraction was not altered. Soya beans appear to be especially valuable. A study in the Netherlands found that rabbits fed soya protein were much less likely to develop atherosclerosis than were those fed animal protein. There were dramatic reductions in their blood cholesterols in only one day. Similar findings have been reported with humans, particularly in vegetarians, who experienced significant rises in total cholesterol after eating beef for four weeks. Other researchers have found that vegetarians who don't eat eggs or dairy products have lower LDL and total cholesterol levels than do meat eaters or vegetarians who do eat eggs and dairy products.

- Eat less cholesterol. This is somewhat contentious because various studies conflict on whether or not it is worth while restricting the intake of such foods. Egg yolks, butter and liver are especially high sources. The NACNE report on healthy eating recommends no curtailing of cholesterol-rich foods but anyone eating a lot of any of these three and who has a high blood cholesterol would probably do well to cut them down or out.

- Polyunsaturated oils used for cooking or as spreads also have an effect on blood cholesterol levels. In one study in Minneapolis twenty-four healthy volunteers were put on a high-cholesterol diet. When polyunsaturated fats were added both total cholesterol and the harmful LDL component fell. HDL remained high. Of the oils tested, unhydrogenated soya oil and corn were best. Other studies have found that cornflour oil has similar effects.

- Yoghurt may be helpful. One researcher believes that the special bacteria used to ferment yoghurt also produce a substance which blocks cholesterol production in the liver. Eating yoghurt has been found to reduce cholesterol in the blood. Milk (even skimmed) raises blood cholesterol, however.

- Chromium has been found to lower cholesterol levels in rabbits fed on a cholesterol-enriched diet. The rabbits fed with chromium also had only half as many plaques on their coronary arteries as did rabbits in the control group. In humans, brewer's yeast (a rich source of chromium) raised HDL levels in one study.

- Vitamins C and E are valuable too. In a study of forty people with coronary artery disease carried out in India it was found that those whose diets were supplemented with 2 g of vitamin C had an average drop of 12 per cent in their cholesterol levels. In a UK study vitamin C was found to raise the helpful HDL cholesterol fraction. The researchers found that many heart-disease patients had both low vitamin C and low HDL levels. A dose of 1 g vitamin C a day brought both levels up towards normal.

Vitamin E also raises HDLs. A

daily dose of 800 IU increased the HDLs of forty-three volunteers and had the greatest effect in those whose HDLs were lowest to start with.

- Get plenty of exercise. When carrying out the vitamin E study the researchers noticed that joggers and long-distance runners in their sample had very high HDLs before supplementation with the vitamin. Several other studies have found that exercise helps keep cholesterol at normal levels. Even moderate exercise, such as a brisk walk, seems to be effective.

- Stop smoking. A Swedish team found that smokers tended to have low HDL levels. When a group of smokers gave up they all experienced 'rapid and pronounced increases in HDL concentrations'. The levels rose by an average of 29 per cent within two weeks and remained high throughout the observation period.

COLDS AND 'FLU

What are they?

Most of us have a cold or two a year, perhaps when we are run down or when the weather suddenly changes. A cold starts with irritation in the nose and throat, then the nose begins to run and you start to sneeze. Most people also get a headache, have a fever and have generalised aches and pains.

'Flu is different because the symptoms are so much more severe. True 'flu produces pains in the back and legs, redness of the eyes, pain on moving the eyeballs, and a general feeling of weakness and malaise. Most people have a fever and feel fairly ill. Once the illness is over many people feel unwell and even frankly depressed for days or even weeks.

When you get a cold you may not be ill enough to go to bed but most people with 'flu have to rest for at least a couple of days.

What causes them?

Both are caused by viruses which are constantly on the move in terms of the body's immunity so that even when we become immune to one type of virus another, slightly different, one can still attack us.

Just why, in a roomful of people or within a family, certain members will catch a cold or 'flu while others do not is not known, but it is almost certainly to do with the level of that particular individual's immunity at the time. In this context it appears that vitamin C may be crucial. Studies have found that people taking vitamin C at the level of 2 g a day suffer fewer symptoms than those not taking the vitamin. It appears that the vitamin acts in a similar way to interferon – an infection-fighting protein produced by human cells. Unfortunately, the human body does not make vitamin C (as most animals do) so we need to keep on taking it in foods or as supplements. Most of the best sources of vitamin C are fruits and vegetables. These include blackcurrants, strawberries, watercress, cabbage, Brussels sprouts, oranges and lemons. All these are rich in vitamin C when fresh, and raw. The vitamin oxidises on exposure to the air and is destroyed by cooking.

- It is now recommended that as soon as you feel a cold coming on you should take four 500 mg doses of vitamin C spread throughout the day. You need lots of the vitamin to saturate the tissues completely. If you smoke (which reduces the body's vitamin C levels) you could need more than this. Rutin (a bioflavonoid) taken in tablet form helps vitamin C to work.

- Vitamin A is vital for the repair and rejuvenation of cells, especially those of mucous membranes, and so is useful in building up protection against the common-cold virus in the respiratory tract. Good sources of the vitamin are liver, carrots, spinach, margarine, eggs, cheese, milk and apricots. It makes sense to increase your intake of all these foods during the colds season. Most of these foods, however, contain less vitamin A during the winter compared with the summer so vitamin A supplements are also helpful. Yellow fruits and vegetables contain carotene which is converted into vitamin

A in the body. Eat as many yellow and green fruits and vegetables raw as you possibly can and cook the rest lightly so as not to destroy this valuable vitamin.

- When it comes to 'flu the situation is similar but more serious. It is probably best to let the fever take its natural course and not to suppress it with aspirin. Hot, herbal teas are good because of their calming effect whereas ordinary tea and coffee are stimulants. Camomile, lemon balm, coltsfoot, elder and vervain are all useful. Vegetable and fruit juices are good too. Garlic and cayenne pepper both induce sweating and should be used with lemon juice – all rich in vitamins and bioflavonoids.

Go to bed and sweat it out. Rest completely. This is the best cure for the immediate symptoms and a preventive against complications. If your temperature goes over 102°F get someone to sponge you with tepid water and favour cooling drinks rather than hot ones.

Large doses of vitamin C (see above) are also indicated, as is vitamin A. Research from the Massachusetts Institute of Technology found that a folate (one of the B vitamins) deficiency hindered white blood cells multiplying and was associated with an increased susceptibility to infections generally. Vitamin E also plays a vital role in combating infections.

The role of zinc in the functioning of the immune system is now well documented. Even marginal reductions in zinc levels in the body produce quite serious damage to the immune system and it is reckoned that many, if not most, westerners are short of zinc as a result of modern food processing.

Most people do not feel like eating much when they have a cold or 'flu but this does not matter as long as the liquids and vitamin supplements are kept up.

Work done by Dr Szent-Gyorgyi, the Nobel laureate who first isolated vitamin C, suggests that wheatgerm potentiates the effects of vitamin C. In a series of very complex experiments he found that it was the trace element manganese in the wheatgerm that triggered this reaction. He maintains that any plant food will improve the activity of vitamin C in the body but that ideally an ounce or two of wheatgerm per day is needed. This could be of special interest to heavy drinkers, smokers, diabetics and those who take a lot of aspirin because all these people need more vitamin C than average.

Other general preventive measures include:

- Stop smoking. Smoke irritates the lining of the respiratory system with provable ill-effects. Smokers provably have more colds than do non-smokers and also have more sinusitis. Air pollution from many sources destroys vitamin A so it makes sense not to smoke for this reason alone.

- Nitrates and nitrites in foods (especially cured meats, processed and canned meats, frankfurters, salami and sausages) have adverse effects on vitamin A metabolism and so are best avoided or eaten only rarely.

- With central heating and air conditioning, most homes and buildings today are dry, and this predisposes to colds and 'flu.

  A study done in Canadian kindergartens and nursery schools found that those without humidifiers had 40 per cent higher absenteeism than those with them. The workers also found that the staff of un-humidified hospitals had 10–15 per cent more sickness absenteeism for colds and 'flu than did staff at a humidified hospital.

  Domestic humidifiers are not expensive and are well worth buying. An interesting study in a Welsh cheese factory found that those working in a cold, damp room had half the colds of those working in the rest of the factory.

- Research has not proved a link between getting cold or getting wet and suffering from colds and 'flu.

- Undoubtedly, people who are happy and eating well are less likely to suffer from these (and indeed other) infections than are the unhappy or depressed. There is now a considerable body of research proving that stress and unhappiness depress the body's immune systems. The prevention of stress is considered on page 80.

- One bout of a cold gives immunity for only a few days, so keep away from others who have a cold if you can, or you could go through it all again. This is particularly important in the elderly and in those whose resistance to infection is poor.

- If you have more than three or four colds per year you should see your doctor because you may have an underlying condition that makes you more susceptible to infections. Most likely your faulty diet, low in vitamins C and D and zinc, is to blame.

- 'Flu vaccination is not a widely used preventive and is usually only given to those who are at special risk such as doctors, nurses, firemen and policemen and women. Some experts think that the elderly should be vaccinated because they can become so ill with 'flu. If you have a severe chest condition such as asthma, bronchitis or emphysema 'flu can be a much more serious illness. Talk to your doctor about vaccination.

COLIC

What is it?

Pain in the abdomen caused by the spasm of a hollow abdominal organ.

Colic can thus occur in the urinary passages, the uterus or the intestine, for example. The term is not often used of adult pains by lay people but is usually confined to the irritable crying of babies and young children thought to be caused by such muscle spasm.

Three-month colic is a condition so called because it consists of colicky pains (in babies) that disappear by 3 months of age. It is usually worst in the evening. Many babies with so-called colic do not have abdominal organ spasm at all – they are crying for another reason.

What causes it?

Given that the very word 'colic' is used so widely and indiscriminately of crying children it is essential to look at what the causes really are if one is to try to prevent any of them.

- Bottle-fed babies who are fed with a teat that has too large a hole in it can gulp down air and so get abdominal pains as the intestine passes this gas along.

- In breastfeeding mothers with a very large and fast flow of milk much the same can happen.

- Often it appears that so-called colic is not colic as such but is a response to the mother's busyness and preoccupation with other things, rather than the baby, at the time of the day typical for 'colic' (6 o'clock in the evening). Some of these irritable babies may simply want attention.

- A considerable number of so-called 'colicky' babies are mislabelled – they are really bored, lonely or hungry.

- Recent research has found that traces of undigested foods and drinks get through into the mother's bloodstream and thus in her milk. These proteins (mainly from cows' milk) then upset certain susceptible babies and produce colic.

- Other foods a mother eats to which neither she nor her baby are actually 'allergic' can also produce colic. Onions, garlic, Chinese food, cabbage, beans, green leafy vegetables and alcohol can all be culprits. Green leafy vegetables and pulses can make a breast-fed baby very windy.

- A poor breast milk supply, for whatever reason, can produce a baby who is always hungry and cries. He is labelled colicky.

- Cows' milk causes colic in some allergic, bottle-fed babies.

- Some teething babies suffer from 'colic' too.

Prevention

- Change the teat on the bottle to one with a smaller hole. Feed more slowly and 'wind' the baby before lying him or her down.

- If a breastfeeding mother has too much milk she can express the first milk by hand and either keep it to give to a breast-milk bank at her local hospital or discard it. The other way of overcoming the problem of too much milk is to feed from one breast only at a feed. Alternate the one you use. Allow the baby to suck at the empty breast for comfort. In this way he or she gets milk and comfort sucking and yet not too much milk. Express the unused breast if it becomes uncomfortable.

- Relax at the end of the day as much as possible. Spread out household chores through the day and pre-prepare the evening meal, for example. Try to sit down and perhaps have a small drink of alcohol to relax yourself.

- Ensure that your baby is not bored, is played with and gets plenty of stimulation and stays with you wherever you are, whether he or she is awake or asleep.

- If you are breastfeeding try cutting out cows' milk and milk products entirely from your diet for two weeks and see if this does anything to your baby's colic. If things improve, stay off dairy products until you wean and then don't give them to your baby.

- If you are breastfeeding, keep off foods you find from experience give your child colic.

- If you have a poor milk supply, feed more frequently day and night and never let your baby go more than three hours without a feed – if necessary wake him or her up and feed.

- If cows' milk is the culprit in your baby's bottle use goats' milk or soya milk intead.

CONSTIPATION

What is it?

The infrequent passage of stools, which are hard. Severe constipation (less than 3 stools a week) is rare, but 77 per cent of the population pass only 5–7 stools a week and a further 8 per cent only 3–4 a week. Compare this with people living on a non-western diet who may pass two or three stools a day! About 40 per cent of the British population say they are constipated and between 5 and 22 per cent take laxatives.

It is worth taking trouble to prevent or cure constipation because it has the following harmful effects:
1. It is difficult to pass stools and can be painful.
2. The hard masses of stool can tear the delicate lining of the back passage and produce an anal fissure which is excruciatingly painful and bleeds.
3. It can produce piles and make existing ones worse.
4. The straining involved raises the pressure in the veins of the legs and produces varicose veins.
5. The straining involved raises

pressure inside the abdominal cavity and worsens or even creates a hiatus hernia (a rupture of the stomach through into the chest).
6. In elderly people severe straining has been recorded as the cause of strokes as the increased pressure breaks a blood vessel in the brain.

What causes it?

- Too low an intake of dietary fibre. The average UK diet contains 20 g dietary fibre but in countries where constipation is unknown the average daily intake is between 50 and 120 g daily. UK vegetarians eat about 40 g a day.

- Too little water to drink.

- Poor 'bowel habits'.

Prevention

- Increase the amount of dietary fibre you consume by:
  1. Eating wholemeal bread only.
  2. Making most pastry with wholemeal flour.
  3. Changing to a bran-containing cereal for breakfast or eating muesli.
  4. Eating more fruit, vegetables and pulses (peas and beans).

Increase your fibre intake slowly over several weeks or you could get an uncomfortable swelling of your abdomen and a lot of wind. Over two or three months you should be able to greatly increase your dietary-fibre consumption and over a year hit the goals outlined above. You will know when you are taking enough fibre because you will open your bowels at least once a day and will do so easily and without any straining. Most people find that when the fibre content is right their stools float. Once your dietary-fibre intake is right, keep it at that level and don't take more than is necessary.

- Drink at least two or three glasses of water a day to top up what you would otherwise drink. This helps the dietary fibre bulk up and pass through the intestine and bowel easily. If you want to see how important fluid is just drink very little for a day and see how constipated you become.

- Get used to opening your bowels at a regular time each day, preferably in the morning immediately after breakfast. You may find that you open your bowels twice a day if you step up your fibre intake as described above.

COT DEATH

What is it?

The death of an apparently healthy, normal baby in its cot or pram for no known reason. The baby has sometimes had a snuffly nose or other minor symptoms.

In Britain one in every 500 babies dies suddenly and unexpectedly like this. In many parts of the world it is the commonest cause of death under the age of 1 year. It is slightly more common in boys than girls and occurs more frequently in the winter months.

What causes it?

The vast majority of such deaths have to be labelled 'cause unknown'. Occasionally, post-mortem examination shows there is an unrecognised serious condition such as pneumonia or meningitis. Evidence of a minor infection is found in some children.

Prevention

Although the cause of sudden infant deaths (cot death) is not usually known there are certain precautions that can be taken, especially if you have already had one such death in the family.

- Breastfeed exclusively from birth until at least 6 months. Whilst breast-fed babies do die from cot deaths the condition is less common in totally breast-feds.

- Don't give a child under 1 year a pillow unless it is a special non-suffocating type. Most babies who die in this way certainly have not suffocated but it will put your mind at rest and will prevent suffocation in itself.

- Try to protect your baby from coming unnecessarily into contact with people who have coughs, colds and 'flu. Of course, all babies will get these illnesses from time to time but once again, it will put your mind at rest if you have taken such simple precautions.

- Those who have lost one child by cot death, and even some who have not, will probably want to think about the following precautions, which are at least sensible, for a subsequent baby:

1. Tell your doctor if you think your baby is at all ill.
2. Always take seriously fits, blue or grey turns, difficult breathing, and exceptional drowsiness. Tell the doctor urgently.
3. Tell the doctor as soon as possible if your baby has any of the following: croup; can't breathe through nose; cries in an unusual way or for a long time; repeatedly refuses food; vomits repeatedly; has watery diarrhoea; or is unusually cold, hot or floppy. Even if you have told your doctor, health visitor or nurse, if things don't improve tell your doctor again the same day.

- If your baby stops breathing, perform artificial respiration, blowing only the amount of air you can hold in your cheeks into his or her nose and mouth by covering both with your mouth.

- If your baby has a fit lay him or her face down with the head turned to one side, clear the mouth of sick or froth and cool him or her by removing clothes or sponging with tepid water.

- If your baby swallows pills or poisons get expert help at once.

COUGH

What is it?

An abrupt intake of air followed by a forcible, explosive blowing out. Coughing is a protective reflex aimed at ridding the body of mucus or debris that is irritating the breathing passages. Often, though, a cough has no such protective effect and is simply a nuisance. The dry, unproductive cough of tonsillitis and laryngitis is an example of this. If you cough up anything there is usually trouble in the lungs themselves and you need a medical opinion.

What causes it?

Most coughs are associated with colds and other mild respiratory infections. Any long-standing cough should always be reported to your doctor. Some of the more common causes are:

- Going into the cold suddenly.

- Smoking.

- Cold weather.

- A nervous cough.

- Lung diseases.

- Certain digestive disorders.

- Problems in the larynx (voice box).

- Whooping cough (a very specific cough).

- Asthma.

- Bronchitis.

Prevention

Obviously, as there are so many causes of a cough, the individual with a cough must first be sure what is causing it. This can often only be established with medical help. Prevention is clearly aimed at dealing with causes. Some of the causes of coughs are dealt with elsewhere in the book.

When it comes to the common cough for which most people medicate themselves a few things are worth knowing. Recent US research has found that cough medicines taken to cure or prevent coughs often do not live up to their claims:

- *Expectorants* are supposed to loosen phlegm in the nose, throat and upper respiratory passages but they often do not work. Unfortunately, some may actually do harm. Large doses of aluminium chloride, for example, can upset the body's acid-base balance. Syrup of ipecac, commonly used in children, can be toxic to them, and terpin hydrate can cause nausea and vomiting. Some expectorants contain a lot of alcohol too.

- *Cough suppressants* are not necessarily good for you. They inactivate the cough reflex and certainly should not be used if you have a productive cough. The phlegm or pus should be coming up–not staying down. Those with asthma or chronic bronchitis should not take cough suppressants because such people rely on their cough reflex to clear their lungs.

- *Anti-histamines* thicken mucus and so make it more difficult to bring up. Some people who have a 'post-nasal drip' that keeps them awake at night use these medications but this can be harmful.

- *Decongestants* should not be used for a cough. Those with high blood pressure, diabetes, or a heart or thyroid disease, should avoid them anyway. Unless you are severely stuffy stay away from these preparations. They dry up the very places that need moisturising!

- *Cough syrups* are bad for children because they soothe the cough for only a very short time yet bathe the teeth in sugar for hours. Similarly, cough drops cause tooth decay, especially in those who carry them around with them all day and suck them much of the time.

- A condition that is increasingly being recognised is a cough that hangs around after a cold or 'flu. This is now thought to be due to a food allergy in certain individuals. The symptoms of the food allergy are triggered by the cold or 'flu. Going on an elimination diet is the only way of finding out if this is so (see page 218). One researcher has found that within even a week of eliminating the offending food(s) the cough stops. The individual should then stay away from the offending food for a month or so. One British expert thinks that most coughs, if not caused by colds, are allergic in origin.

- A dab of honey on the back of the tongue seems to work wonders.

- Supplement the diet with vitamins C and E.

- If post-nasal drip at night is a problem, sleep on your stomach.

- Drink plenty of fluids.

- Have a humidifier going.

- Use a herbal chest rub.

CYSTITIS

What is it?

Cystitis is an inflammation of the lining of the bladder. More than half of all western women suffer from it at some time in their lives, and some do so repeatedly. Although cystitis is unpleasant it is not dangerous and can be prevented much of the time if you know what to do.

What causes it?

- Bacteria which normally live in and around the bowel opening can find their way up the urinary passage and into the bladder. This happens very easily in women because the passage is very short. The germs multiply inside the bladder, irritate it and make the woman want to pass water frequently, often with a burning sensation.

- Friction along the urinary passage during sexual intercourse. A woman who is insufficiently aroused produces only a very small quantity of natural secretions in her vagina. Her partner's penis then causes too much friction and 'milks' germs up her urinary passage and into her bladder. Also, some women's bladders are directly bruised by their partner's penis in certain intercourse positions.

- Allergies are an uncommon cause. Some women are allergic to vaginal deodorants, perfumed talc and so on.

- Irritable bladder. A few women have exceptionally sensitive bladders.

- Anxiety or depression. Some women who are depressed or who are having relationship or sexual problems develop cystitis. This often removes them from the sexual arena altogether – which may be what they unconsciously desire.

- Coffee, tea and alcohol can cause cystitis in some women.

Prevention

- Eat a healthy, balanced diet low in refined foods and high in fruit and vegetables and cereal fibre. This, in itself, will help prevent infections.

- Drink plenty of fluids–about 3-4 pints a day. This flushes out germs and keeps your urine dilute.

- Don't wait until you are bursting to pass water. Get into the habit of going before you leave on a journey or go somewhere where you will not have access to a lavatory. Avoid hanging on until you can't wait any longer.

- Ensure that you empty your bladder fully. Don't rush off the lavatory–give yourself time.

- If you think your cystitis is related to sexual intercourse here are some things to do.
  1. You and your partner should wash your genital areas beforehand.
  2. Your partner should spend more time in foreplay to arouse you better.
  3. Pass water before and after sex.
  4. Use KY jelly or a similar bland lubricant if you don't produce enough natural secretion yourself. These are available from chemists.
  5. Avoid intercourse positions that seem to cause bruising of your bladder.

- Get into the habit of wiping your bottom from front to back, to avoid dragging germs from your bowel opening to your vaginal area.

- Wash your vaginal and anal area every morning and evening, even if you don't plan to have sex. Get into the habit.

- Never use vaginal deodorants, perfumed soap or talcum in the vaginal area.

- Avoid coffee, tea or alcohol if they seem to make you worse or drink them very dilute.

- Avoid wearing tights–change to stockings. Never wear jeans or tight, airless trousers. Wear cotton, rather than man-made, panties.

DENTURE PROBLEMS

What are they?

There are many problems connected with wearing dentures, many of which are related to the fact that they are not nearly as stable as natural teeth. Advertisements suggest that denture fixatives are the answer and they certainly do work, but even the best false teeth are clumsy and cannot match up to natural teeth. Surveys have found that between 15 and 45 per cent of denture wearers are unhappy with them, and that 20 million people wear dentures in the

US alone. This amounts to a very large number of individuals worldwide. One study found that about 30 per cent of denture wearers thought they needed refitting, or that they needed new dentures.

What causes them?

Some problems with dentures are inevitable because they are not fixed structures like natural teeth. They are only as good as the bony ridge or foundation on which they sit. In a fair percentage of denture wearers the bony ridge shrinks away. As this happens the dentures fit less and less well. This bone loss can be prevented.

Prevention

- Take more calcium. One study of people with denture problems found that those with good underlying bone were consuming about 900 mg calcium a day and that those who had jawbone problems were getting only about 500 mg calcium. Another trial looked at dummy tablets versus vitamin D (which helps with calcium absorption and better bone formation) for jawbone loss. After a year those taking the supplemental calcium had lost 34 per cent less bone from their upper jaws and 39 per cent less from their lower jaws than had the unsupplemented group. This study also found that the ratio of calcium to phosphorus the person consumed was important too. As levels of phosphorus rose

jawbone resorption speeded up. The ideal ratio of calcium to phosphorus is 1:1. In red meat, though, there is twenty times too much phosphorus and in refined cereal products six times too much. They found that meat, bread and potato eaters experienced more of this bone loss than did other people. Also, soft drinks contain lots of phosphorus. Even teenage girls have been found to have started losing bone abnormally as a result of their soft-drink intake. This study recommended taking Dolomite, a phosphorus-free calcium and magnesium supplement. It can be bought at health-food shops and chemists.

All of this is interesting even to those of us who still have our teeth, because the breakdown of tooth support is seen in gum disease. A study of people with bleeding, inflamed gums found that taking 1g of supplemental calcium for six months produced considerable improvement. X-rays of the jawbones showed that bone loss reversed in 70 per cent of the cases.

DEPRESSION

What is it?

Depression is a highly complex condition that can be defined in many ways. To the man or woman in the street it is often taken to mean 'the blues' or 'feeling low', but at the other end of the scale doctors see people who are really ill with depression, which is still the biggest single cause of suicide.

However we define it, depression is extremely common – in fact it is the most common psychiatric condition in the western world. Between 8 and 15 million Americans are being treated for it at any one time, and it is the biggest single cause for admission to mental hospitals in the western world. Women seem to be more commonly affected than men, but this assumption is being seriously questioned as it now appears that men may simply show their depression in other ways – the main ones being anti-social behaviour, alcoholism and sexual misdemeanours.

There are two types of depression. The most common by far is the 'endogenous' kind. This occurs for no apparent reason though as we learn more about the condition more and more causes are being recognised. The second type is 'manic' depression. In this disease the individual suffers bouts of being highly active and sleepless and bouts of deep depression.

The signs and symptoms of depression are many, and surprisingly it can be a difficult diagnosis to make when the picture is not clear-cut. Many depressives have few mental or psychological symptoms and go to the doctor with physical complaints which are in fact a manifestation of their depression. The main signs of depression are: sadness; a slowness of thought; feeling worse in the morning and brightening up as the day progresses; trouble getting off to sleep, and waking early in the morning (4 or 5 a.m.); a poor appetite for sex and food; a loss of interest in life generally; a lack of interest in things that used to be of value (e.g. hobbies); self-neglect; loss of self-confidence; a sense of guilt and worthlessness; anxiety; irritability; a tendency to cry easily; a fear of being left alone; a fear of death; a sense of hopelessness; extreme weakness and tiredness; delusions; and suicidal thoughts.

Some of the commonest physical symptoms are: tiredness; itching; weakness; dizziness; palpitation; blurred vision; a tendency to drop things; burning pains in the limbs; abdominal pains; nausea; constipation or diarrhoea; 'can't draw a good breath'; facial pain; excessive sweating; food 'sticks' in the throat or gullet; aches; and pains and cramps in the legs. In one study of people complaining of symptoms for which no cause could be found one in ten were clinically depressed and half had been ill for more than ten years. Many had had numerous operations and investigations – most of which were quite unnecessary.

Treatment takes the form of drugs, psychotherapy, or electro-convulsive therapy (ECT). Each has its place but all the treatments have drawbacks and the best way of handling depression is clearly to prevent it, if at all possible.

What causes it?

- Normal sadness. If someone

close to us dies it is natural to grieve over the loss. For some people this will go on to a true depression with many of the symptoms outlined above. This kind of depression is called 'reactive' because it occurs as a perfectly understandable reaction to a life event. People suffering from reactive depression usually get better within a few weeks, perhaps with the help of a short-term course of drugs as a crutch.

- Genetic vulnerability. There is little doubt that certain personality types are more prone to depression – circumstances that would not produce depression in others do so in them. The predisposition to depression is often the result of the loss (real or imagined) of an important person early in life. This can make the individual especially sensitive to psychological pain later in life. Manic-depressive illness is probably inherited, at least to some degree. One sort of depression (which appears early in life) is almost certainly inherited.

- Psychological events in life that so stress a person that he or she simply cannot cope.

- Psychological causes of depression. Given that depression is a psychological illness it makes sense to look at psychological causes for the condition. Unfortunately, this is not easy and ironically the psychological causes of depression remain one of the more controversial areas of the whole subject. The psychoanalysts see depression as an inward turning of self-hate and aggression that should really be directed elsewhere. Being made to feel worthless early in life (often as a baby) also contributes to a depressive type of personality. Other analysts have focused on the helplessness side of depression, and claim that it is a condition that occurs when people feel they have no control over life events, and that depression occurs when individuals cannot live up to their expectations of themselves and others. Another group of psychologists believe that people become depressed because of the way they think of themselves. Such people see little good in life (often quite rationally) and then go on to expect less and less. So it is that helplessness and hopelessness become a part of depression.

- The breaking of close bonds is a potent cause of depression. Both animal and human research shows that breaking close bonds even very early in life can produce depression in both the young and adults. Adults who become depressed for the first time in adulthood are more likely to have lost a parent (usually a mother) early in life than adults who are not depressed. Even a long stay in hospital can be seen by a baby or young child as a 'loss' in this context.

- Biochemical causes of depression are still hotly debated. Certainly it is possible to detect and even measure biochemical events in the brains of depressed people, but whether the chemical differences between depressed and non-depressed people are the cause or the effect of the depression is impossible to say. Lowered serotonin seems to be important in both depression and mania. Tryptophan, the essential amino-acid, is known to be linked to depression. One study found that the most common cause of post-natal depression was linked to shortages of tryptophan, and several other studies have confirmed the effectiveness of this amino-acid in the treatment of depression. Vitamin B_6 also seems to keep people from being depressed. A study of fifteen depressed pregnant women found that those with the worst depression had the lowest blood levels of vitamin B_6. This vitamin is also linked to the depression experienced by a certain number of women who take the Pill. This drug lowers B_6 levels, but the depressive effect can be reversed by giving the vitamin with the Pill.

  In another study doctors gave tryptophan and niacin to eleven patients with depression. They did this because they noticed that some people given tryptophan did not get better. After a month on the two substances the patients' blood levels of tryptophan rose about 300 per cent and their depression fell by 39 per cent. Tryptophan has also been tested against a standard anti-depressant drug and found to be effective but to have fewer side-effects.

  Hypoglycaemia (see page 248) is another biochemical cause of depression – some experts claim it is the most common.

- We now know that many things in our environment (including foods and environmental chemicals) can affect the production of certain natural chemicals in the brain to alter mood.

- Social causes of depression are many and varied. Doctors think of depression as a 'medical' condition but sociologists see it as a condition associated with social malaise. At least a quarter of working-class mothers with young children living in central London suffer from a condition which, if they went to a psychiatric clinic, would be labelled depression. Women with no close, confiding relationship (boyfriend, spouse or similar) also fare badly when the going gets tough, as do women with three or more children at home under the age of 14.

  Sociologists, then, claim that some people – and there are millions of them throughout the western world – are born into, or find themselves in, social and economic conditions which predispose to depression. This does not mean to say that depression is solely a social disease but that it can be caused or perpetuated by social factors. The vast majority of things that are wrong with society and which predispose to depression cannot be influenced by doctors at all.

- Drugs. More than 200 drugs have been claimed to cause depression but only a few do so with any frequency. Some drugs cause depression as a side-effect of their use and others do so only if they are withdrawn too rapidly.

  Alcohol is the commonest drug to produce depression and it is often involved in suicides. Sedatives and anti-anxiety drugs, pain-killers and anti-rheumatics, stimulants, the contraceptive pill, blood-pressure drugs, steroids, certain antibiotics, and a host of other drugs, can all be culprits.

- Infections can cause depression, especially those caused by viruses. Meningitis and encephalitis (in which the brain is directly affected) produce serious brain-centred symptoms early on and depression later. It can often last for several months. Influenza, hepatitis and glandular fever are especially likely to cause long-lasting depression.

- Surgical operations can cause depression too but no one knows why. Operations that involve the loss of a part of the body (such as the removal of a breast or the uterus) are obvious causes but many people having quite minor

and non-disfiguring operations can be depressed for months.

- Serious physical disease is a common cause of depression. In the acute phase of a serious disease at least a quarter of patients become depressed, according to one US study of 150 people in hospital for physical ailments. Several studies have found a high correlation between suicide and physical illness. Rheumatoid arthritis, peptic ulcer, and high blood pressure, were found to have the greatest 'suicide' potential in one study.

  Chronic illness and disability can, undoubtedly, make people depressed. For some such people depression becomes a way of life.

  Talking of chronic disease, several surveys have found that people who are depressed stand a much greater chance of dying prematurely of cancer than do others of the same age.

- 'Glandular' problems can sometimes cause depression. Thyroid disease is a fairly common cause.

- Food allergies and intolerances are an increasingly recognised cause of depression. Foods especially likely to be at fault are cows' milk, eggs, nuts, and wheat and its products. Elimination diets can be useful in detecting the culprit but results can take several weeks (as opposed to days with other food-allergy manifestations) so one has to be very careful in the early stages to be sure that the diet is not so poor that this adds to the clinical problem. Taking plenty of water, minerals and vitamin supplements will definitely help.

- Babies and children are a major source of depression. One of the most depressed groups of people in the West are mothers of young children. Post-natal depression is extremely common, with eight out of ten women complaining of at least some 'baby blues'. Women who deliver at home have much lower levels of depression post-natally, as do those whose babies are exclusively breast-fed.

- Success. We have been conditioned into thinking of depression as caused by failure and negative life events but a small minority of people become depressed when they achieve goals and are successful. Some see their success as undeserved or a hollow sham and yet others fear it will be taken away from them. Some fear what success will bring and back away from it just as they are about to achieve it. Many people unconsciously (and sometimes even consciously) fear the effect that their success has on others and fear the rivalry it produces. Rather than provoke such rivalry (which may remind them of childhood rivalry) they fight shy of success even when it stares them in the face.

- Mental or physical fatigue is a little-discussed cause of depres-

sion but most of us can easily slide into true depression if either or both strike. This could be at the heart of much of the depression seen in young women with small children.

- The menstrual cycle causes depression regularly in a proportion of women. About half of all women have at least some premenstrual symptoms, and depression can be a real problem for a few. Admission to mental hospitals, suicide attempts, child battering, and depressive episodes are all more common premenstrually than at any other time of the month in the female population generally. Clearly there is a hormonal effect but recent thinking suggests that dietary imbalances too play a vital role.

- Retirement, divorce, separation and loneliness are powerful sources of depression in our culture today. Divorce and separation are especially likely to make people depressed, particularly if children are involved. Admission to mental hospital and all kinds of physical illness (including cancers) are much more common in the divorced and separated than in the married. Marital problems themselves are potent and common causes of depression. One large study compared various different forms of therapy for depression and found that of all those tested (including drugs) marital therapy was the most successful.

Prevention

Obviously the prevention of depression is a vastly complex subject and involves many different facets of life.

- Prevention begins in the cradle by breastfeeding totally and by ensuring that a child is brought up to feel wanted and loved for itself. The more stable a home life the child has the better, though some instability is inevitable and certainly will not necessarily produce depression later in life. Preventive measures are especially valuable in any family in which there is a history of depression or suicide, if only because clinical experience shows that both are more likely once they have been 'sanctioned' already within a family. Attending to a baby's needs for food, comfort and attention as soon as he or she expresses them makes the baby think well of the world and tends to produce a less frustrated personality.

- Healthy eating right from weaning will help too, especially in the prevention of hypoglycaemia, premenstrual tension and certain other biochemical causes of depression.

- Social causes are often unpreventable except with endless money, other resources and social engineering, but much can be done to alleviate loneliness and isolation in the young mother. The other social remedies are beyond the range of a book such as this.

- Keeping off drugs unless absolutely essential is a very good preventive, simply because so many people are on one drug or another that promotes depression. Find other ways (perhaps from this book) of dealing with the underlying problems. Come off the Pill or try adding vitamin B$_6$ if you are depressed while taking it.

- Understanding what is going on during pregnancy and labour and a feeling that you have a say in what happens to you and your baby will help prevent post-natal depression. Try to choose a hospital that invervenes as little as possible, if only because it has been found that women who have forceps deliveries, Caesarean sections, and so on, have higher levels of post-natal depression than those who do not.

  Keep your baby with you all the time, day and night, right from delivery. If at all possible the baby should be exclusively breast-fed for at least six months or so. This reduces post-natal depression in you and sets your baby up for the future both psychologically and nutritionally. Food allergies (now known to be a cause of depression) are less common in breast-fed babies than in bottle-feds.

  Lastly, watch that you don't become overstretched physically and mentally. Take care of yourself and don't push yourself too hard. Learn to relax (see page 87), eat well (see page 70) and look at the list on page 79 to see how you rate in organising your life.

By no means all depression can be prevented, but with some long- and short-term planning such as this it could be a greatly reduced burden on society and on families.

DIABETES

What is it?

Diabetes is a condition in which the pancreas gland fails to produce sufficient insulin and in which the insulin that *is* produced does not have its normal effects. Because of the poor insulin supply, too much sugar remains in the bloodstream and spills over into the urine.

There are about 3.5 million diabetics in the US alone, and it is estimated that there are half as many again undiagnosed. Diabetes is a family of conditions but there are two main types. Type 1 (formerly called juvenile diabetes) can occur at any age but is more frequently seen first in children and young people. Such diabetics need insulin for the rest of their lives. Type 2 diabetes is a disease of obese middle-aged people (usually women)–it only rarely occurs in children. In this latter condition there is probably a normal amount of insulin being produced but there is not enough to go round such a large,

overweight body, and an apparent shortage occurs and produces symptoms.

Both types of the disease are seen mainly in westernised countries and are rare among peasant agriculturists and other traditional-living people. Recent theories suggest that this difference is all to do with the food the different cultures eat. By and large it appears that a diet low in fat, low in sucrose, high in unrefined starches and high in fibre protects against the disease.

Diabetes is worth preventing because it produces a considerable number of illnesses and if untreated can be fatal. Before the discovery of insulin, all sufferers who would now be called insulin-dependent diabetics died. Now such early deaths are rare, though many diabetics die younger than they should because of their complications.

The earliest symptoms of diabetes are considerable thirst, excessive urination, feeling hungry, and–in spite of the latter–weight loss. There is a generalised weakness, a tendency to get infections (especially vaginal thrush in women), boils, blurred vision, numbness, dry mouth, tingling, cramp in the legs and, later on, impotence.

The diagnosis is easily made today and treatment means that most diabetics live nearly as long as anyone else.

What causes it?

No one knows what causes Type 1 diabetes. Undoubtedly genetic, environmental and immunological factors play a part. It is currently thought that certain genetic abnormalities make particular individuals more susceptible to outside agents that affect the insulin-producing cells in the pancreas.

- Several experimental findings are not easily explained by this hypothesis, though, especially the fact that there are such different incidences of the disease in genetically very similar populations–for example, different generations in Scandinavian countries. If a population is genetically stable yet has very different variations in incidence over the years, it suggests that an environmental factor must be involved.

  All of this led a team of doctors in Denmark to look at the link between breastfeeding and childhood diabetes. They found that when breastfeeding rates were low in a population the babies subsequently went on to have more diabetes than when breastfeeding rates were high. So, breastfeeding appears to protect against childhood insulin-dependent diabetes. The peak onset of diabetes was nine years after the low-point in the breastfeeding-popularity graph and this figure coincided with the average age of onset of diabetes in Oslo children (9.3 years).

  The authors of this study propose that breast milk (already known to contain many protective factors) contains certain anti-infective agents that prevent viral infections that would otherwise affect the insulin-producing cells in certain people. Another possibility is that cows' milk formula actually changes the pancreatic cells because of the abnormal protein or chemical load it contains. Whatever is the case, it is clear that children from susceptible families would be more vulnerable if bottle-fed.

- It is current practice to give sugar water very early on–often in the nursery of the post-natal ward. I feel that this must be harmful and it is proven that such slugs of sugar (which are of no physiological value) produce surges of insulin production way beyond normal. Perhaps such overstimulation of the insulin-producing cells of the pancreas also damages them early in life. No one knows if this is so but it seems a reasonable hypothesis.

- Diet has always been seen as a major factor in the control of diabetes of both types. Since the end of the eighteenth century low-carbohydrate diets have been advised on the basis that diabetics, being low in insulin, could not handle the glucose produced by high levels of ingested carbohydrate. A study carried out in 1974 found that the majority of diabetic clinics were recommending a diet providing 40 per cent of daily calories as carbohydrates. In reality such diets usually yield only about 30 per cent of calories in this way and about 50 per cent of all the calories come from fat. There is now substantial evidence that diabetics should be advised to eat a high-fibre diet rich in unrefined, complex carbohydrates. This is an intrinsically slimming diet (if such carbohydrates form 60 per cent or more of total daily energy), which helps middle-aged Type 2 diabetics, whose treatment depends mainly on losing weight. But more excitingly research has found that insulin-dependent diabetics also prosper on the diet and that some can even come off insulin entirely. It seems likely that bulk-forming fibres smooth out the absorption of sugar from the intestine. Such a diet also alters various risk factors for heart disease (namely lipoprotein levels and blood-clotting factors), which is good news because diabetics are especially liable to suffer from heart disease. In fact heart disease is a main cause of death.

- There is no doubt that Type 2 diabetes is caused by obesity, especially in middle age.

- Chromium is a trace mineral increasingly thought to be vital in the production of diabetes, but so far the work has mostly been done on Type 2 diabetes. Early research in rats found that abnormal glucose metabolism could be corrected by adding chromium (as brewer's yeast) to the diet.

The biological significance of this trace element has only recently been recognised, but now that it has been there are signs that many people are short of it. Chromium is physiologically active in the body in only one inorganic form (the trivalent form). This inorganic (non-living) type of chromium is very inactive in the body compared with another chromium-containing compound – the organic complex called the glucose tolerance factor (GTF). It is not known exactly what this is but it appears that animals have only a limited ability to produce it themselves and so need external sources. GFT is the only known form in which chromium can cross the placenta. When trivalent chromium is given orally less than 1 per cent is absorbed.

Chromium's main function is to help insulin control the body's sugar levels. Experiments with animals have found that glucose (sugar) metabolism is quickly impaired if the animals are fed diets poor in chromium, and that giving the element soon returns the situation to normal. Because animal work has found that chromium-deficient animals develop diabetes-like symptoms, it was natural to ask whether a similar mechanism could be at fault in human diabetics. Several reports have suggested that giving chromium has had beneficial effects on diabetics and in one study four out of six maturity-onset diabetics improved with a dose of 250 micrograms of chromium a day. Other studies have found that diabetics put out more chromium in their urine than do non-diabetics. Studies of poorly-nourished children in Jordan, Turkey and Nigeria found that they grew faster when given extra chromium. In spite of this circumstantial evidence there are no definite indications that diabetes is *caused* by a deficiency of chromium, and it is certain that many diabetics will not be improved simply by taking chromium.

Unfortunately, the refining of foods removes a very substantial part of their chromium. Blackstrap molasses, honey and raw sugar are rich in chromium but white sugar has almost none. This is especially unfortunate since chromium is needed if the body is to handle sugar effectively, as we have seen. White bread contains only one third of the chromium of the original whole wheat and this, of course, goes for anything made from white flour.

The food richest in chromium is brewer's yeast but whole-grain bread, nuts, shellfish, liver, kidneys, grape juice, beef and beer are also rich sources.

As with many other trace elements, absorption is very poor, especially from tablets. Overall, only about 3 per cent of the chromium in our food is absorbed, so with our relatively chromium-deficient diet there is not much of a safety margin.

The recommended daily intake of chromium varies from 5 to 100 micrograms a day. Given that the body needs to absorb about 10 micrograms a day and that only 3 per cent is absorbed, perhaps the amount we consume should be even higher than 100 micrograms.

Prevention

- If at all possible, breastfeed from birth on demand and give no other food or drink at all until at least 4–6 months. A useful handbook on the subject is *Breast is Best* (Pan Books 1978).

- Never allow a baby to be given sugar water. It is better to give him or her the breast, or water if absolutely necessary. This will correct any low blood sugar condition naturally.

- Give a diet rich in complex, unrefined carbohydrates, low in fat and high in fibre, right from weaning off the breast.

- If you are middle-aged and overweight, and therefore at risk regarding Type 2 diabetes, eat in the way outlined above and lose weight slowly but evenly. If you already have the disease, the diet may mean that you could come off all your drugs, and will also prevent further complications of diabetes occurring.

- Take brewer's yeast daily if you

have a family history of diabetes or if you are diabetic.

- Eat foods rich in the following:
1. Vitamin A–diabetics are especially susceptible to infections and this vitamin helps fight them.
2. Vitamin B_1–increases insulin production and helps prevent diabetic nerve troubles developing.
3. Vitamin B_2–especially good for diabetics who have difficulty controlling their condition with drugs and diet.
4. Vitamin B_3–insulin-dependent diabetics have a particular need for this vitamin. It prevents swings in blood sugar in Type 1 diabetics. Vitamin B_3 is also an important part of the glucose-tolerance factor (see above).
5. Vitamin B_6–can become low in diabetics because they lose so much in their large volumes of urine. Studies have found that diabetics often have a shortage of B_6 in their blood.
6. Choline and inositol–are B-vitamins that affect fat metabolism. It has been proposed that the large, fatty liver of the diabetic is caused by the urinary loss of these vitamins. They are also useful in controlling high blood pressure and liver and gall-bladder activity, and are of great importance in diabetics.
7. Vitamin C–usually low in diabetics. The therapeutic effect of insulin is increased when this vitamin is taken, and the side-effects of several drugs (including aspirin) can be reduced by taking it. Diabetics often suffer a heavy toll of infections, and vitamin C is of proven value in combating infections. A daily dose of 1–2 g is not at all excessive, especially as this water-soluble vitamin is lost in the urine of diabetics in greater amounts than in normal people.
8. Magnesium–six out of the nine enzymes involved in sugar metabolism need magnesium, and a deficiency of magnesium is found in diabetic ketosis. There is also evidence linking diabetic eye disease to magnesium deficiency.
9. Manganese–diabetics have only half the manganese in their blood that healthy people have. This element is vital for insulin metabolism and the stabilisation of many vitamins, including vitamin C.
10. Zinc–is one of the many substances that diabetics lose in their copious urine. Zinc is added to insulin to prolong its action. As long ago as 1938 it was found that the pancreatic tissue of diabetics contained less than 50 per cent of the zinc in the tissue of healthy control subjects.

- Don't smoke. This is exceptionally harmful for diabetics because it reduces vitamin C by 25 mg per cigarette; releases adrenaline, which increases blood-sugar levels; and narrows the diabetic's already damaged arteries.

- Drink very little alcohol. Beware

of these drinks containing large amounts of sugar (Martini, brandies, liqueurs, champagne, beer and sweet wines).

- Cut down on coffee and tea. They both stimulate the adrenal glands to produce adrenaline which, in turn, raises blood sugar.

- Use sucrose alternatives such as fructose, sorbitol, manitol and xylitol.

- Eat less salt. This is especially harmful to diabetics given their particular liability to develop kidney and eye problems and high blood pressure.

DROWNING

What is it?

Drowning occurs when a person's lungs become affected by water so that he or she cannot breathe. It is often fatal. Although only a few hundred people drown each year in all western countries almost all are preventable. Three-quarters of all drownings occur in inland waters (lakes, streams, brooks and ponds), and domestic paddling pools are a real hazard. Three-quarters of those who drown are males.

Although the lives of many are saved because they can swim the ability to swim is not enough to prevent drowning. Many people who drown had no intention of going anywhere near water.

What causes it?

- Ignorance or disregard of danger. Water can be much deeper than it looks and conditions in open water cannot be compared with those in a swimming pool. Even a confident swimming-pool swimmer can find such water a surprise.

- Access to danger is a constant problem. Fences are broken, warning notices pulled down, and home pools unfenced.

- Poor supervision. Young children should never be left alone near water–they can drown in a couple of minutes and in a few inches of water.

Prevention

- Never let young children out of your sight when you are near water or deep mud.

- Empty paddling pools after use.

- Keep swimming pools fenced off and covered in the winter.

- Never leave a child alone in a bath while you go away to answer the phone, or the front door.

- Fence off garden ponds and check that a child can't get into water butts.

- Never change or remove warning notices to do with water.

- Leave life-buoys alone in their proper place–you never know when they will be needed.

- Always wear a life-jacket when boating, even if you are a strong swimmer.

- Never fool about near, or run around, swimming pools.

- Never dive into the shallow end of a pool.

- Learn to swim really well and confidently.

- Look before you jump into a pool.

- Ensure that cess-pit covers are safe from small children.

- Beware of home-made rafts and boats – they usually sink quickly and are very dangerous.

- Don't play in or around gravel-works, excavations or reservoirs.

- Keep off frozen reservoirs and lakes.

- When at the seaside find out the times of the tides and be sure you don't get trapped.

- Never swim immediately after a heavy meal.

- Don't sleep on inflatables – you could drift out to sea.

If you think someone is drowning

- Think first before you do anything or you too could end up dead.

- Reach with a stick, a scarf or anything else available. Lie down and anchor yourself to avoid being pulled in too.

- Throw a life-buoy or rope if you have one. Always throw a life-saver well in front of the person, not at them – the last thing they need is to be hit on the head.

- Wade out to help if the water is shallow enough.

- Never touch the person him- or herself – he or she could pull you under. Even very strong swimmers and life-savers have been pulled under water and put at risk by a panicky, drowning person.

- If someone is in trouble in the water either perform proper life-saving techniques, if you know how, or drag him or her to shallow water.

- If the person is having great difficulty in breathing (not simply choking, in which case he or she will probably clear his or her own airway adequately), or has stopped breathing, start mouth-to-mouth resuscitation (see below) at once, as soon as you have a foot on the bottom or can hold on to a boat, for example – don't wait until you get to dry land. Don't worry about emptying water out of the lungs – even in someone who has drowned, there is remarkably little water actually in the lungs.

- Go on with mouth-to-mouth resuscitation for an hour if the person does not revive before – drowned people can be revived after a much longer time than most people who have stopped breathing.

- When breathing re-starts, put the person into the recovery position (on their side) with a slight head-down tip.

- Get him or her to hospital as soon as possible.

Mouth-to-mouth resuscitation

How to tell if breathing has stopped
1. Put your cheek against the person's mouth and feel for breaths.
2. If breathing is not obvious, purse the person's lips and try your cheek again.
3. Look for chest movements (though these may be difficult to see because of bulky clothes).

If breathing has stopped
1. Lay the person on the ground.
2. See if there is anything in the mouth (vomit, false teeth, foreign body, etc.) that might be causing obstruction. If so, remove it and lay him or her on his or her back. Kneel on the ground on his or her left side.
3. Pull the chin upwards so that the person's neck is bent backwards. With your left hand pulling the chin up, push the top of the head down with your right. This simple procedure opens the airway at the back of the throat and may re-start breathing. If it does, put the person into the *recovery position* and stay with him or her.

If breathing does not re-start at once
Start artificial respiration while someone else gets a doctor or an ambu-lance. The best method by far of re-starting breathing is the 'kiss of life' (mouth-to-mouth resuscitation).
1. Put the person on his or her back.
2. Tilt head back as far as possible (nostrils then point directly upwards at you), using both hands together.
3. Cup one hand under the chin.
4. Put the heel of the other hand on his or her forehead so that the fingers of that hand can pinch the nose.
5. Pinch the nose shut.
6. Make sure the mouth is open.
7. Take a full breath yourself.
8. Apply your mouth to the person's, ensuring that there is a good seal all round.
9. Breathe into the open mouth firmly and slowly – don't puff out hard. As you do this, the person's chest will rise.
10. Take your mouth away, breathe in fully while the air escapes from the person and repeat the procedure.
11. While you are taking a breath in, the person will breathe out spontaneously.
12. Repeat the breathing into his or her mouth and watch for spontaneous re-starting of breathing as you turn your head away to breathe in yourself.
13. Try to 'blow' a breath into the victim about every six seconds. Be guided by common sense on this. For example, the first few breaths can be given much more quickly to get some oxygen into the individual.
14. Stop when the person shows clear signs of re-starting to breathe, but even then keep a close eye on his or her chest movements until professional help arrives.

Some useful hints

1.   Don't blow too hard as this may send air into the stomach and make the person vomit, which is dangerous for him or her and unpleasant for you.

2.   Should vomiting occur, turn the person's head to one side and let the vomit dribble out of the mouth. Clean out the mouth and carry on with resuscitation.

3.   If a child is the victim, seal your lips over both nose and mouth after positioning the head as before. *Only blow gently.* Be guided by what produces a rise and fall of the chest wall. In babies, use only the amount of air you can hold in your cheeks – *don't blow from your lungs.*

4.   If the abdomen starts to swell up, you will know you are blowing air down the gullet into the stomach instead of down the windpipe. Stop resuscitation for a moment, turn the child to one side and press firmly over the swollen stomach. This will probably force the air out.

5.   Check that the person's heartbeat has not stopped by feeling in the neck beside the Adam's apple for the carotid pulse from time to time.

How long to continue
Either:
Until the person starts to breathe easily again. Never try breathing into someone who is already breathing spontaneously. It can be helpful, though, to give the odd helping breath if he or she is gasping or breathing irregularly.
Or:
Until professional help arrives. This may take time, so get others to help you. Keep going until a doctor says the person is dead. Don't give up too readily, especially in cases of drowning. People have been revived after an hour of resuscitation. Once breathing re-starts try not to let the victim die of hypothermia. Remove wet clothing, and wrap him or her in blankets or a sleeping bag. Never give alcohol (which will increase heat loss).

DRUG ABUSE

What is it?

A condition in which an individual, often a youngster, takes drugs of addiction which he or she then cannot do without.

'Drugs' can include all sorts of substances – from prescribed medications to alcohol, cigarettes and glue – but here we will talk about the drugs that are used illegally. This includes LSD, heroin, cocaine, amphetamines, barbiturates and cannabis.

Drug-taking starts young, often in the teens. Most youngsters start on drugs in much the same way as they start to smoke – to keep in with their friends. Some like the risks involved and others probably do it as part of their general adolescent rebellion against their parents. Others take drugs because they are depressed, unhappy at home, bored, don't like school, and so on. Sometimes starting on drugs is a cry for help or attention from parents who seem to have no time or inclination to care.

It is not easy to tell whether or not your child is taking drugs but here are a few signs that might help. Remember that just because a youngster shows any or even most of these signs it does not necessarily mean that he or she is taking drugs.

- Sudden mood changes.

- Irritability or aggression.

- Poor appetite.

- No interests in hobbies, friends or school.

- Drowsiness and sleepiness.

- Telling lies.

- Shifty and furtive behaviour.

- Unusual smells, stains or marks on the body or clothes.

- The disappearance of money or belongings from around the home (to pay for the drugs).

None of these things is particularly hazardous, of course, but drug abuse can lead to three which are. First, accidental overdose is an ever present problem with any form of drug addiction, and can lead to unconsciousness and even death. Many users of illegal drugs mix them and this can render the dosage totally unpredictable. Drug overdose is now a major cause of death in the under 25s in New York State and there are signs that things are going the same way in the UK.

The second hazard of drug abuse is the increased risk of accident. Accidents of all kinds are more com-

mon in those taking illegal drugs. Some, such as road accidents, can easily be fatal to the drug-taker or to an innocent party.

Finally, addiction or dependence is the most worrying problem for parents because they see their child trapped in a habit that is extremely difficult to get out of.

On a day-to-day basis drugs can make the youngster confused and have hallucinations, and can cause serious emotional and psychological disturbances. First-time heroin users may be sick, and regular users become constipated. Girls stop having periods. Eventually more serious emotional and physical disorders set in.

The injection of drugs can cause hepatitis (a potentially lethal infection of the liver), sores, abscesses, blood poisoning and jaundice.

The social consequences are equally horrifying as the individual becomes desperate for the next fix and steals and resorts to all kinds of other crimes to fund the habit.

Prevention

Prevention is more difficult than for most of the subjects covered in this book because so often the drugtaking adolescent has become involved as a result of a complex mixture of personality, social and parental factors. Many of these are deeply rooted in the past, even in the pasts of the parents, and most of the problems are inaccessible to all but the most skilled professional. There are, however, a few preventives that are worth trying:

- Discuss between you as parents what your views on drugs are. Sort out what you both feel so that should a problem arise you will deal with it more sensibly and compassionately and won't make it worse by panicking.

- Give up smoking and drinking yourselves. Research shows that a youngster whose parents are addicted to legal drugs is much more likely to use *illegal* ones. This also goes for medications from your doctor. Keep all medicines out of the reach of children and youngsters.

- Make time to create a relationship with your children, from very early on. Give them confidence in the future and show that you care. If they feel that they can turn to you when things get tough you will have done the very best for them. The alternative is that they turn elsewhere and that could involve drugs. Youngsters who can trust their parents and like them as human beings will also be less likely to turn to drugs.

- Try, when discussing the subject with your children, to steer a course (however difficult it is) between making drug-taking seem acceptable and creating a 'no-go' area. When talking about drugs it is best not to talk about it in too dramatic or horror-inspiring terms because if the child knows people who take drugs and enjoy them they simply will not believe you. This will reduce your credibility all round which will be a loss. This is somewhat parallel to scare stories about VD when discussing sex with youngsters.

- Don't be suspicious of your children, because if they are not taking drugs this could drive them to do so.

- Calmly tell your youngsters of the legal problems with drugs. Possession of heroin, cocaine and LSD can lead to prison sentences of up to seven years and trafficking in drugs can put someone in gaol for up to fourteen years. Even possessing fairly 'harmless' drugs such as cannabis, amphetamines and barbiturates can result in a five-year sentence.

- There is no guarantee that any of these preventive measures will in fact stop a youngster from taking drugs–the only sure preventive is a loving, caring, non-judgemental family in which the parents treat their youngsters with respect. This is a way of behaving that cannot just be started in the child's early teens when you think you might begin having problems with sex and drugs– this is almost certainly too late. Preparation for this kind of relationship starts in the cradle with prolonged breastfeeding whenever the baby or mother wants to feed. The closeness this kind of behaviour produces is a sure foundation for good parent-child relationships and is likely to help the children withstand the certain knocks that life will bring.

DYSENTERY

What is it?

Dysentery is the name given to a serious infectious illness affecting the bowels. It occurs all over the world and used to be a major killer in western countries. Swallowed germs breed in the bowel and produce vomiting, diarrhoea and pain. Tell your doctor at once if anyone in your household has an illness like this. He or she will tell the local health authorities who are responsible for halting the spread of such highly infectious illnesses.

Prevention

If you are to ensure that dysentery does not spread outside your house you will have to take the following preventive action:

- Wash your hands well with soap under running water before preparing food or drink, before handling a baby, and before leaving the house. Also, you should wash your hands thoroughly after using the lavatory, after doing anything to the person with dysentery; after changing the baby's nappy, and after washing clothes or bedding.

- Don't use towels – use paper tissues. Wash children's hands for them.

- Serve food fresh and always keep uneaten food in the fridge. Don't have visitors into the house until the infection is cleared up. Keep pets' food separately from yours.

- Don't send the infected person's washing to the laundry or launderette. Put it in a plastic bin liner or bag separately. Set the washing machine to hot, or boil the bedding and clothes. Use a disinfectant if you are not able to wash this thoroughly.

- Clean the toilet thoroughly using rubber gloves kept in the toilet for this purpose. After each use the door handle, the flush handle, the seat and if need be the floor must be cleaned (in this order). If you use a lavatory brush do so with scouring powder and flush the water away at once. Always wash your hands on leaving the lavatory.

ECZEMA

What is it?

Eczema is an itchy dermatitis that is usually allergic in origin and occurs in families. It usually starts with patches of dry, itchy skin which in babies and young children (the commonest sufferers of the condition) are behind the ears and knees, in the body creases at the elbows and the neck, on the face and on the trunk or scalp. When the eczema is bad the skin is red, raw, weeping and crusted and may become infected.

Eczema is not infectious and most babies grow out of their infantile eczema. For a few, though, allergic eczema can persist throughout life. About three children in a hundred suffer from it and many of these have a family history of eczema, asthma, hay fever or other allergies.

What causes it?

- There is no doubt that there is a familial susceptibility.

- As ezcema is much more common in bottle-fed as opposed to breast-fed babies there is little doubt that an allergy to cows' milk plays a part in many children. Some children are allergic to other foods too.

- Scratching makes it worse, so it is best to avoid wool and nylon next to the skin because these make the skin hot and sweaty.

- Feathers, down and wool bedding make it worse.

Prevention

- The single greatest preventive measure is undoubtedly to breastfeed a baby right from the very start and not to give him or her even *one* bottle of cows' milk. This will need very careful super-

vision because it is still the practice in many maternity hospitals to take babies away from their mothers at night and to feed them the odd bottle of cows' milk formula.

- The way round this is to talk to your family doctor and midwife before the baby is due to ensure that everyone knows that you have a baby that is 'at risk' and is to be totally breast-fed from birth. If eventually you find breastfeeding impossible (which is rare with good advice) then you will have to use a soya-based milk. There are several on the market.

Aim to feed your baby breast milk exclusively for at least four months and preferably longer. The protective effect is greater the longer you continue but after about six months you should add in other (non milk-containing) foods.

Unfortunately, even this way of feeding a baby may not prevent all eczema. This comes about for two reasons. First, the child may be allergic to some other allergen, such as the house-dust mite; and second, antigens in the mother's diet may be transmitted to the baby via her milk. Recent research suggests that eating large quantities of certain allergens during pregnancy can sensitise a susceptible child *in utero* . The answer here is to take all foods in moderation during pregnancy, especially foods that are likely to induce allergies in children. These include cows' milk and all its products, eggs, wheat, nuts, fish, tomatoes and colourings and preservatives. If you have a family history of allergy, and especially of eczema, it makes sense to avoid these foods as much as possible during pregnancy and breastfeeding, or at least certainly never to binge on them. Don't worry about the calcium you will be missing–it can be eaten in other forms, and you can take zinc and calcium supplements (Sandocal effervescent tablets are good) which more than compensate for the calcium loss in dairy products. Start weaning your solely breast-fed baby at about 5-6 months and be sure to breastfeed after each meal until the end of the first year of life. Introduce vegetables and fruit first of all and then add milk-free margarine. Over a few weeks add in foods that are 'safe' (not on the above list of common culprits) and see how it goes. If ever a food seems to precipitate eczema stop giving it and don't try it again until the child is 2. If a child is allergic to eggs he or she might also be allergic to chicken, so beware.

- Having done your best to prevent eczema at source dress your child with soft cotton next to the skin – never wool or nylon. These latter will make him or her hot and sweaty, which makes any early eczema likely to progress further than it otherwise would. Choose loose clothing styles that keep the child neither too hot nor too cold.

- Disposable nappies may irritate – use soft terry nappies. Change nappies frequently and clean the child's bottom well. Avoid plastic pants if there is any sign of nappy rash. Never wash nappies in biological detergents because very allergic babies are allergic to the enzymes in them. Drying clothes out of doors helps destroy house-dust mites and bacteria. Avoid feather, down and wool bedding because these can irritate eczema. Use duvets filled with synthetic filler and cotton cellular blankets and cotton sheets. Change bedding twice a week at least, and damp-dust and vacuum the child's room daily.

- Join a self-help group to help you cope with the day-to-day problems and prevent family discord. Having a baby or child with severe eczema can be exhausting for all the family and you will be grateful for tips on how to cope.

EPISIOTOMY

What is it?

A cut made surgically during the later stages of labour to enlarge the birth canal and so let the baby out more easily.

There are few subjects that cause so much concern to women having babies–many episiotomies are done uncaringly and the after-effects on the woman and her sex life can be far greater than is often realised by the medical and midwifery professions.

Episiotomies are very commonly performed–in some units in the US about 90 per cent of women have one, especially for a first birth. There is evidence that they are slowly being used less.

Clearly there *are* medical and obstetric reasons why an episiotomy should be done but a book such as this is no place to discuss these. Usually, though, the reason the procedure is performed is that the doctors or midwives are inexperienced in delivering women without doing one and because with modern birthing positions many women are in labour in a position that makes an episiotomy more likely. Women who labour and give birth in an upright position do not have prolonged labours and rarely need an episiotomy at all because in such positions the pelvic tissues stretch slowly and evenly.

Why are they done?

- Habit–most modern midwives and obstetricians see an episiotomy as 'normal' and so continue to perform them.

- Impatience–many hospitals set a time limit on the length of the second stage of labour, and if the baby has not arrived by this time (usually about 1½ hours) an episiotomy is ordered to get the baby out.

- Because women who labour on their backs *are* actually in danger of having prolonged second stages of labour. The answer is to labour and give birth upright.

- Many obstetricians and midwives believe that tears that occur naturally as the baby is born are more difficult to repair than cuts made surgically. There is no truth in this.

- Most midwives have lost the art of 'guarding' the woman's perineum to control the emergence of the baby's head to prevent the vaginal opening from being stretched too wide, too fast–an age-old midwifery technique that worked. Many medical and paramedical people actually believe that a woman's vaginal opening is too small and so needs surgical help during birth. Such people argue (quite without factual evidence) that a woman who has a birth without an episiotomy goes on to have a flabby vagina that is unpleasurable to her partner and that she will eventually have more gynaecological problems, such as uterine prolapse.

Prevention

As with so many things about birth, prevention is better than cure–so how can you ensure that you have the least possible chance of having to have an episiotomy?

- Decide well in advance that you will not have an episiotomy except for one of the very specific medical reasons that you have been able to discuss well ahead of time at an ante-natal visit, or if your experienced midwife is fairly certain that you will have a bad tear if you do not have one. Get the staff to write it in on your notes, and ensure that your husband or partner understands your feelings precisely. Then it will be understood that the midwife or obstetrician will have to justify the episiotomy to you before doing it. This should dramatically reduce the likelihood that you will have one as a matter of routine. Of course, ideally you should choose a unit where episiotomies are done rarely and only for good medical reasons, but such units are rare.

- Practise pelvic-floor muscle and perineal stretching exercises (see below) during pregnancy.

- If you arrange in advance to labour in an upright position of some kind, and to keep changing position as you feel best, it will probably reduce the likelihood of your needing an episiotomy.

- If you do end up on your back because it is deemed obstetrically necessary, ask the midwives to hold your legs so that your knees are only a foot or so apart, not widely apart as in lithotomy stirrups. This will reduce the stretching of the perineal tissues and so reduce the likelihood that an episiotomy will need to be done.

- It is worth learning *perineal massage* , even from quite early on in

pregnancy. In this the woman lies flat on her back on the floor or on a bed with the soles of her feet flat together. Her husband or partner then uses his fingers, well lubricated with vegetable oil or baby oil, to massage the whole of the lower vulva and the area between the vagina and the anus. It is this area that stretches so much during the birth of the baby, and a supple, relaxed perineum is far less likely to tear or to need an episiotomy than is an unprepared one. This form of massage can easily develop into sexual foreplay as the man inserts his fingers into the vagina until, towards the end of pregnancy, the woman will be able to take four fingers quite easily. Don't forget that from quite early on in pregnancy a woman's vagina becomes more relaxed and will, by twelve or fourteen weeks, be able to take two or three fingers easily. Using sweeping movements around the lower vagina, the man can often feel the deep pelvic muscles relaxing as pregnancy progresses, and the woman will learn to relax her perineum and sense the stretching of her perineal tissues in a controlled, loving setting before the real thing takes place in the labour ward.

The idea early on is to stretch the woman's vulval opening to the point where she complains of tingling or pins and needles, or simply says it's enough. The man then holds his fingers in this position for some time until the stretching sensation passes. Over subsequent sessions the couple can gradually increase the amount of vaginal stretching until the woman can easily take four fingers. Any woman who has had this kind of perineal preparation is unlikely to need an episiotomy, especially if she gives birth in an upright position. When it comes to experiencing the strange bursting sensations as the baby's head stretches her vulva during the last stage of labour she will not be alarmed or think she is going to burst open (as many unprepared women fear) because she will have experienced similar (though less intense) sensations.

Some American midwives use perineal massage as the baby's head comes down the birth canal, massaging the tight, whitened and thinned areas of the vaginal opening with oil as the baby's head emerges. They also massage the pelvic muscles to relax them via the vaginal walls. Such midwives rarely use episiotomies however big the baby.

- It can also be a useful preparation for the birth to master *pelvic exercises*, and they can be of considerable value after the birth of the baby too, to both you and your partner. Here are three ways of exercising your deep pelvic muscles. Do any or all of them, several times a day, perhaps while driving the car or watching TV.

Start off by sitting on the lava-tory and, while passing urine, stop in mid-flow. Start and stop; learn to control the stream at will. The muscles you are using are the deep pelvic ones that you will need to be aware of, both during the birth and afterwards when you are getting back to normal. Once you have conquered this to your satisfaction, start on the exercises proper.

1. Tighten and relax your pelvic muscles, holding them in a tightly contracted position for several seconds, then relaxing them. Try to increase the length of time you can hold the muscles contracted.
2. Tighten and relax the muscles quickly, in a sort of fluttering way, gradually increasing your control.
3. Pull up your entire pelvic area as if your vagina were a pump drawing up water, then force the 'water' out of the 'pump'. This exercise uses some abdominal as well as pelvic muscles.

If you put a finger or two inside your vagina (or get your partner to do so) you can gauge how well you are progressing with your muscle control. Early on it may well feel flabby and rather weak, but after a few weeks the muscles will be so powerful that they will feel as if they could squeeze your fingers off.

These exercises are also very useful post-natally to get your pelvic muscles back to strength after being stretched by the baby coming down the birth canal.

FAINTING

What is it?

A condition in which a person has a reduced blood flow to the brain, causing him or her to feel faint, weak and eventually even to lose consciousness. On falling to the floor the person becomes horizontal and the blood flow to the brain is restored. Sometimes people who feel they are about to faint feel giddy, sweat a lot and have a fast heartbeat. When a person faints they look pale, breathe rapidly and have a feeble pulse. After a few minutes consciousness usually returns.

What causes it?

- An emotional upset.

- Sickening for an acute infection.

- An overheated, ill-ventilated room.

- Prolonged standing, especially on an empty stomach.

- Severe pain.

- Pregnancy.

- Severe anaemia.

- Severe bleeding.

- Adolescence (notably in girls).

- A minor epileptic attack can be mistaken for a faint.

Prevention

The prevention of most of the above is fairly obvious and needs no elaboration. However, if you feel faint or likely to faint here are a few simple preventive hints.

- Always have breakfast if you know you are going to have to stand up for any length of time.

- Ensure that your environment does not become too hot and stuffy.

- As soon as you feel at all like fainting sit down, loosen your tie, belt or any other constricting clothing; get someone to open a window or to take you to an open window or outside the stuffy room. If you feel worse, lie down flat. Within a few minutes you should feel normal again. Look for the cause of the faint and take steps to prevent similar occurrences.

FITS (Convulsions)

What are they?

Sudden spasms of the muscles caused by an abnormal burst of activity in the brain. Convulsions are common in babies and young children. Epilepsy, which causes one kind of fit, is relatively rare, so you should not jump to the conclusion that your child's fit is epileptic in origin.

What causes them?

- The most common cause of fits

(in children) by far is a raised temperature. These so-called febrile convulsions occur most often between the age of 6 months and 3 years old. They are rare after the age of 5 years.

The most usual causes of such high fevers are tonsillitis, acute ear infections, urinary infections and measles. There is often a family history of febrile convulsions during infancy.

- Epilepsy. This is a condition in which a person has repeated losses of consciousness. There are more than 100 causes for such attacks but for the vast majority of people with epilepsy there is no known, provable cause as such. Epilepsy starts at any age but usually during infancy. Most epileptic children are normal mentally and physically when the attacks start and most lead happy and normal lives with the help of drugs.
Epilepsy can be triggered by late nights, too much alcohol, a high fever, flashing lights, and many other things. It can now be controlled in the vast majority of both adults and children.

- Hypoglycaemia (see page 248).

- Infections of the brain such as encephalitis, rabies and tetanus.

- Shortage of vitamin B_6 in children.

- Brain tumours.

- Certain poisons and intoxica-

tions, including lead, arsenic and alcohol poisoning.

- Head injuries.

- Hysteria. Some hysterical people (usually women) have convulsions but only in front of an audience – they never occur when they are alone.

Prevention

The preventive measures that can be taken against the above causes are obvious and some, such as hysteria, cannot be prevented. The two main causes of convulsions – fevers in children and certain precipitating factors in epilepsy – can, however, be prevented.

- If a child has a high fever the parent is in a difficult dilemma because there is no doubt that the fever is valuable in killing the bacteria or virus that caused it in the first place. It used to be thought that fevers should be lowered by using aspirin or similar drugs but this is now disputed. A substance called endogenous pyrogen produced during fevers enhances the body's immunity to disease. Once this pyrogen is produced it circulates in the blood to the brain and stimulates the body's thermostat to produce substances called prostaglandins which set the body's temperature to normal. Endogenous pyrogen increases the mobility of white blood cells and stimulates the production of proteins to fight infection. Antibiotics, it appears, also work better at high temperatures.

However, high fevers have damaging effects too, especially over about 104° or 105°F. The secret then is to start lowering the child's temperature before it gets this high – say at 102°, or earlier if the baby or child is irritable. Take all the clothes off the child and lay him or her on a waterproof sheet on the bed. Cool his or her face, trunk and limbs with tepid (just warm) water so as to make the surface blood vessels dilate and lose heat. Cold water makes them contract and conserves heat. Wrap cloths soaked in tepid water around the child's groin and neck, and check his or her temperature every 10 minutes until it is normal. Don't give aspirin unless the fever is very high (over 103°F/39.4°C). Give the child plenty of drinks (preferably water or dilute fruit juice).

The above procedure will prevent the vast majority of feverish fits. If ever your child has a fit, don't panic but do tell the doctor.

● Prevention of epileptic fits is far more difficult because the cause is rarely found. If you find that tiredness, alcohol, flashing lights or TV bring them on, you will have to avoid these things. You can avoid the TV problem by watching in a light room and not going near the set to switch it off or to adjust it. Most photosensitive people can overcome their problem by covering one eye with the palm of their hand. The effects of flashing lights on water can be reduced by wearing polarised spectacles. Sometimes psychological treatments can prevent attacks. The majority of preventive measures for true epilepsy centre around adequate drug control.

FLUID RETENTION

What is it?

The accumulation of tissue fluid in the body. It is most noticeable in the fingers (rings become tight), around the eyes (eyelids look and feel puffy), and in the abdomen (belts become tight). It is a condition that affects millions of women, often around their period times.

About 60 per cent of the body's weight is water, which is distributed in the various fluids inside and outside the cells. The average person takes in about 2–3 quarts of fluid a day and the body's balancing mechanisms ensure that the loss through urine, sweat and on the breath keep the total body water steady. A healthy person can handle at least 8 quarts of fluid a day without retaining any but people with heart disease, liver disease, kidney disease and certain hormonal problems retain fluid abnormally. Water is retained in places that offer least resistance, particularly around the eyes or where gravity exerts its main influence (such as around the feet and ankles). If, when you poke your fingertip into a swollen ankle it leaves a depression, you have about 8–9 lb of water too much in your body overall.

Immediately before a period many women, because of their hormonal changes, retain water–sometimes putting on up to a stone in weight. This produces swollen, tender breasts, pelvic pain, headaches, stomach swelling, nervousness, irritability, a feeling of mental dullness, insomnia and poor concentration. Even the eyeballs can swell and make the wearing of contact lenses impossible. During pregnancy ankle swelling is also common.

What causes it?

- Hormone changes in the premenstrual phase of a woman's cycle.

- Long periods of standing and walking can cause foot and ankle swelling.

- Pregnancy causes ankle swelling as a result of the pressure of the heavy uterus on the pelvic veins, which reduces their ability to collect fluid from the legs.

- Heart disease (especially heart failure, in which the reduced pumping efficiency of the heart means a smaller blood flow to the kidneys to produce urine).

- Steroid hormones (which cause salt to be retained by the body along with water to dissolve it in). This includes the contraceptive Pill, of course.

- Kidney diseases in which the capability of the kidney to put out normal amounts of urine is impaired.

- Certain allergies cause local fluid retention. This is especially seen in urticaria (hives). The swelling may be generalised, or may affect only the hands, feet and face.

- Too much sodium in the diet. Water always goes hand in hand with sodium so if you eat too much sodium (salt) you will automatically retain too much water.

- Stress and emotional conditions can cause (in men as well as women) too high a production of anti-diuretic hormone which causes the retention of water.

- Very hot weather, especially if humid too, can make some people retain water.

Prevention

- Wear elastic stockings if your legs swell.

- Do the same in pregnancy and in both cases use every opportunity to take the weight off your feet. This greatly helps reduce the swelling.

- Come off the Pill and use another method of contraception.

- Prevent allergies by eliminating foods and other allergens from your diet and surroundings.

- Take vitamin B$_6$. This seems to affect the balance between oestrogen and sodium. Taking 200 mg a day premenstrually has been shown to prevent fluid retention. B$_6$ is especially good in pregnancy. Never take more than 200 mg a day.

- Take vitamin C–it seems to enhance the action of vitamin B$_6$. It also has a diuretic effect of its own.

- Drink more water–an additional 4–6 glasses a day on top of what you currently drink. This increases the excretion efficiency of the kidneys.

- Take less salt. Some people are exceptionally sensitive to salt and as little as 1 g can produce swelling in them. One large pickled cucumber, for example, contains 2 g salt.

- Eat only complex carbohydrates (as found in fruit, vegetables and whole grains)–no refined ones. Sugar is a major culprit when it comes to water retention, and we consume quantities of sugar without being aware of its presence. Look for anything with the suffix 'ose' on the label (fruct*ose*, lact*ose*, dextr*ose*, malt*ose* etc) and avoid it.

- Include in your diet natural diuretics, such as pineapple, cucumber, parsley, alfalfa, strawberries, apples, grapes, beetroot and camomile tea.

- Ensure that you eat plenty of calcium-containing foods, especially if your fluid retention is a part of your pregnancy symptoms, as there is a link between the amount of calcium in the diet and fluid retention during pregnancy.

- Take more exercise. Any exercise that improves the tone of blood vessels will help.

- Try to lie down flat at least once a day for twenty minutes or so, as urine production is increased in the horizontal position.

FOOD ALLERGIES

What are they?

Food allergies, like other allergies, occur when the body's immune system produces an exaggerated response to a particular substance. In this case the culprit is a food or foods. Food allergy is a physiological response of the body that occurs even if the person is fed the offending food in a disguised form. In other words it is not a form of food avoidance by someone who simply does not like a particular food. Food allergy causes a variety of very tangible physical reactions including some serious ones, such as asthma–in which an allergen affects the lungs and produces illness.

Food allergy is much more common than is generally supposed, and studies have found that anything from 1 to 20 per cent of children show signs of food allergy at some time or another. One study found that tartrazine, a very commonly used food dye, produced positive skin reactions (indicating that the individual was allergic to it) in up to 46 per cent of those tested. Out of every 10 million people 40,000 will be intolerant of aspirin, for example, and a sensitivity to aspirin seems to be linked to a sensitivity to certain foods.

When an individual develops an immediate swelling of the lips, tingling in the mouth or throat, vomiting or abdominal pain, after consuming a certain food, it is not difficult to link the food to the symptoms. The connection can be fairly easily established even if the symptoms such as diarrhoea, constipation, bloating of the abdomen or fatty stools, are apparent only after some hours. The problem is that many food allergic people develop problems such as asthma, hay-fever symptoms or eczema perhaps only some days after eating the offending food. This can make tracking down the culprit very difficult indeed.

Food allergies are very much more common in children than in adults, and can produce colic, vomiting, hyperactivity, epilepsy, migraine, altered moods, poor growth, diarrhoea, nappy rash, generalised rashes and respiratory infections. Many paediatricians feel that food allergy is grossly under-diagnosed. A sensitivity to foods is commonest in children who come from families who have a history of allergy, probably involving asthma, eczema or hay fever. On testing, some such children are found to be allergic to many foods (often up to twenty).

What causes them?

No one knows why certain people overreact to certain foreign proteins or chemicals that they eat, just as it is not known why some people get hay fever when exposed to pollens and others do not.

- Undoubtedly there is a familial tendency to be allergic. Though people can't choose their parents, there are preventive measures families can take to lessen the chances that a new member of the family will inherit the problem.

- Some foods, including wine, yeast extracts, avocado, bananas, cheese and chocolate, contain substances called vasoactive amines. These substances release adrenaline and noradrenaline from nerve endings. Many, children especially, have immediate sensitivity reactions to such foods as soon as they eat them.

- During storage and handling some foods become infected with fungi and mites, and during storage a number of foods become rich in histamine – a substance known to produce allergic effects.

- The commonest foods to cause allergy and intolerance are: cows' milk; fish and shellfish; wheat, cereals and flour; yeast; chocolate; nuts; pork, bacon and tenderised meat; tea and coffee; preservatives and artificial colours. Almost any food *can* cause problems in a sensitive individual but these are the typical culprits. Often a highly allergic child will have problems with many of them.

Prevention

- There has been considerable debate as to whether the tendency to be allergic to things (atopy) can be prevented. It is certain that atopy runs in families – or at least that the predisposition to atopy does. By no means all children of atopic parents will be allergic to anything, let alone to foods, but they stand a higher chance of being so.

  One way to prevent a child from becoming allergic, when one or both of the parents has a history of allergy, is to ensure that the mother is very careful about what she eats. It has been found that babies can be sensitised *in utero* if the mother eats large amounts of particular foods. It is probably not wise to avoid certain foods totally (unless they make the mother actually ill, of course) – the most important thing is not to binge on a particular food at any stage of pregnancy.

- Breastfeeding totally and exclusively seems to have some protective effect against allergies generally, and recent work suggests that even one bottle of cows' milk formula can sensitise the highly susceptible baby to other allergies. It seems to 'turn up' the sensitivity of his or her immune system so that it subsequently overreacts to many things. It certainly makes sense, given current evidence, to breastfeed exclusively for at least 4–5 months, during which time the baby's own immune system can mature sufficiently to be able to cope with allergens he or she meets later in life. Having said this, allergies *do* occur, though much less commonly, in totally breast-fed infants. This can come about because the mother eats large amounts of a particular food, microscopic particles of which get through into her milk and so to the baby. The lesson here is to be sure not to eat large amounts of any one food, especially of those listed above.

- Preventing problems once a child has a food allergy can usually only be achieved by eliminating the offending food or foods from the child's diet. Discovering what the offending substance is may involve putting the child on a very simple diet of a single vegetable, a single meat (lamb, for example) and water. If the symptoms have disappeared after a week on this type of diet, one food at a time can be added into the diet, with a careful watch being kept for any symptoms of the allergy. A new food is added every 1 or 2 days, until the one that produces the trouble is found. This substance is then totally avoided until the child is much older. Continue to add in foods one at a time even after you have found one that causes an allergic reaction because you will probably find more problem foods as you go along.

All this is very tedious and takes a lot of time and patience. It also needs great care early on so that the child does not become malnourished from eating such a restricted diet. When the child is eating only a vegetable or two and a single type of meat and water it makes sense to give a vitamin and mineral supplement as well. As the items are added back the diet approaches normal and the danger of malnutrition disappears. Don't forget as you add back foods only to add those the child would normally eat–not strange ones. This is all rather less trouble than it at first seems because children, especially very young ones, eat only a limited range of foods.

- If at any stage your child becomes ill or loses weight, see your doctor to have him or her referred to a specialist who can supervise such an elimination diet with the child in hospital. Also, when adding foods back in go gently, especially when it comes to eggs and nuts. Some children are so highly sensitive to these that they become really ill and need medical help. Common sense is the key. Do everything gently and slowly

and you could well end up curing your child of troublesome symptoms that have previously defied diagnosis.

- Avoid 'junk' or processed foods.

- Ensure that your diet is still substantially adequate even when you have cut out the offending food.

- Stop smoking–smoking stresses the body's ability to cope with allergies. Stopping will make you better able to cope with foods to which you are borderline allergic.

- Come off the contraceptive pill. A few women start to have food allergies when they go on the Pill.

- Take a general nutritional supplement of vitamins and minerals (see page 73). Once again this helps the body to combat the stresses of the allergy. Try such a supplement for at least three months before deciding whether or not it is doing you any good.

- Take measures to reduce the level of stress in your life (see page 87).

FOOD POISONING

What is it?

Food poisoning is a loose term applied to any disease carried by food. Sometimes it is caused by the presence of disease-producing bacteria and sometimes by the toxins they produce.

The potential for food-borne disease has never been greater, if only because we all rely so much on massive, centralised food production, processing and distribution. Any contamination along the chain could involve hundreds or even thousands of individuals, whereas food contaminated in the home affects only the members of the household.

Although we all assume food to be safe it does not take much to make it unsafe and then for it to cause disease. The commonest food poisoning organisms are salmonella, staphylococcus, viruses such as hepatitis, and tapeworms. Of course, food can also be contaminated by chemicals and poisons but these are less common.

Most people who eat contaminated or infected food will simply become ill with diarrhoea and vomiting but a small proportion become seriously ill and even die. Food poisoning causes large numbers of deaths around the world and thousands a year even in sophisticated westernised countries.

What causes it?

- Poor personal hygiene.

- Sloppiness in the kitchen and other food preparation areas.

- Faulty storage of food.

Prevention

- The prevention of food poisoning starts with good personal hygiene. Before doing anything with food wash your hands thoroughly with soap and water. Wash your hands after going to the lavatory, using a nailbrush to scrub both hands and nails thoroughly. Never wash your hands in a sink used for food preparation. Make sure your overall or apron is clean. Keep your fingernails short and clean. If you work in a commercial food-preparation area wear a hat or hair net if you have lots of hair.

  Never comb your hair in the kitchen; don't pick your nose and handle food; don't smoke while preparing food; and don't cough or spit over food.

  If ever you cut or burn yourself make sure the wound is covered at once and then kept covered with a waterproof dressing or a plastic finger-stall.

  If you are personally ill, and especially if you have any diarrhoeal illness, don't prepare food for others. This is especially important if you work with food that is eaten by the general public.

- Don't handle food more than you absolutely have to. Never dip your fingers into things to taste them. Keep all the utensils and the surfaces you use really clean. Wipe up spills as soon as they occur because germs breed quickly in a warm kitchen. Keep scraps in bins with lids so that flies can't get to them and germs can't get out.

  Use really hot water for washing up. Use a detergent for greasy things and then be sure to rinse off the bubbles thoroughly. Using properly hot water also means that things will dry quickly which is more hygienic.

- Once you have cooked food allow it to cool and then always keep it in a refrigerator. Be sure especially never to leave meat out in the open – it is a breeding ground for germs. Never store cooked meat alongside raw meat in the fridge. If this is unavoidable ensure that the cooked meat is totally covered. By and large try to cook only as much food as you will eat at that meal unless you are pre-cooking deliberately to freeze some for later. Subsequent reheating of most foods, especially meats, needs to be as thorough as the first cooking.

Poultry is a potent source of food poisoning. Always thaw frozen birds properly before cooking. A large turkey can take forty-eight hours to thaw out completely. Egg products, including custards, artificial creams, fillings and trifles, are especially prone to bacterial growths, so be especially careful with these. Ice cream should be used at once and if there is too much for one meal put the rest back in the freezer immediately. Ice cream that has gone liquid and been refrozen is a dangerous source of food poisoning.

Store food in a refrigerator or chiller cabinet to keep flies off it during the warm months. Empty dustbins regularly and keep them clean so that they don't breed maggots and flies. Keep hot foods hot and cold foods cold!

GALL-STONES

What are they?

Bile is a fluid produced by the liver and stored in the gall-bladder ready to be squirted into the duodenum (the first part of the intestine) to aid the digestion of fats. After a meal, unused bile is stored in the gall-bladder for some time.

Gall-stones arise when the cholesterol in bile starts to crystallise out. The stones slowly increase in size until eventually they are so large that they can't escape with the bile into the intestine. They then start to cause infections in the gall-bladder and other symptoms. Most gall-stones are made of cholesterol.

Gall-stones appear to be a disease of western culture and are seen only rarely in traditional-living peoples around the world.

What causes them?

We still don't know the exact answer to this question but modern research is getting very close to the heart of the matter.

Under normal circumstances nature's own bile acid, chenodeoxycholic acid, dissolves any stones formed in this way, and synthetic versions of this natural chemical are now used to dissolve gall-stones. Clearly the answer should be to try to raise the level of this normal protective substance. This can be done by eating fewer fats and refined carbohydrates and by increasing the amount of fibre and complex carbohydrates. According to one study, people eating like this and taking chenodeoxycholic acid dissolved their gall-stones in a third of the time taken by a group using the drug alone.

Interestingly, gall-stones are often associated with certain other diseases, especially hiatus hernia and diverticular disease. Obesity is the factor common to all three diseases and obesity is also linked to diabetes and high blood-fat levels. The link between all of these conditions is the overconsumption of refined foods and fats, leading to a surplus of energy.

It is said that gall-stones are commonest in women who are fat, fertile, flatulent, fair and forty, but they can occur in anyone of any age and are increasingly common in children.

Wild animals very rarely have gall-stones but they can be induced to do so if they are fed artificial diets such as we eat in the West. A lack of dietary fibre seems to be especially potent in this respect.

Prevention

- Eat fewer refined foods, less fat, and more dietary fibre. Eat less sugar. A study in Italy comparing 160 gall-stone patients with a group of healthy subjects found that the stone patients ate much less fruit and vegetable fibre and significantly more sugar and refined foods generally. Eating sensibly will tend to reduce your weight which is the best preventive against gall-stones. Even being 20 per cent overweight doubles your chances of having gall-stones. Don't worry about reducing your cholesterol intake, though, as there is no real evidence that it matters. The important point here is to eat more dietary fibre as this provably reduces the amount of cholesterol in bile and puts out more in the stools. A recent study of French women who skipped breakfast, having only a cup of coffee, found that they had a much greater risk of gall-stones than would be expected.

GLAUCOMA

What is it?

Glaucoma is an eye disorder in which the eyeball becomes harder and the area of vision is narrowed down. It occurs in about one in 100 people over the age of 40. About 20,000 people are blind as a result of glaucoma in England and Wales alone. It is about ten times as common in close relatives as it is in the general population, and it is not catching. It can be treated, and loss of sight prevented, if it is caught early. Treatment is by eyedrops, tablets and operation. Glaucoma usually affects both eyes, though frequently one more than the other.

What causes it?

Watery fluid is normally formed in the eye and then drains back into the bloodstream through a sieve-like area of tissue. If this becomes partly blocked the fluid gets dammed up in the eye and presses on the sight nerve. Parts of this nerve go out of action and this causes a loss of vision around the edge of the field of vision. Eventually, if untreated, only the centre of the field of vision is left, and it can even blind you.

Prevention

- Vitamin C can lower the pressure and stem the disease. Research has shown that healthy people who consume about 1.2 g vitamin C a day tend to have lower pressure inside their eyes than those who consume only 75 mg of the vitamin a day. Take 1 g a day to be sure.

- Thiamine (vitamin B_1) may also help glaucoma sufferers. A recent Californian study found that people with glaucoma usually have lower amounts of thiamine in their blood. A study in Guyana in the 1950s found that East Indians living there who ate a largely vegetarian diet, rich in B vitamins, rarely suffered from glaucoma while their fellow countrymen living on a different diet often developed the disease. This researcher relieved the effects of glaucoma with large injections of thiamine (100 mg a day for ten days) and followed this up with oral supplements.

- Modern medicines prevent the glaucoma from getting worse, even making an operation unnecessary, and saving sight. Possible side-effects of the drops are an increase in urine passed and a tingling in the fingers and toes. They generally work for only a limited time and have to be repeated every six hours or so, though the latest drops last longer and only need to be used twice a day. Tablets boost the effects of the drops and are needed in some patients.

  This 'medical' treatment may make your eyes a little better and will certainly stop them getting worse. If you take certain tranquillisers or steroid drugs (including the contraceptive pill) you will have to be aware that your glaucoma could get worse and get your optician to measure your eye pressure more frequently than he otherwise would.

- Regular testing of your eyes for glaucoma is a simple and painless procedure which should be done every two years if there is glaucoma in the family and every three years or so as part of a regular eye check-up for anyone over 40. This enables the condition to be caught early before irreparable damage is done to the eyesight. Screening for glaucoma, especially among 'at risk' groups, is an example of preventive medicine at its best.

There are about 100,000 people diagnosed as having glaucoma in the UK but it is estimated that there are about 150,000 people who have the disease yet don't know it. Given that this is a major preventable cause of blindness, as soon as you are diagnosed as having the condition do every-thing you can to ensure that your close family all have an eye test.

GUM DISEASE

What is it?

A condition of the gums that causes them to become inflamed, resulting in the loosening and eventual loss of teeth.

Three-quarters of those over the age of 35 have gum disease, at least to some degree, and nearly half of all 60-year-olds have lost teeth as a result of it. Tooth decay is what wrecks children's teeth but in adults gum disease is to blame.

What causes it?

Gum disease, like dental caries, is caused by a bacterial coating of plaque. This collects all the time along the gum line and, if it is not removed

once a day, builds up to produce inflammation of the gums. Gums that are affected in this way bleed on brushing (healthy gums never bleed) and start to recede, making the teeth look longer. The fibres that tether the teeth into the jawbone weaken and eventually the affected tooth falls out.

The problem with gum disease is that you often do not even realise you have it until you start to notice bad breath, bleeding gums or loose teeth. Treatment is uncomfortable and time-consuming.

There is one specific cause of gum disease:

- Poor, or insufficient, cleaning of the teeth. Plaque has to be re-moved at least once a day if it is not to build up and cause gum disease.

Other contributory causes are:

- A lack of vitamim C. There is evidence that this vitamin pro-tects against gum infections but no one knows why. Certainly vitamin C is known to play a vital role in combating infection gener-ally but it seems to be exception-ally valuable in gum disease.

- Certain foods produce a transi-tory inflammation of the gums which can be very painful indeed. These are usually nitrate-contain-ing foods (preserved meats and other meats that have large amounts of preservative in them). The condition is self-limiting when you stop eating the foods.

- Stress. Some people have serious

gum inflammation at a time of high stress in their lives. Drugs and oral surgery can cure the condition but obviously prevention is better.

Prevention

- After the age of 30 or so regular brushing of the teeth becomes more valuable in terms of what it can do to promote healthy gums than in the battle against tooth decay. Brush your teeth at least once a day with a fluoride toothpaste, ensuring that you have a good-quality nylon brush. Always brush from gum to tooth and never scrub *across* the teeth. Work systematically around your mouth so that no area is missed. Don't forget the inside surfaces of the teeth.

  Now return to where you started and, using small circular motions with the brush at the junction of tooth and gum, work around your mouth from tooth to tooth 'massaging' the gums gently. If you notice that your teeth trap food between them (this is especially likely with meats) see your dentist to have this area looked at. A piece of food caught between two teeth even for a day or two can make your gum very sore and start up an infection.

- If you do get a sore gum, don't panic. Simply start the above routine and within days it should be better. In other words, thorough brushing can actually *cure* early gum disease, provided your technique is good.

- Take more vitamin C on a regular basis—1 g a day and double this when you have a sore area of gum. Animal research has proved that vitamin C helps reduce the risk of gum disease, and experiments in Yugoslavia have found that the vitamin can reverse the kind of gum breakdown seen in gum disease. When the volunteers were given as little as 75 mg vitamin C daily for six weeks the cells in the gums became observably healthier.

  But vitamin C alone may not be enough—calcium too may be vital. Certainly it is true that calcium deficiency can weaken the jawbone into which the teeth are set, but in addition this is now thought to make the bone more liable to infection. After the menopause women especially lose calcium in large amounts and many a woman first notices loose teeth at this time of life. Repeated pregnancies also cause a substantial loss of calcium into the fetuses. This plus slimming diets that involve eating no milk or dairy products can leave a lot of women calcium-deficient.

  One US study used folate (the B vitamin) too with great success. After sixty days of gargling with folate-rich water the subjects' gums were examined. They had soaked up folate 'like a sponge' and were much less inflamed than those of a control group who had been gargling with plain water for the same sixty days.

- There is some evidence that gum problems are linked to emotions. Trench mouth, for example, is a very rampant type of gum disease. Sufferers have higher levels of the natural steroid cortisol in their urine than normal. One study found that these patients had experienced more negative, unsettling life events in the previous year than had other people. They also demonstrably had higher levels of anxiety, depression and emotional disturbances. Clearly, preventing these life events is one way to combat at least this cause of gum disease.

HAIR PROBLEMS

What are they?

There are many types of hair and scalp problem but the most preventable ones are: dry, flaky scalp; hair loss; greasy hair; and split ends and hair that breaks easily. Most other scalp and hair conditions are not preventable and so will not be considered here.

What causes them?

- A diet high in dairy produce can lead to a dry, flaky scalp. Dietary deficiencies generally affect both

the hair and scalp but understandably affect the scalp sooner because hair is an 'old' part of the body. The ends of long hair could be several years old and the content of these ends reflects what the person's diet was like when that hair was emerging from the scalp.

- Incorrect washing. Most people with flaky scalps wash their hair too infrequently. A flaky scalp is often greasy too. Washing removes the flaky cells and keeps grease down.

- Stress. It has been said in trichology circles for many years that dandruff is a cry for help.

- Shortage of vitamin B. Anecdotal evidence suggests that some people with flaky, dry scalps do well when adding vitamin B supplements to their diet.

- Poor hairdressing. Too harsh a treatment during perming, or the combination of a perm and tinting, weakens each individual hair and makes it more susceptible to split ends and breaking generally. Pulling hair–especially hair that is not particularly strong anyway–into tight plaits etc., can cause an inflammation of the scalp, and can even lead to hair falling out because of the pull on it.

- Poor hair care. Most people overbrush their hair, in line with the old wives' tale that a hundred strokes a day are desirable. Research shows that this damages many people's hair and breaks it unnecessarily.

- Heated rollers, heated tongs and hot hairdriers all make the hair weaker and more likely to break and split.

- Overuse of elasticated bands, especially to hold pigtails in place. These cause the hair to fracture at the tension point of the elastic band.

- Crash diets. These make some women lose their hair, even when they are taking mineral and vitamin supplements.

- Pregnancy and childbirth are a cause of hair loss in some women, but regrowth starts again within a matter of months. Many women say that the condition of their hair greatly improves during pregnancy.

Prevention

- Eat a healthy diet low in dairy products if you have a dry, flaky scalp.

- Wash your hair every other day if it is short and once a week if it is long. Too frequent washing of long (old) hair can damage it and cause it to split.

- Reduce stress (see page 87).

- Try a course of vitamin B complex if you have a flaky scalp.

- Keep perms and tinting to a minimum. Always let your hair have a recovery period between perms.

- Comb your hair rather than brush it.

- Wrap a paper tissue around each heated roller and don't use tongs on permed or tinted hair because the heat will damage the hair further. Don't dry hair with too powerful a heater.

HAY FEVER

What is it?

An allergic condition affecting one person in ten in which the sufferer overreacts to pollens, moulds or spores in the air.

Hay fever–a seasonal form of allergic rhinitis–is really an inflammation of the nasal passages. The sufferer complains of sneezing, an itchy, blocked or runny nose, itchy eyes (which may also be red, watery and sensitive to light) and an itchy throat.

The condition can easily be confused with perennial allergic rhinitis which occurs year-round and is caused by an allergy to house-dust mites which live in carpets and bedding. Some people who appear to have allergic rhinitis are in fact sensitive to the weather, a deodorant spray or indeed one or more of many other things. This is not a true allergy but simply an oversensitivity.

Most people who have hay fever

start having trouble before the age of 15 and some grow out of it. Hay fever, like all allergies, tends to run in families. You don't need to live in the country to be troubled with hay fever but if you live at the seaside you will be protected to some extent by winds that are pollen-free coming off the sea.

What causes it?

- An oversensitivity to pollens, moulds or spores. Tree pollens are most plentiful in April and May; grass pollens in June and July; and moulds and spores in August and September.

- Allergies run in families. We can't choose our parents but a couple one or both of whom has a family history of allergy can take certain steps to reduce the chances of their children suffering from allergies.

Prevention

- Do all you can to avoid producing allergic children (see page 218).

- Take preventive medications prescribed by your doctor or have a series of desensitising injections. Discuss these with your doctor.

- Try an 'alternative' therapy. Homoeopathy, acupuncture and hypnotherapy all claim to prevent hay fever.

- Buy a car that has a ventilation system that can filter out pollens.

Only one European car does this (Saab). Sneezing when driving can be very dangerous because if your eyes are shut for half a second, say at 60 mph, you will travel 'blind' for 44 ft.

- If you have to drive start early in the day or late at night when pollens are not so plentiful in the cool air. Keep your car windows shut and the ventilators closed.

HEADACHES AND MIGRAINE

What are they?

Pain in the head from any cause. Migraine is a very specific type of headache and is relatively uncommon, whereas headaches are extremely common – one of the most familiar of everyday pains.

Migraine is characteristically a one-sided headache and more than half of all sufferers have their first attack before the age of 20. Most people who have true migraine know when it is about to start. Often sufferers say that they feel exceptionally well a day or two before the attack. The senses are often generally sharpened at this time. Shortly before the headache itself begins there may be a sensation called an aura. This often takes the form of difficulty with or changes in vision. You might see flashing lights and you might even go blind for a while. There may also be peculiar smells, a feeling of nausea and you might even vomit. Some people lose their voice and have altered sensations of touch. The aura lasts for up to half an hour and then fades.

Next comes the headache, which can last from an hour up to a few days. It starts above or behind one eye and spreads to the back of the head on the same side. Many people feel nauseated and may even vomit. For many, sleep cures the headache but others wake with the headache still there.

Cluster headaches are not at all uncommon and are a sort of face-headache migraine. They come in bouts (clusters) with an attack every day for weeks and then nothing for months. This complaint is much less common than ordinary migraine and men have it more often than women. The individual attack starts at the same time each day (or more often, night) often in the spring or autumn. When an attack is at its peak it is very painful, usually being worst in the eye and the cheek. The eye on the affected side becomes red and watery and the nostril on that side blocked. Anti-migraine drugs can be useful but often the condition persists.

What causes them?

- The causes of migraine are many. Some people are exceptionally sensitive to particular foods (typically cheese, citrus fruits, fried foods, chocolate, seafood or red wine). Others are sensitive to: stress; not enough or too much sleep; noise; certain smells; missed meals; excitement; bright and flickering lights; changes in daily routine; or the weather (especially thunderstorms and snow-storms). Migraine, and indeed all types of headache, are three times more common in women than in men. Perhaps a fall in oestrogen triggers an attack. Women taking the contraceptive pill often have headaches, and taking the Pill can make migraine worse.

- Dehydration (too little fluid) is a common cause of headaches. Most people drink too little fluid and easily become dehydrated in hot surroundings or if they miss a drink or two.

- Tension headaches are produced by anxiety and stress. They are often seen in people who are meticulous and fussy. Unlike with migraine the pain of tension headaches lasts all day. The sensation is described as being 'like a weight pressing on the head' or 'a tight band around the head'. Sometimes the pain goes to the back of the head and down the neck. People who concentrate for long periods of time (such as lorry drivers) often get this kind of headache. A variation of this is the tense-jaw headache which is caused by the individual clenching the teeth.

- Hangovers are a very common cause of headaches. They are the results of consuming too much alcohol, which overloads the body's ability to detoxify the alcohol.

- Foods cause headaches in certain susceptible people. Ice cream and very cold foods can cause pain in the head and throat. Cured meats often contain nitrates which make blood vessels around the skull wider and cause headaches. Monosodium glutamate (especially plentiful in Chinese food) causes a headache in some people—often accompanied by nausea, abdominal pains and dizziness.

- Poor vision does not cause headaches but if you sit with your eyes screwed up, frowning to see better, you can easily get a tension headache.

- Headaches are often a sign of an impending infectious illness or fever. A simple pain-killer usually tides the person over until the cause becomes obvious.

- Head injuries are, undoubtedly, a cause of headaches but the cause is usually all too apparent and cannot readily be prevented (except for the obvious measures of driving carefully, and wearing seat-belts in cars and crash helmets on motorcycles).

- Very high blood pressure can cause a severe, pounding headache which is worse in the morning and improves during the day. The pain improves with the head up and is worse when lying down.

- Brain tumours certainly cause headaches and many people worry that they might have a tumour, especially if they have repeated headaches. However, brain tumours are very rare indeed. If your headache is worse on waking in the morning or if it is worsened by sneezing, bending down or exertion then you should see a doctor to discuss it. If you have double vision, vomiting, drowsiness or weakness in a limb and are not a migraine sufferer you should seek medical help at once.

Prevention

Helpful things to prevent headaches and migraines include:

1. Stop smoking.
2. Come off the Pill.
3. Stop drinking tea and coffee.
4. Cut out alcohol.
5. Stop eating sugar.
6. Cut out tyramine-containing foods such as chocolates, yeast extracts and yeast products, liver, sausages, broad beans, pickled herrings and cheese.
7. Cut out histamine-containing foods such as sauerkraut, salami and sausage meat.
8. Don't eat oranges—they contain substances that can precipitate migraines in some people.
9. Avoid foods containing additives such as tartrazine, benzoates and sodium glutamate.

10.   Avoid wheat-containing and milk-containing foods.

- Noise and annoying surroundings can also cause headaches.

- True migraine can often *not* be prevented, unfortunately, as many sufferers know. Look through the triggering factors above and see if you can avoid at least some of them in your life.

- If during the summer months or in hot environments you tend to get headaches, be sure to drink more watery fluids. Aim to keep your urine pale yellow.

- Cluster headaches may be helped by anti-migraine medications. See your doctor.

- The answer to tension headaches is to learn how to relax (see page 87).

- Hangovers can be prevented by following this list of tips. Drink a pint of water or other non-alcoholic drinks for every two pints of beer or two 'shorts' you take. Take an antacid in the morning to settle your stomach. Take 1 g vitamin C with the water you drink last thing at night–the vitamin will help your liver to cope with detoxifying the alcohol. Take a simple pain-killer if you have to. Don't mix drinks. Don't drink alcohol to cure a hangover ('hair of the dog') because this only makes the final effects worse.

- Avoid foods that give you headaches. See page 217 for the foods to which people are most often allergic and work out if any of these are affecting you.

- Have your eyes checked by a good optician just in case poor eyesight could be giving you tension headaches.

- Have your blood pressure checked if you are over 40 and have repeated headaches for which you can find no explanation.

- Massage your scalp. A US researcher has found that he can prevent headaches by a special hair-brushing technique. It involves massaging the scalp, which could, of course, be done with one's fingers, but he found better results using a hairbrush. Use a natural brush which is stiff but not as rigid as a typical hairbrush. Synthetic bristles are too sharp when moved across the skin. Ideally the brush should be one that can be held in the hand comfortably. When buying a suitable brush use it on the skin on the back of your hand to test it. Move it in small circles to make the skin move but not so as to cause an abrasion or irritation to the skin.

  The next thing, having found a good brush, is to make the scalp massage a regular part of your everyday routine, spending 90 seconds on it, morning and night. Starting at the temple just above the eyebrow, press the brush against the skin and rotate it in small circles so that the upper part of the circle goes towards the back of your head. Move up the skull with each pass from front to back of your head so that after three circles you are at the top of the head. Continue these small circles all over the scalp right down to the hair line.

HEARTBURN

What is it?

A burning pain behind the breastbone, sometimes accompanied by watery acid coming back into the mouth. The reflux of acid from the stomach into the gullet is usually prevented by a valve at the junction of the two. This valve can become faulty in several medical conditions, or excessive amounts of acid may be produced by the stomach. Smoking reduces the effectiveness of the valve and, like alcohol, increases the amount of stomach acid produced.

What causes it?

- Hiatus hernia – a condition in which the top end of the stomach ruptures through the diaphragm into the chest.

- Heavy meals before retiring.

- Lying flat in bed.

- Smoking.

- Alcohol.

- Being overweight.

- Tight, constrictive clothing.

- Eating too heartily.

- Stress.

- Pregnancy.

- Stooping.

Prevention

- Hiatus hernia is common in obese women, and slimming generally helps cure the condition. Prevention of hiatus hernia therefore includes keeping slim (see page 290). Hiatus hernia is also thought to be caused by excessive straining to pass hard, sticky motions caused by eating highly refined, low-fibre foods. Probably the best preventive for hiatus hernia is a high-fibre diet with plenty of fruit and vegetables, wholemeal-flour products and fluid. This keeps the motions soft and means that the individual does not have to strain to pass stools. When straining at stool the pressure inside the abdominal cavity rises dramatically and forces the top end of the stomach to rupture into the chest.

- A large meal before retiring means that the stomach is full and triggered to produce a large amount of acid. The full stomach will also force food up the lower end of the gullet if there is any weakness of the valve there. The acid will produce pain because it will come into contact with gullet lining that is sensitive to acid.

- Raising the head of the bed on books or a couple of bricks and keeping several pillows behind you is a good way of keeping the upper part of your body upright. This in itself can help cure and prevent heartburn.

- Cut down on or stop smoking (see page 332).

- Cut down or stop drinking alcohol (see page 134).

- Reduce your weight–this alone can work wonders (see page 290).

- Don't wear tight belts, corsets or even tight skirts or trousers. This can have the effect of forcing the abdominal contents upwards and making heartburn worse.

- Eating too heartily can produce indigestion and an over-production of gastric acid. Chew food well before swallowing and eat several small meals rather than having a smaller number of big blow-outs.

- Stress is a powerful producer of acid in the stomach. If acid travels from the stomach into the first part of the intestine it can cause a duodenal ulcer but if it flows into the gullet it can cause a lot of pain and a condition known as reflux oesophagitis. This can be prevented by taking medications that stop acid production in the first place (available on prescrip-tion from your doctor) or you can take antacids or stomach powders to mop up the acid. Milk does not help as it actually increases stomach-acid production after a while. The best preventive is to sort out the causes of stress in your life and learn to relax (see pages 87–9).

- Pregnancy causes heartburn because the greatly enlarged uterus forces the abdominal contents upwards and encour-ages the reflux of gastric acid into the lower end of the gullet. The best preventives for this are: to sleep upright in bed at night; to adopt love-making positions that keep the woman upright; and to take antacids and frequent, small meals.

- Stooping can usually be avoided. Sit down to put on shoes, etc. Kneel down to pick things up. In short, avoid bending double for any reason.

HEART ATTACKS

What are they?

A heart attack occurs when the mus-cle of the heart cannot get sufficient oxygen-containing blood for it to function. Angina pectoris (a tight chest pain that comes on exertion and goes) is often the earliest sign that something is wrong. In this condition there is insufficient blood getting to the heart muscles, especially on exertion, and the person complains of tightness in the chest as the heart muscle goes into cramp.

A heart attack is like a very severe bout of angina. Sometimes the loss of blood supply is sufficiently severe to kill off a part of the heart's muscle, and less commonly the damage from a shortage of blood is so severe that it causes almost instant death.

The heart finds itself in this lethal condition as a result of a lifetime's abuse which causes a progressive narrowing of the arteries (atherosclerosis) that supply the heart with oxygen. Blood clots may obstruct the arteries further.

Heart disease is now the prime killer in the western world, although in the US death rates have fallen by a quarter over the last fifteen years. Given that much of this improvement is caused by lifestyle changes it makes sense to look at heart attacks as substantially preventable. Historic evidence and evidence from populations who migrate from one country to another also strongly suggest that mankind doesn't *have* to suffer from coronary artery disease and heart attacks.

There are compelling reasons for rejecting a fatalistic view that heart attacks cannot be prevented. We still have a lot to learn about heart disease, but it does seem clear that it is affected by lifestyle. We have seen that the coronary-artery death rates in the US and Australia have fallen dramatically over the last fifteen years. This improvement pre-dates the widespread use of coronary care units and coronary bypass surgery and even the widespread use of drugs for combating high blood pressure. The fall in heart disease *has*, however, coincided with a considerable reduction in both cigarette consumption and consumption of saturated fats. However, things are not quite as simple as this suggests, because heart-attack rates are still high in Sweden despite their wealth of medical technology and falling cigarette and fat consumption, and rates in American women are falling despite their rise in cigarette consumption.

What causes them?

No one knows exactly what ultimately causes heart attacks but several fairly clear-cut 'risk factors' have been established after vast and complicated studies worldwide.

- Smoking. Several studies have shown the link between smoking and heart disease. A study of particular interest looked at British doctors who stopped smoking between 34 and 55 years of age. It found that their coronary death rate fell by half over five years compared with doctors who continued to smoke. Stopping after 55 appeared to make much less difference. The degree of risk with smoking is related to the number of cigarettes smoked. Filter cigarettes are probably not protective. Cigarettes act along with the contraceptive pill to increase the risk of heart disease in young women twentyfold. We look at stopping smoking on page 332.

- High blood pressure. Many studies have found that reducing raised blood pressure, provided the treatment is begun in middle age, reduces mortality from strokes, heart failure and kidney failure. There is some evidence that anti-hypertensive drugs reduce mortality from heart attacks. We see how to reduce blood pressure on page 242.

- High blood fats. The fats in the blood are many and take different forms. They all come originally from the digestion of dietary fat. The fractions of fats that seem to be of greatest significance in heart disease are the lipoproteins. High density lipoproteins (HDLs) appear to protect against heart disease, whereas low density lipoproteins (LDLs) seem to be harmful in this respect. The balance of these two types of lipoproteins can be altered by what we eat.

- Exercise. Studies show that those who take regular, vigorous exercise tend to have fewer heart attacks, though the evidence is not so clear-cut as is that on smoking, high blood pressure and dietary fats.

Prevention

It is probably fair to say that more research has been done on ways of preventing heart disease than on any other condition, with the exception of cancer. It is impossible to do more than briefly summarise the vast literature in the medical journals, so here is a brief list of measures that seem to have proved helpful in prevention.

All of the measures below make sense as preventives against a major killer (in the western world) but they are especially worth while for anyone who has a history of high blood pressure or heart disease in the family.

- Eat less sugar. Studies at the US Department of Agriculture's Human Nutrition Center have found that people who are unable properly to metabolise carbohydrate (especially men) have a greater likelihood of having a heart attack. Sugar also provably elevates serum cholesterol and blood fats as well as insulin levels. This is not to say that sugar *causes* heart attacks but that unrefined carbohydrates, rich in dietary fibre, are more healthy. But cutting down on sugar and sugary foods also helps to keep weight down, which is good for preventing high blood pressure and obesity, two other risk factors for heart disease.

- Stop smoking. This is no longer a debating point. Your chances of dying of coronary artery disease reduce sharply after the first year of stopping smoking and continue to fall over the next few years. A recent Swedish study of men who survived a first heart attack found that only just over half as many of those who stopped smoking died from coronary-artery disease as those who continued to smoke. The longer you stay off cigarettes the closer your risk level comes to those who have never smoked.

- Take more exercise. See page 74 to see how much you need to do.

- Whilst on the subject of exercise – many men consciously (let alone the many others who do so unconsciously) avoid sex after a heart attack or even if they have severe angina. Yet research has shown time and again that the actual amount of physical energy expended during intercourse is equivalent to such everyday household activities as scrubbing the floor or climbing several flights of stairs. In one study of 100 heart-attack victims, 90 returned to work yet only 40 resumed normal sexual activity.

- Don't allow yourself to get overweight. A number of studies have linked obesity to heart disease. High blood pressure, a risk factor, is more common in fat people and fat people take less exercise.

- Relax. The aggressive, competitive personality (called 'type A') is at greater risk than the phlegmatic personality ('type B'). Acute stress and adverse life events can also be associated with increased

risk. Look at page 87 and see what to do to relax.

- Don't add salt to your food. This is a potent contributor to high blood pressure (see page 242).

- Cut down the amount of saturated fat you eat. This means less butter, meat, cheese, cream and whole milk, replacing them with polyunsaturated fats and semi-skimmed milk. There is no evidence that cutting out or down on cholesterol-rich foods does any good at all. Ways of reducing blood cholesterol levels are considered on page 174.

- Eat more fish oils. Studies of people who consume large amounts of fish (notably the Japanese and the Eskimos) show that they have very low heart-disease rates. Both groups have low blood-fat levels, high levels of high-density lipoproteins (the good, helpful kind) and a reduced tendency for their blood to clot. These people also have a high level of a particular type of fatty acid called eicosapentaenoic acid (EPA). This and its close relative, DHA, are found in fish, fish oils and the fat of marine animals. Many research groups have now looked at the role of fish-oil supplements and found that various risk factors for heart disease can be altered beneficially. The main advantage appears to be that the blood becomes less sticky and so less likely to form clots. This must reduce the risk of heart attacks because they are so often triggered off by a clot in one of the arteries that supply the heart. It is especially encouraging to find that the higher the blood fats before taking fish oil, the more they are affected by the treatment. So far there do not seem to be any drawbacks to taking fish-oil supplements – for example, the blood does not go on getting thinner and thinner. So, by increasing your fish consumption and possibly taking a food supplement of EPA, you can almost certainly reduce your chances of having a heart attack.

- Eat more magnesium-containing foods. Recent work suggests that it is brief spasms of the coronary arteries rather than clots that trigger a significant number of heart attacks. It appears that a deficiency of magnesium could be behind this problem. Eat more fruit, whole grains, vegetables and pulses to enrich your diet with magnesium.

- Make friends and be sociable. Social isolation has been found to be a factor in heart attacks, according to a study of 4,000 men in the US. The most sociable people had fewest heart attacks. In parallel with this an Israeli study found that men who had a good sex life were much less likely to have a heart attack. There is also evidence that loving care reduces the arterial disease that makes a heart attack more likely by narrowing the coronary arteries.

- Control your diabetes if you have Type I (insulin-dependent diabetes) and cure it if you have middle-age onset diabetes. These are considered on page 195. Diabetics have a very much increased risk of having a heart attack and this preventive measure is very worth while.

- Don't take the contraceptive pill if you have a history of heart disease in the family. It is not known why women have so much less heart disease than men – the hormonal differences are not an adequate explanation – but taking the Pill definitely raises the risk unacceptably for susceptible women, especially after the age of 35.

- The weather, particularly the invasion of cold fronts and rapid falls in barometric pressure, has been linked to admissions to hospital with heart attacks. Things you can do to prevent heart attacks occurring in these circumstances are to avoid exposure to cold, especially the combination of vigorous exercise and cold. It is no coincidence that so many men die from heart attacks every year shifting snow from in front of their homes. The use of a light face-mask helps maintain temperature and humidity and can be a useful preventive.

HEAT RASH (Prickly heat)

What is it?

An itching skin condition caused by heavy sweating (usually in hot climates). Little red pimples occur in sweaty areas.

What causes it?

Inflammation of the sweat ducts.

Prevention

- In hot and sweaty climates reduce your physical activity and hence the amount you sweat.

- Don't drink hot drinks.

- Wear as few clothes as possible, preferably made of light, natural fibres.

- Shower in tepid water and use no soap. Dry carefully and use a dusting powder.

- Soothe the bad areas with calamine lotion.

HEAT STROKE

What is it?

Heat stroke is a condition in which the body is unable to lose heat, for example in extremely hot climates in which the air is hotter than the body so that the body does not lose heat into the air. It can also occur in very humid conditions in which the body is unable to sweat and so lose heat.

The skin is hot, dry and red, and the sufferer has a rapid pulse and a high temperature and may also vomit and be irritable. If severe, it can lead to a coma.

What causes it?

An inability of the body to cool off by normal heat loss or via sweating (which also reduces body temperature).

Prevention

- Avoid extremely hot situations.

- Drink ice-cold liquids to lower the body temperature. NB This is *not* a treatment. No one with this condition should be cooled quickly.

- When in hot climates wear thin, natural-fibre clothes and keep out of the direct sun.

HERPES

What is it?

A viral disease which produces cold sores on the lips, a venereal disease that is difficult or impossible to cure, and a potentially fatal infection in newborn babies.

Although many think of herpes as a new disease this is not so–it has been around since ancient times. What *is* new is the extent of the disease in society and this was almost certainly brought about by the sexual revolution of the 1960s. The larger number of sexual partners that this social change has brought about has meant that any venereal infection spreads more quickly than before. Coupled with this is a greater readiness to experiment with new sexual techniques. Thirty years ago oral sex was considered a perversion but over the last twenty years it has become fashionable. Now the transfer of the virus from the mouth to the genitals is a major source of the disease. Lastly, as with polio virus, about fifty years ago most children would have contracted the herpes virus and would have built up at least some resistance to it. Today this is less likely. Having had oral herpes (cold sores) affords at least some protection against the genital variety but the level of such protection is not great.

Herpes became the media scare story of the 1970s, and understandably so, with stories of an 'incurable' disease which killed babies of affected mothers, produced intermittent, long-term infections in adults, might be implicated in cancer of the cervix, had serious harmful effects on people's sex lives, and so on.

Herpes is caused by the herpes simplex virus that is related to the chickenpox virus, the glandular fever virus and cytomegalovirus. Although, as with other viral infections, the virus can affect many different parts of the body, the real scare (and what this piece is about) is genital herpes.

In a man herpetic sores can affect any part of the penis and scrotum but they are most often seen on the head of the penis. The sores are painful and the glands in the groins enlarge. Herpes can also affect the area around the anus and can cause extreme pain on opening the bowels.

In women the same pattern occurs as in men but with certain differences. One is that there are more ulcers and they are much more painful. Passing urine can be 'agony' and there can be considerable difficulty in passing urine at all in some women. The virus may attack the neck of the womb and such women have a temperature and pain in the lower abdomen as well as the other signs. An attack of thrush can also occur alongside the herpes as the woman's local defence mechanisms break down.

Between 40 and 70 per cent of all herpes sufferers have recurrent attacks and some people go on having them for years.

What causes it?

Genital herpes is caused by two viruses, HSV1 and HSV2. The vast majority of infections with the virus are subclinical, that is they produce no effects of which the sufferer is aware. That an infection *has* occurred can be detected by finding antibodies to the herpes virus in the individual's blood. The first attack of the virus tends to occur in childhood or adolescence–just as with other viral illnesses. Such attacks produce a 'flu-like illness with relatively few local symptoms.

Herpes virus is transferred from person to person by close body contact between wet areas of the body. This is why the lips, genitals, mouth and gut are affected. The virus enters the cells and some enter sensory nerves up which they travel to clusters of nerve cells close to the spinal cord. Here they remain to produce recurrent infections over the years.

Prevention

- Keep the number of sex partners you have down to a minimum. You can never tell if someone has herpes–until it's too late.

- Avoid public lavatories if possible. Some recent work has shown that herpes virus can survive on lavatory seats for a number of hours and on cotton gauze for 72 hours.

- If someone has sores of any kind, skin contact should be avoided. The sufferer from recurrent herpes should not have intercourse during an attack. Many people with recurrent attacks have a warning when one is about to occur. This varies from individual to individual but can be an itch, tingle or burning in the genital area. This type of sensation rules out sex until the sores have healed. These precautions also apply to kissing (not just on the genitals) someone with a cold sore on the lips.

- Oral sex increases the risk of getting genital herpes because the mouth is such a reservoir for the virus. Some people overcome this by using a sheath on the man before fellating him. Unfortunately, although this confers some protection it is not totally safe because the pores in the latex of the sheath are larger than the herpes virus and some could pass through.

All of this may sound daunting but in fact the risks involved in sexual activity between individuals who have no sores are very small indeed. Unfortunately, lesions inside the woman's vagina or on her cervix are not visible and it can be impossible to know if she is 'safe'.

- Vaccines are being researched but so far the outlook is not very encouraging and experts think that a safe, effective vaccine is a long way off, and possibly may never be found.

- Wash your hands thoroughly with soap and water after touching the sores.

- Don't share towels – it is just possible to pass the virus to someone else via a towel.

- Never use saliva to wet your contact lenses.

- Not everyone who has one attack of herpes goes on to have another – about half of all sufferers never get another attack. Keep a record of when you have your attacks (if you have them repeatedly). You may find that you get them under specific conditions. These can be avoided, at least to some extent, to prevent more attacks. Here are some conditions that some people find make their herpes worse or brings on an attack:

1. Tiredness or stress.
2. A particular time of the menstrual cycle.
3. Friction from intercourse or masturbation.
4. Sunlight and sunbeds.
5. Tight clothing.
6. Nylon knickers.

The avoidance of any or all of these will help prevent herpes in at least some people.

HYPERTENSION (High blood pressure, see also page 91)

What is it?

When the heart beats it pumps blood around in surges. When the pressure of these surges is measured (say at the arm) there is a high and a low point. The high point registers the pressure at the peak of a pulse of blood and the low point the trough in between two successive heartbeats. The 'ideal' blood pressure is generally held to be 120/80 (120mm of mercury/80mm of mercury – mercury is used in the blood-pressure machines because it is heavy and the column height needed is small; if a watery liquid were used the column would be many feet high).

The upper recording is called the systolic pressure, and the lower the diastolic pressure. Systolic blood pressure can vary greatly with exercise, emotion, stress, excitement and so on. The diastolic pressure is much more stable and is usually considered to be of greater significance if it is raised. As we stand up our blood pressure falls slightly as blood pools under gravity in the lower half of the body. This is why a doctor will always take your blood pressure with your arm at the height of your heart.

Hypertension (high blood pressure) is the commonest of all chronic ailments in the western world. About 60 million Americans suffer from it.

If you are between the ages of 45 and 74 and you have high blood pressure your chances of having a heart attack are three times greater than normal, and those of having a stroke are seven times greater. In the US nearly a million people a year die of the effects of high blood pressure.

You may not realise you have high blood pressure and many people have no symptoms at all. Headaches, dizziness and lightheadedness are common symptoms. Some people with hypertension blush very easily and some are very tired all the time.

The diagnosis is usually easy but treating the condition is not so easy. Drugs certainly have a good record of helping hypertensive people but they also have drawbacks. Many people on them complain of drowsiness, dizziness, depression, nausea, headache, a dry mouth, feeling faint when standing up suddenly, impotence, palpitation and many other side-effects. This is the main reason why so few people take their blood-pressure medicines regularly and reliably. Many studies show that these drugs are especially likely to be left on the medicine-cabinet shelf.

Hypertension is an excellent illustration of the potential of the preventive approach: it is a major killer and is often difficult to treat successfully, but the individual can significantly reduce his or her chances of suffering from it.

What causes it?

- Being overweight.

- Too much salt.

- Too much sugar.

- Stress.

- Caffeine.

- Too little exercise.

- Noise.

- Speaking too fast.

- Genetic predisposition.

- Several 'medical' conditions including pre-eclamptic toxaemia of pregnancy, Cushing's syndrome, certain hormonal diseases, abnormalities of the blood vessels and certain neurological diseases.

- Alcohol.

- Saturated fats.

- The contraceptive pill.

- Toxic minerals, especially lead and cadmium.

- Too little dietary potassium.

- Too much dietary calcium.

Prevention

- Although no one knows quite why it should be, hypertension is much more common in fat people. One study of 10,940 hypertensive patients found that 60 per cent of them were overweight. Hypertension does, of course, occur in thin people but it is almost unknown in cultures where all the population is thin. Often, mild blood pressure can be treated simply by losing a stone or two. Certainly preventing obesity also helps prevent high blood pressure. This starts at the cradle. Breastfeeding exclusively for at least six months and then weaning on to unrefined, wholefoods rich in dietary fibre will prevent many children from becoming obese. It is during these rapid-growth early years that obesity sets in, mainly because of poor eating habits and even an addiction to sweet, refined foods. These habits are difficult to change later in life and almost inevitably produce obesity.

A study in California looked at twenty-five obese hypertensives and after only a twelve-week weight-reducing diet found a significant decrease in blood pressure to within the normal range. Furthermore, few (only about a quarter) of the subjects reduced to their 'ideal' body weight but the reduction they did achieve was enough to reduce their blood pressure to normal. They found that a 10–30 per cent reduction towards ideal weight was enough to lower blood pressure significantly. Interestingly, such losses in weight reduced the blood pressure of all the obese subjects whether or not they started out with high blood pressure.

- The subject of too much salt is discussed more on page 91. Several studies have suggested that salt added to food during cooking or at the table is responsible for much of the hypertension we see in the West. However, a great deal of salt (probably the majority) is added during food manufacture and processing and we have little direct control over this hidden salt (especially in cured and processed foods). This is a real danger. Get used to reading labels and avoiding products where salt comes high on the list (ingredients are listed in order of weight in the product). Buy salt-free products if possible. Unfortunately, even drinking water can be very rich in sodium (salt). A Massachusetts study found that a particular town had a very high level of sodium in the drinking water. Even high-school students in this study had raised blood pressures, and it was found that the water they drank accounted for 40 per cent of the difference in total salt intake between these children and those of a neighbouring town.

- When cutting down salt do it slowly over a month or two, first by not adding salt during cooking. Use a salt shaker with smaller holes for adding salt to food at the table, and over 6–8 weeks use less and less. Once again, prevention starts in the cradle. Discourage children from eating salty foods and wean them on to salt-free foods whenever possible. Research suggests that children have already acquired a

243

taste for salt by the age of two.

Interestingly bound up with the salt story is potassium – another essential mineral. Potassium is vital for the transmission of messages in nerves, aids digestive enzymes, and is essential in muscle function. Sodium and potassium are intimately interlinked within and outside cells, and the balance has to be finely maintained if we are to remain healthy. A study at the London Hospital Medical School showed that potassium seemed to act as a shield against sodium-induced hypertension. In the first study sixteen people with mild hypertension and a group with normal blood pressure ate one diet for a twelve-week period, and then a different diet for the next twelve weeks. During the first twelve weeks both groups ate their normal diet plus sodium tablets. During the second period the normal diets were supplemented with potassium and they were asked to avoid salty foods and not to add salt.

The high-sodium diet produced a slow rise in blood pressure in both groups. But with potassium and a low-salt diet both systolic and diastolic pressures fell sharply and significantly in the hypertensive group – in contrast to an insignificant rise in the normal group! A month after the study ended both groups went back to normal eating. The hypertensive blood pressures shot back up again. This rise was explained by the researchers as due to the poor levels of potassium in their food rather than the marginal rise in sodium (salt).

Other research found that if you have a family history of blood pressure you are especially likely to be sensitive to the blood-pressure-lowering effect of potassium. Such people develop the condition when the potassium in their diets falls below a certain essential level. Fruits and vegetables are among the best sources of potassium so this could be yet another advantage of a high-fibre diet. Particularly rich sources are potatoes, Brussels sprouts, broccoli, wheatgerm, dates, chicken, salmon and halibut. A banana contains 350 mg potassium and only 1 mg sodium. A glass of pure orange juice contains 180 mg potassium and only 2 mg sodium.

- Too much sugar has not been proved harmful to the blood pressure in humans but it has in animals. One experiment in monkeys found that adding sugar to a high-salt diet made the blood pressure jump even higher. (Refined sugar definitely has an adverse effect on cholesterol metabolism – putting up the levels of harmful blood fats which also predispose to heart disease. Unrefined, complex sugars do the opposite.)

- Stress undoubtedly plays a part in producing at least some cases of high blood pressure, and almost certainly keeps it high in others. Many studies have now proved that biofeedback (see page 88, autogenic training and self-hypnosis can all be used to reduce blood pressure in hypertensives. Simple meditation can reduce blood pressure both at the time and long-term. Read pages 87–9 for some ideas. In a study reported in 1981 one group of hypertensives were taught how to relax, while a parallel group were left alone. The relaxation group had a three times greater drop in blood pressure than the others. On checking six months later the difference in blood pressures was still the same.

It appears that if you expect relaxation techniques to be successful they are more likely to be so. A study of thirty patients under medical treatment for high blood pressure divided the patients into two groups. The first group were told that the muscle-relaxation exercises they were to do could produce immediate results which would persist with increased practice, and the second group were told that the value of the relaxation could be delayed and that they might even expect a small rise in blood pressure. The 'expectant' group achieved a 17 point fall in systolic blood pressure but the 'delayed' group had only a 2–4 point fall.

- We see on page 164 how dangerous caffeine can be. A study in Nashville found a 14 per cent rise in blood pressure in volunteers who consumed the equivalent of about two cups of coffee. This made the researchers conclude that habitual coffee drinkers keep their blood pressures artificially high and that some will push marginal blood pressures into the seriously hypertensive range that needs treatment.

- Exercise can provably reduce blood pressure. A study in Florida looked at 370 hypertensive patients and measured their blood pressure before and after several twenty-minute rides on a stationary bicycle. About 96 per cent of the volunteers had a fall of blood pressure (of between 10 and 50 points) after three months' exercise.

- Noise can produce blood pressure and removing it prevents it. Monkey experiments found that after nine months of exposure to a noise level typically experienced by industrial workers the animals' blood pressures went up by an average of 27 per cent. After the end of the experiment the monkeys' blood pressure remained high for over a month even in the absence of noise. Investigations at the Volvo car factory in Sweden checked the effect of industrial noise on the blood pressure of their workers. Because some people are thought to be more sensitive to noise the researchers selected out all those with noise-induced hearing loss. All 414 men with hearing loss turned out to have significantly higher blood pressures than the 74 men with normal hearing.

Further evidence of the strain of noise comes from studies done on people who live near airports. A study of those living around Los Angeles International Airport found that people living within 3 miles of the airport had 29 per cent more admissions to mental hospital than those living 6 miles away. A similar study of London's Heathrow Airport found the figure to be 31 per cent.

- Simply slowing down the pace of one's life can help prevent hypertension. According to one US expert, people who talk fast tend to have high blood pressure. 'Such people don't put commas into their sentences,' he claims. As a result they breathe poorly and this also contributes to their high blood pressure. This researcher uses a piece of equipment that can measure blood pressure very accurately during talking and other routine social interactions. He found that virtually everyone's blood pressure goes up (by about 10–15 per cent) when speaking. Hypertensives, however, are more reactive–the higher a person's blood pressure when quiet, the more it goes up when speaking. This statement is based on a study of 2,000 people from the cradle to old age. The researcher teaches people to speak more slowly and to put commas back into their sentences. Just using this method

alone he has had formidable success in curing hypertension without drugs.

- Take your blood pressure every day. It used to be thought that people taking their own blood pressure would be made anxious or neurotic about it but twenty years of clinical experience shows that this is not the case. Rather, research has found that people get reassurance from measuring their own blood pressure. This may account, at least in part, for the positive results achieved by people monitoring their own levels.

  A study in Seattle asked sixty hypertensive people to measure their own blood pressure at home twice a day for a month. At the end of the month there were significant reductions in blood pressure (10 points or more) in 43 per cent of the sixty. Clearly the actual taking of the blood pressure had acted as a sort of simple biofeedback mechanism.

- Getting a pet appears also to help with high blood pressure–even a tankful of fish can be beneficial! A researcher at the University of Pennsylvania thinks that 'companion animals in particular provide an access to intimacy'. You talk to your pet more slowly, you smile a great deal, your voice becomes gentle and the cadence of the speech changes. It is a much more relaxed dialogue, characterised by a combination of touching and talking! Pets exert a calming effect through the day. He found that the presence of pets reduced their owner's blood pressure by 10–15 per cent. Anything that turns your attention outwards to the natural environment around you is a powerful way of controlling tension.

- Eat onions and garlic. The Bulgarian Academy of Sciences in Sofia tested extracts of garlic on forty-six hypertensives. Most showed a drop in blood pressure of about 20 points as well as a decrease in physical symptoms. Onions are now known to contain prostaglandins, natural hormone-like substances that lower blood pressure.

- A recent study at the Oregon Health Sciences University has found that there is a link between calcium and high blood pressure. A study of computerised records of 10,000 people in the US aged between 18 and 74 found that there was a direct link between the amount of calcium they ate and their likelihood of suffering from hypertension. People suffering from the disease were on average eating between 18 and 22 per cent less calcium than those with normal blood pressures. Conversely, those who had a high calcium intake had low blood pressure. Clearly much more research needs to be done on this. In any event, the finding does not mean that we should all go out and drink large amounts of milk (which contains calcium),

as milk (whole milk at least – skimmed milk is better) contains unwelcome levels of fat.

The role of calcium in blood pressure is complicated and not yet totally worked out, but there is now considerable interest in calcium-antagonist drugs. Epidemiological evidence suggests that there is a link between low dietary calcium and high blood pressure as we have seen, but large trials have yet to be carried out. Some studies giving one gram of calcium to people with normal blood pressure have shown a substantial lowering of blood pressure. There is epidemiological evidence linking high blood pressure in pregnancy with calcium deficiency.

- There appears to be a link between alcohol and high blood pressure. Withdrawal of alcohol from someone who is used to drinking produces a rise in blood pressure before there is a fall. The re-introduction of alcohol then produces a rise in pressure within a few days. It is best to avoid alcohol altogether, if you have high blood pressure.

- Saturated fats may play a part. Research in Finland suggests that reducing the ratio of saturated to polyunsaturated fats in the diet may reduce blood pressure. This is independent of the effects on cholesterol and unrelated to dietary salt intake.

- There are several studies which

suggest that the Pill causes a small but significant rise in blood pressure. It probably makes sense to use another method of contraception if you are at all worried about your blood pressure, if there is a history of blood pressure in your immediate family, or if you are over 35.

- Lead and cadmium are dangerous to those who work with them. They should be avoided in the workplace whenever possible.

- One of the main features of modern food processing has been to reduce the amount of potassium we consume. Cooking vegetables in large volumes of water also reduces their potassium content and the adding of salt during cooking does the same. Giving potassium to people with normal blood pressure reduces the blood pressure. It is also well proven that vegetarians (who consume more potassium than the rest of the population) have lower blood pressures than do omnivores. It thus seems sensible, if you have high blood pressure, to include potassium-rich foods in your diet and to cook carefully so as to retain the potassium you buy. Also, restrict salt intake to help the potassium do its job.

HYPOGLYCAEMIA

What is it?

A condition in which the pancreas produces too much insulin (usually in response to a high sugar load in the diet) which in turn produces a host of mental, emotional and physical symptoms.

Hypoglycaemia is a normal phenomenon too. When our stomachs get very empty the level of glucose (sugar) in the blood falls and makes us feel hungry and faint. We remedy this by eating. The sort of hypoglycaemia we are looking at here is somewhat different.

All the cells of our bodies need glucose for energy but this is especially true of the brain. It cannot function normally for long without its supply of glucose. Some parts of the body store glucose but the brain needs a reliable ongoing supply. This is why any shortage of glucose in the brain's blood supply can cause so many symptoms related to the brain. Nervousness, anxiety, irritability, depression (even suicidal feelings), forgetfulness, poor circulation, poor decision-making, nightmares, weepiness, and sensitivity to noise, are just some of the mental and emotional symptoms that have been reported in hypoglycaemia.

The physical symptoms of hypoglycaemia are just as real and just as disturbing as are the mental and psychological ones. Palpitation, weakness, dizziness, shaking and sweating, blurred vision and headaches are all common. Some people black out altogether if their blood sugar falls very low.

What causes it?

- If the brain is starved of blood sugar, it may appear that the answer must be to eat more sugar and sweet foods. The answer is in fact exactly the opposite. Hypoglycaemia is caused by an overindulgence in sugary foods. The average westerner eats or drinks more than forty teaspoonsful of sugar a day. He or she also eats large amounts of refined carbohydrate foods – all of which are converted into sugar by the body. The pancreas, faced with this overload, is forced to produce abnormally large peaks of insulin. This effectively sweeps away the excess glucose from the blood but often there is an over-supply of insulin, which causes the blood glucose to plummet. The result is low blood sugar – hypoglycaemia with all its symptoms.

- Two interesting studies bear this out. In the first a doctor researcher in the field gave a glucose-tolerance test to 220 neurotic patients with obvious symptoms of low blood sugar, such as fatigue. In fact 205 of them had low blood sugar. When these depressed, anxiety-ridden people were put on to a sensible diet, both their physical and psychological symptoms disappeared.

Next, the same researcher did a hypoglycaemia blood test on 700 people who had *no* physical symptoms of hypoglycaemia yet had all kinds of odd psychological signs and symptoms. The test showed that 600 had the condition! When put on to the right diet they all regained their mental health.

A study of 144 children with 'learning disability' found that 78 per cent had hypoglycaemia, and many other studies have produced similar findings.

Many experts in this field now see hypoglycaemia as a source of marital and family problems that is almost entirely overlooked.

When the blood sugar drops, the adrenal glands pour out their hormones to release sugar from the body's stores, but unfortunately caffeine, alcohol and nicotine also stimulate the adrenal glands in this way, so triggering the pancreas to produce more insulin. This produces hypoglycaemia. The cigarette or drink of coffee makes the person feel good for a while but once the blood sugar plummets they are forced to go back to the cigarettes and coffee to give them a lift again. And so it goes on.

- Chronic stress seems to predispose people to hypoglycaemia.

- There is now evidence that certain specific foods can produce an abnormally low, or indeed high, blood sugar, irrespective of their actual carbohydrate content.

Given that wheat and dairy products are two of the most commonly offending foods in adults, it is hardly surprising that a high-protein, low-carbohydrate diet is of provable value in managing hypoglycaemia.

- Deficiencies of certain nutrients, such as magnesium, chromium, potassium, manganese, zinc and the B vitamins can all produce the condition.

- Certain drugs, notably metronidazole (Flagyl) used to treat vaginal thrichomoniasis and parasitic infestations of the gut, can cause hypoglycaemia.

- Missed meals are a common cause, in children especially. Tea and coffee increase the release of insulin from the pancreas and can produce hypoglycaemic symptoms.

- Smoking causes both insulin and glucagon to be released with resulting hypoglycaemia. Often a smoker then needs to 'top up' his blood sugar with another cigarette.

- Alcohol can produce profound hypoglycaemia and alcoholics coming off alcohol should always be given an anti-hypolglycaemic diet.

Prevention

- Change your diet to remove all added sugar and unrefined carbohydrates.

- Eat six small meals a day rather than three large ones. Don't eat more food–simply eat the same amount spread out more evenly.

- Eat more unrefined, complex carbohydrate foods and plenty of fruit and vegetables.

- Take brewers' yeast tablets–the chromium these contain helps sugar metabolism.

- Cut right down on caffeine-containing drinks, alcohol and cigarettes.

- Be sure to keep up your level of animal-protein intake. This provides a substance known as carnitine–a deficiency of which can produce hypoglycaemia and heart disease.

- Take a vitamin and mineral supplement containing the following:
  Vitamin B complex, 100 mg daily
  Tryptophan, 500–1500 mg daily
  Chromium GTF, 200 mcg daily
  Zinc, 15–25 mg daily
  Manganese, 5–10 mg daily
  Magnesium, 250–300 mg daily
  Potassium, 500–1000 mg daily
  Vitamin C, 2–3 g daily

- Talk to your doctor about stopping metronidazole if you are on it.

HYPOTHERMIA

What is it?

A condition in which a person, usually elderly, becomes very cold and can die. Technically speaking it occurs when the body temperature falls below 35°C (95°F)–the normal is 37°C (98.6°F). Obviously this is a some- what arbitrary cut-off point as many individuals will be able to live at this temperature whilst others will be severely ill.

The outward signs of the condition are drowsiness, slurred speech, unsteady movement, a pale and puffy face, mental confusion, a slow pulse and breathing, and cold-feeling skin. Treatment involves slow, gentle, re-warming. A doctor should always be called because the condition is usually much more serious than at first appears.

What causes it?

Younger people can tolerate very wide swings in ambient temperature without any danger to their bodies. Their natural thermostat keeps the body temperature steady at around 98.6°F. Their skin temperature may fall but the 'core' of the body remains at the correct temperature. For vari- ous reasons to do with the ageing process, and as a result of inactivity, poor food intake and poor clothing, many older people easily get ex- tremely cold so that even the very core of their bodies cools down.

The condition often goes undiag- nosed because the standard clinical thermometer does not go down as low as 35°C. This can be a very serious hazard because the condition is fatal–killing as it does nearly 1,000 old people a year in the UK alone.

Prevention

- Move the individual's bed into the warmest room of the house– usually the living room–and keep that room at 70°F. Ensure that all heating appliances give sufficient heat, and are safe, easy to manage, and economical.

- Draughtproof the room.

- Check for rising damp and damp coming through the walls (from blocked drains and gutters). Ensure that there is adequate ventilation to combat condensa- tion.

- Arrange for frequent, small meals throughout the day–meals on wheels if necessary. Take fre- quent, small, hot drinks through- out the day from a thermos flask.

- Ensure that at least one meal a day is hot.

- Use an electric blanket but ensure that it is switched off when you are in bed.

- Wear several layers of thin clo- thing made of closely woven fabric. Air is the best insulator so the principle is to trap as much air as possible between the layers of clothes. Down-filled clothing is the most effective insulator. Wearing long underwear does not actually make much difference to how much heat we lose but it does make us *feel* warmer. It is also amazing how much warmer putting on a hat can make you.

- The body acclimatises to the cold by producing more heat and scientists can measure this. On exposure to cold the fingers of a person who has adjusted to the cold have a greater blood supply and warmer temperature than those of one who has not adjusted. One of the best ways to adjust to cold is to exercise. Riding a stationary bicycle or 'conducting' an imaginary orchestra perhaps to the accompaniment of the radio or record player works wonders. This activity creates heat. When sleeping or sitting in a chair the body burns about 100 calories per hour but just standing up raises it to 140 and doing gentle household chores raises it by another 40.

- Fats and carbohydrates are the best fuel for the body to use to make heat. Healthy sources are wholemeal bread, nuts, grains and fruit. Eating hot meals and drinking hot drinks raises the core temperature of the body and so works wonders in warming it up where it matters most.

- Low levels of vitamin C are related to a decreased resistance to cold, as is a low level of vitamin B. Supplementing both these in full doses therefore helps prevent hypothermia.

IMPOTENCE

What is it?

A condition in which a man is persistently or recurrently unable to obtain or maintain an erection of sufficient rigidity to have intercourse. It can have a partly physical basis or can be a form of unconscious sex avoidance.

What causes it?

Most impotent men believe that there is a physical cause for their impotence but this is probably not so, and psychosexual therapy can often do much to cure them. However, there is little doubt that zinc deficiency, for example, is much more common than is realised and this provably contributes to the problem. There are scores of causes for impotence – here are just a few of them.

- Any painful condition of the penis, such as a tight foreskin.

- Diabetes is a common cause – about half of all middle-aged insulin-dependent diabetics have sexual problems, the most troublesome of which is impotence.

- Any arterial disease that produces a reduced blood supply to the penis is a well-recognised cause.

- Certain diseases of the nervous system such as multiple sclerosis and paralysis.

- Certain operations, including prostatectomy and pelvic surgery for cancer.

- Certain hormone deficiencies.

- Psychological illnesses such as depression.

- Alcohol.

- Zinc deficiency.

- Smoking.

- Drug abuse.

- Medical drugs, especially those for high blood pressure, and anti-depressants.

- Various psychological reasons, including: the man unconsciously thinking of his partner as his mother; guilt about sex; such a degree of anxiety that he is unable to relax and let an erection occur; a fear of women and their 'purity'; a fear of VD or unwanted pregnancy (this is especially common in extramarital impotence); misperceptions of women's sexuality generally; and many more.

- Earlier failures – leading to the belief that he will always fail.

- Old age. As men age they tend to become less potent. Few men in their nineties are potent.

- Any of the reasons that cause a loss of sex drive (see page 317).

- Doubts about the relationship with the partner.

- Hostility towards the woman (often not recognised consciously).

- Fear of being detected (in the parental home or in a public place, for example).

- Tiredness, either mental or physical.

- Latent homosexuality – the man would unconsciously rather be with another man and not his partner.

- Fear of hurting his partner, especially after a baby or an operation on the woman.

- An overdemanding woman.

- Stress – from, for example, work, money, home, business problems, or worries about children and parents.

Clearly these causes are many and complex and will often need to be sorted out with the help of a professional who is expert in the area. Having said this, there *are* some preventable causes so we shall now look at these.

Prevention

As with any sex problem, prevention starts in the cradle with parents bringing up their children to have a natural, uninhibited view of their sexuality as a normal part of life. Let's look now at the preventable causes of impotence:

- Any painful condition of the penis should be treated – see your doctor.

- Ensuring that your diabetes is well controlled can prevent any sexual problems getting worse (see page 198 for the prevention of diabetes).

- Recent French research found that most of the men they studied who were impotent improved on a diet low in animal fats. The researchers also took the men off cigarettes (see below). Both of these practices benefit the arteries in such a way as to improve the blood flow to the penis. In many middle-aged men who have been smoking and eating a diet heavy in fats for some years the calibre of the penile arteries is reduced. In the heart this narrowing produces angina and even a heart attack but in the pelvis it produces impotence.

- Alcohol can undermine sexual drive because it tends to reduce the production of sex hormones. Even those who take only one or two alcoholic drinks a day can suffer the harmful effects of alcohol. Unfortunately, a fair proportion of impotent men use alcohol to overcome their fears of failure and at the same time to give themselves an excuse for failing.

- Zinc deficiency. This condition is much more widespread than is generally recognised and the effects of a reduced level of zinc are now well documented. Too little zinc results in a low sperm count, poor development of the testes and penis in young men, and prostatic problems in older ones. Recent research has found that it does not take much of a zinc deficiency to play havoc with potency. Studies at the Wayne State University in Michigan have found the zinc deficiencies artificially induced by feeding men zinc-deficient diets made their sperm counts and their testosterone levels fall. Testosterone is the hormone that is responsible for sex drive in both men and women, so clearly zinc is vitally important.

  Another study found that men complained of diminished interest in sex when fed a zinc-restricted diet. After they received several meals fortified with 30 mg zinc a day their sexual appetites returned to normal within 16–20 weeks. The cadmium in cigarette smoke interferes with zinc metabolism and accumulation in the testes. Alcohol makes the body excrete too much zinc. This causes a loss of appetite which in turn makes it more likely that the man will drink more rather than eat more. The same effect is seen in men with severe kidney disease. About 70 per cent of renal patients have some degree of impotence but studies have found that these can usually be reversed by giving zinc supplements. In one study twenty men aged 28–65 who were on dialysis machines all had low sperm counts and low testosterone levels. A study was carried out giving 50 mg zinc twice a day to some subjects, and a placebo to others – without either group knowing which they were getting. After a year every zinc-treated man showed biochemical improvement and reported restored potency. In some cases the potency returned in six weeks. The placebo-fed group stayed as they were.

If you are on drugs for high blood pressure, follow the regime on page 242 and reduce your drugs under your doctor's supervision. This will reduce the impotence-producing effects they have.

- Keep up a healthy diet in old age, ensuring especially that you take vitamin and mineral supplements. As we age our intestines absorb nutrients less efficiently, and because of poor appetites and low exercise levels many old people eat poorly anyway.

- If you have tried all the 'treatable' causes of impotence and still have no result, perhaps the problem is 'in the mind'. The ideal starting point is to discuss the whole subject with your partner, being careful not to apportion blame.

Stop having intercourse. Once the threat of having to perform is removed, many impotent men can erect perfectly well and, with the help of their partner, can get used once more to having full and spontaneous orgasms, by masturbation. By alternately stimulating

and not stimulating the penis the partner of such a man can often train him, over a few weeks, to have long-lasting, good-quality erections.

During all this the couple should go back to courtship behaviour (see page 319) with the emphasis on closeness, loving, kissing, mutual pleasuring, massage and so on. When the genitals are brought into play the emphasis can be more on looking and admiration (like children) than on performance. The woman can be of great help by sharing her fantasies and intimate sexuality with the man. This helps him see her as a real woman with earthy needs and appetites and not as an untouchable virgin who is too 'nice' to want sex. This works wonders in many such cases. The woman can also help by making a conscious effort not to behave in a 'motherly' way that reminds the man of his mother. Few men can function well in this situation because sex with one's mother (and by extension anyone who behaves in a 'motherly' way) is forbidden. On the other hand, quickly switching to sexy underwear and becoming a sex siren can also be intimidating and could appear to the impotent man to be a demand for performance which can set back his progress.

Along with all this the man should re-establish self-masturbation so that he eventually learns that the 'uncontrollable' is in fact not so. Sex aids can be useful at this stage. Progress towards intercourse should be slow and controlled, or good gains made over several weeks can be lost in one love-making episode.

- Lastly, give yourself a chance to have an erection. Too many men bring their worries and overactive mind with them into the marriage bed. Give yourself a chance to unwind before sex. At work a man is generally non-sexual and few men can change instantly from this mode into the lover role. Get changed into comfortable clothes, relax, have a small drink. Spend time together just talking or reading something erotic. Get the lead-up to sex right, spending time showering or bathing alone or together, then cuddle and kiss before even trying to have intercourse or produce an erection.

INDIGESTION

What is it?

Indigestion is a vague term used to describe pains or discomfort in the abdomen after eating or drinking. Dyspepsia is a discomfort in the uppermost part of the abdomen after food. Some people's indigestion is caused by a peptic ulcer (see page 362).

What causes it?

- Peptic ulcer (see page 362).
- Smoking.
- Alcohol, tea and coffee.
- Specific foods (often spicy ones or sugar).
- Fatty foods.
- Stress.
- Too little gastric acid.
- Hypoglycaemia (see page 248).
- Thrush (see page 348).
- Reflux oesophagitis or hiatus hernia (see page 232).
- Irritable bowel syndrome (see page 271).
- Gall-bladder problems.
- Angina.

Prevention

- Smoking stimulates the production of gastric acid and can cause quite severe indigestion in some people. Smoking also reduces the efficiency of the valve of the top of the stomach, so allowing acid stomach contents to flow into the lower end of the gullet (oesophagus) and cause pain there. Other substances that do this are chocolate, alcohol, spearmint, and peppermint. Stopping smoking brings relief in days to many people with indigestion. Any treatment being given for indigestion is made less effective in someone who continues to smoke.

- Alcohol, tea and coffee stimulate gastric-acid production. Experiment with leaving out all of these for a few days and see the results. If the indigestion goes completely reintroduce one drink at a time (weak if it is tea or coffee, and infrequently in the case of alcohol) and stop as soon as you get indigestion again. It may be that there is one (or more) of them that you will never be able to drink without feeling ill.

- Research has found that certain individuals improve when they go on to a low-carbohydrate diet. Sucrose increases pepsin secretion by the stomach by 200 per cent. The same study found that eight out of nine people with hiatus hernia did better when they went on a similar diet, low in refined carbohydrates. Five out of eight people with duodenal ulcer also improved.

- Fatty foods often produce pain or discomfort in the upper abdomen (if the individual's gall-bladder is not working well) partly because of gall-stones. If fatty foods regularly bring on your indigestion, see your doctor.

- Stress is a potent stimulant to gastric acid, and many people complain of odd discomforts and uneasiness in the stomach when they are stressed. Stress also affects the rate at which the stomach digests food and passes it on to the intestine, and this can cause indigestion as well. Ways of preventing stress are looked at on page 87.

- Although many people with indigestion have too much gastric acid and improve when taking antacids, some do not. These people have *too little* acid in their stomachs and the antacids make them worse. Prevention here involves taking pepsin and hydrochloric acid supplements regularly. A good way to take hydrochloric acid is in the form of 1–3 tablets of betaine hydrochloride before each meal.

- The yeast *Candida albicans*, which causes thrush, can infect the stomach and produce a sense of burning after the ingestion of food. This type of indigestion can only be cleared up by treating the infection.

- In the irritable bowel syndrome the colon (large bowel) goes into spasm after food (see page 271). The middle part of the colon lies in the upper abdomen very near the stomach and this pain can be mistaken for indigestion. Prevention of this condition is discussed on page 272.

- Angina pectoris can often mimic indigestion. If you have any history of heart disease in your family or have any of the risk factors known to be important in heart disease (see page 234) always take 'indigestion' seriously. The prevention of indigestion in your case might be to treat your angina.

- If you have indigestion *don't* take a sloppy diet or drink lots of milk as neither have been proven to reduce indigestion, except temporarily. Unfortunately, they often worsen it because milk produces a rebound *over*production of acid once its initial buffering effect has passed.

INFECTIOUS DISEASES IN CHILDREN

What are they?

Almost any infectious disease can occur in children, just as in adults, but some diseases are very much more dangerous than others if contracted early in life. For this reason immunisation schemes are in operation to prevent such diseases. Diphtheria, whooping cough, tetanus, measles and poliomyelitis are still very serious diseases which are better prevented, and immunisation against them is recommended. Although tetanus is rare in the UK it is commonest in children and it is conveniently prevented by a vaccine given along with that against whooping cough and diphtheria.

The five diseases mentioned above are serious but are all preventable.

Whooping cough

A very common and highly infectious disease. It is caught from other children and causes long and exhausting bouts of coughing. They can be so severe that the child can't breathe and vomits a lot. As a result, the child becomes ill, loses weight and can suffer severe medical complications, which can include ear infections, hernias, pneumonia, collapsed lungs, bronchitis and even convulsions. Over the last five years prior to writing forty children have died from whooping cough in England and Wales.

Diphtheria

This starts like a sore throat but can last for weeks as a serious illness. It blocks the nose and throat, making breathing difficult or impossible. The toxins produced by the bacteria attack the heart and nervous systems. Diphtheria is very rare in the UK but is still a killer worldwide.

Tetanus

This disease is caught by germs in the soil getting into an open wound. The bacteria produce a toxin which attacks the nervous system, causing painful muscle spasms. Because they occur in the jaws on occasions, the disease has become known as 'lockjaw'. Tetanus is uncommon but people still die of it every year in the UK.

Polio

Now uncommon in the UK, polio is still seen worldwide, even in quite sophisticated countries. It attacks the nervous system and causes muscle paralysis. If the breathing muscles are affected the child can die. If it affects the legs they can become weak, and permanent disability can result.

Measles

The most common infectious disease in the world, measles starts like a bad cold and the child has a fever and rash. Red spots appear behind the ears and spread to the face and body. Whilst measles *can* be trivial it can also be very serious.It causes an inflammation of the brain in some cases and a few children are permanently braindamaged as a result. It can also cause ear infections and convulsions. About twenty children a year die from measles in the UK.

Immunisation

There is a different schedule of immunisation times from country to country and there is a good case to be made for delaying immunisation against diphtheria, whooping cough and tetanus until the second half of the first year of life in children in industrialised countries. The reasons for this are as follows. First, infections of these diseases are rare in babies under 6 months in developed countries, and second, the presence of natural antibodies masks the antigenic effect of certain vaccines. If a mother has immunity to a disease she will usually transmit it to her baby. This interferes with the effec-

tiveness of the vaccines if given in the first three months of life. Most natural antibodies disappear over the first few months of life but measles antibodies from the mother can protect the baby up to one year old. This is one reason why measles vaccine is not given until the second year of life. The third reason is that young babies are not immunologically mature and do not respond to antigens by producing antibodies in the normal way. Lastly, reactions to vaccines are more common in very young babies. Not only are reactions to vaccines unfortunate for the baby in whom they occur but the bad news spreads and makes other parents less likely to immunise their children.

Immunisation against the five diseases outlined above not only protects the child who is immunised but also reduces the risk within your family if you have another child later. A new baby is always at risk from infections carried by older children, and if your older children are immunised your baby will be at less risk.

Every vaccine is hazardous to some people in certain conditions. The danger or inconvenience of such reactions has to be weighed against the dangers to life and health if the baby subsequently suffers from the disease itself. Normally reactions are minimal or non-existent, but babies who come from allergic families need special care. Discuss the whole subject with your doctor before having your baby vaccinated if the baby: has had a reaction to a previous vaccination; is sensitive to egg; has just had or is recovering from any illness; is sensitive to antibiotics; is taking any medicines; has fits; or comes from an allergic family.

Here is a recommended schedule of routine immunisations that will suit most people.

During the first year of life

Combined diphtheria, tetanus, whooping cough and oral polio vaccine–a second dose is given 6–8 weeks after the first, and a third dose follows after a six months' gap.

The earliest the first dose can be given is at about three months but it is better to wait until 6 months in order to get the best immunological response in the baby.

During the second year of life

Measles vaccine. Delaying this vaccination until the third year reduces the risk of occasional severe reactions which occur in children under the age of 3.

At the age of five

A booster dose of diphtheria/tetanus/whooping cough/polio vaccine.

Between the ages of 10 and 13

BCG vaccination to all those shown by the skin test to need this protection against tuberculosis.

All girls ages 11–13

Rubella (German measles) vaccination. This should be offered to girls whether or not they have a history of German measles, to ensure that they enter their childbearing years protected against this disease which, if caught early in pregnancy, can produce such devastating effects on the unborn baby. Be sure to leave at least a month between the BCG and rubella vaccinations.

On leaving school

Polio vaccine and tetanus toxoid booster. The tetanus booster should then be repeated every ten years throughout adulthood to be safe.

Vaccinations against influenza and infectious diseases you are likely to come into contact with when travelling abroad should be discussed with your doctor. Remember that polio and TB are still very common worldwide, even in relatively advanced countries. Be sure to keep your vaccination levels of these up if you are travelling anywhere other than to highly westernised cities.

INFERTILITY

What is it?

Primary infertility (as opposed to secondary infertility which occurs in a couple who have already had a baby but have trouble conceiving again) is present when a couple cannot conceive after a year of unprotected, unlimited intercourse. Almost one in seven of all couples in the West are infertile and the number is growing.

What causes it?

- Putting off having babies until the woman is past her peak fertility. The average couple are at peak fertility in their early twenties and most don't start trying to have children until five to ten years after this. A woman's eggs (ova) are all present at birth and age along with the rest of her body. By the time she is 30 some of the eggs are already of poor quality and so do not result in a fetus, or are aborted spontaneously very early. About seven or eight out of every ten conceptions in human beings end up being wasted naturally. Well over 30 per cent of women aged 40–45 are infertile and one UK study found that three-quarters of mothers having a baby when they were 30 or more had been having unprotected intercourse for two years or more before they conceived.

- VD is now a real epidemic, especially in the form of gonorrhoea. Its growth is exceptionally high among teenagers. A substantial proportion of females with gonorrhoea have no symptoms and by the time they know they have it their fallopian tubes have been irreparably damaged and so cannot allow an egg to pass from the ovaries to the uterus.

- Prolonged use of the Pill can delay the return of ovulation after stopping the drug in about 2 per cent of women. This is a very small proportion but the number of individuals is large because of the numbers of women on the Pill–nearly 3 million in the UK.

- The IUDs (intrauterine devices) currently used can delay the return of conception and older women seem to fare especially badly in this respect. Also, IUDs are often associated with subclinical pelvic infections which can cause infertility in their own right.

- Abortions are followed by infections and damage to the cervix in a small number of women. These effects are very uncommon, but given the increasing numbers of women involved the numbers of individuals with such problems are building up.

- Exposure to drugs, pollutants, food additives and so on is rising and some undoubtedly play a part in the increasing toll of infertility.

- Not making love around the time of ovulation. Many infertile couples attending clinics are having intercourse only once a month and then not around ovulation time.

- Using lubricants, jellies, etc. All such creams, jellies and lubricants kill sperms, at least to some extent.

- Women who get up immediately after sex, so allowing the semen to run out. This is fine if the man has a large volume and she is very fertile but this may not be the case.

- The couple have sex problems which means they rarely make love.

- The man's scrotum is too hot. Sperms need to be kept at 2–3°C lower temperature than the rest of the body or they die or don't even form properly. This is why the testes lie outside the body.

- Gross obesity.

- Smoking, drinking and hard drugs all reduce sperm counts.

- Stress can inhibit ovulation in a woman and sperm formation in a man.

- Ovulation problems are the most common cause of infertility in women. Usually the cause is unknown but the post-Pill syndrome has been mentioned above.

- Endometriosis is a common cause of female infertility. Some of the lining tissue of the womb finds its way into the pelvic cavity and embeds there to produce pain and bleeding every month with a period.

- Varicocele is the name given to a vein that supplies a testis (usually the left one) when that vein is varicose. About 30 per cent of male infertility is thought to be caused by this.

- Zinc deficiency. Zinc is known to be necessary for many parts of the male genital system and is found in greater concentration in the male prostate gland than in any other part of the body. Zinc deficiency definitely reduces sperm quality.

- Low sperm volume is an uncommon cause of male infertility.

- Some women become allergic to their partner's sperms and so never conceive.

- Certain drug allergies cause a temporary shutdown of sperm production if the drug is taken.

- Really poor nutrition undoubtedly reduces sperm production. Vitamins A, B and C have been found to be vital in human sperm formation and function and vitamin E is vital in rats at least.

- Drugs can affect fertility in two ways. First, they may affect a man's sex drive so that he wants to have sex only very infrequently (alcohol, sleeping tablets, tranquillisers, anti-depressants and some anti-blood-pressure drugs are examples). Second, several drugs actually affect sperm production. (Examples of these are sex hormones, anti-malarial drugs, certain anti-cancer drugs and Depo Provera.)

- Impatience. Some couples are not really infertile but expect to conceive almost immediately and worry when they do not.

Prevention

The list of causes of infertility is long and there are many more causes for which there is no known preventive. Let's look at each of those listed above in turn and see what can be done to prevent it in the first place.

- Have babies younger rather than older. Ideally a woman should (from the fertility point of view) have completed her family by the time she is 30. Of course, there are other constraints – social, financial, etc. – which could make this difficult or undesirable.

- Prevent VD (see page 378). Treat suspicious symptoms early.

- Have breaks from the Pill every two years and use another method for a few months. Today's young woman may well have been on the Pill for a decade before trying to conceive – a consequence may be that she does not start to ovulate again as soon as she would like.

- Don't use an IUD if you are at all worried about your fertility.

- Do all you can to prevent unwanted pregnancies (see page 365) so that you never have to have an abortion.

- Take as few drugs and highly coloured and adulterated foods as possible.

- Make love around ovulation. This usually occurs fourteen days before the onset of a period, and you can time your love-making using a calendar or by charting the temperature rise that occurs at ovulation. Make love on alternate days (to allow the man time to build up a good stock of semen) around ovulation to stand the best chance.

- The woman should lie down on her back after sex, preferably with her hips on a pillow. This gives the sperm the best chance of swimming up into the uterus.

- Go to a professional to sort out any sex problems you may have.

- The man should wear boxer shorts and not Y-fronts or similar tight-fitting pants. He should avoid hot baths and showers.

- Lose weight if you are obese.

- Stop or drastically cut down on your smoking, drinking and the use of hard or soft drugs.

- Learn how to relax and reduce stress in your life (see page 87).

- If you have any pain on deep penetration see your doctor and get him or her to rule out or treat endometriosis if necessary.

- Abide by the advice for preventing varicose veins (see page 377) to prevent a varicocele.

- Take zinc supplements and eat zinc-rich foods (seafoods, bran, cows' milk, peas and carrots).

- Have sex at most every other day and preferably every third day. Some men with poor semen volume have sex with a frequency that means they deposit so little semen in their partner's vagina that she stands little chance of conceiving.

- If it is proved that the woman is allergic to her partner's sperms the man can wear a sheath for a year so that her body becomes desensitised to the sperms. Drugs are also used in this condition.

- If you ever have an allergic reaction to a medication or drug, keep off it for good. Only take drugs that are absolutely essential if you are trying to conceive – find ways of dealing with the problem other than using drugs.

- Don't be impatient. It takes an average of 5.3 months for a couple who are normally fertile to conceive. Twenty-five per cent will have conceived in the first month; 63 per cent by the end of six months; 75 per cent by the end of 9 months and 80 per cent after a year. Getting impatient and worrying about not conceiving is counterproductive because a woman who is worried tends to be less likely to ovulate normally, and a man who is worried may have difficulty erecting.

INFLAMMATORY BOWEL DISEASE

What is it?

Inflammatory bowel disease is a blanket term that covers two major conditions, Crohn's disease and ulcerative colitis. They are very much more common than they used to be, hospitalising more than 100,000 people in the US every year.

At first symptoms are so mild that you ignore them: a bout of diarrhoea every few months and occasional abdominal pain. As the years pass the symptoms get worse. There is either diarrhoea or constipation and the stools are bloody. Fleeting abdominal pain turns into chronic pains and the person feels ill and lacking in energy.

The vast majority of medical efforts are useless in these conditions though drugs can help a few and surgery a few more.

What causes it?

No one knows for sure but there are several plausible theories.

- Food intolerance. A group of researchers in Cambridge have found intolerance in Crohn's disease (see page 216 for more on food intolerance).

- Crohn's disease was unknown until the 1930s, but now it affects one in every 3,000 westerners. Because there have been such profound dietary changes over this period research has been aimed at dietary factors. A German study found that patients with Crohn's disease 'consumed large quantities of refined carbohydrate'. Another survey of the breakfast habits of Crohn's disease patients found that they usually ate refined breakfast cereals such as cornflakes. In a survey of sugar intake Crohn's patients were found to eat the equivalent of ten teaspoons a day while those without the disease ate seven. Other studies have found that Crohn's patients add 26 per cent more sugar to tea and coffee, and 13 per cent more to cereals than do people without the disease.

- Zinc deficiency is now well recognised as part of the problem. Crohn's patients have many dietary deficiencies, partly because they lose their appetite and eat so poorly and partly because the disease itself reduces the intestinal absorption of nutrients. Crohn's patients have insufficient levels of protein, iron, folate, calcium and vitamin B_{12}. Recently, though, zinc deficiency has been found to be the most important of all. Zinc controls many body systems but in Crohn's patients its lack further heightens the poor appetite and loss of taste for food. Many Crohn's patients have no desire to eat. Zinc is also vital for healthy skin and some people with this condition have severe skin rashes. Normal eyesight needs zinc and some Crohn's patients have night blindness. Zinc is vital for wound healing and Crohn's disease never fully heals.

  Adults with Crohn's disease have been found to have zinc levels 15 per cent lower than normal, and their sense of taste has been found to be 65 per cent duller than normal. Studies giving patients with Crohn's disease zinc supplements have found that several of the abnormalities associated with the condition are eliminated.

- Vitamin C deficiency can also cause some of the symptoms of Crohn's disease. One study found that Crohn's patients had vitamin C levels 32 per cent lower than normal. This led the researchers to suggest that all patients with Crohn's disease should supplement their diet with vitamin C.

- There is some evidence of a link between Crohn's disease and psoriasis and monilia. Though there is little true scientific evidence to support it, anecdotal evidence shows that some people with inflammatory bowel disease improve on nystatin–the antifungal drug–combined with a low-yeast, low-refined-carbohydrate diet.

Prevention

There is probably no way of preventing inflammatory bowel disease from occurring in the first place but under-standing the causes suggests some valuable ways of preventing the disease getting worse once it is present.

- If you are allergic to or intolerant of any foods, don't eat them (see page 216). This could prevent unseen and unrecognised damage being done to the large bowel.

- Eat a diet low in refined carbohydrates and rich in unrefined ones.

- Eat less sugar.

- Eat more dietary fibre.

- Take zinc supplements once you start to suffer from any of the symptoms of the disease.

- Take vitamin C in large doses – 1 g twice a day – if you have the condition.

- Talk to your doctor about trying nystatin and go on to a low-yeast diet (see page 349).

INSOMNIA

What is it?

The inability to get to sleep or to get as much sleep as we think we should have. Many people troubled by insomnia believe they need more sleep than they actually do. This is especially true of the elderly, who are often immobile or take very little exercise, snooze on and off through-

out the day, and then worry that they don't sleep for eight hours at night as well.

Research has found that most people sleep too much and could manage just as well with far less. Certainly it is true that prolonged sleeplessness is harmful but it has also been found that most healthy adults could function perfectly adequately on four or five hours' sleep.

There are many unhelpful myths about sleep that make people feel bad about perfectly 'normal' insomnia. Some imagine that they are being punished for some evil deed by not being able to sleep; others equate insomnia with madness; and from the perfectly reasonable notion that some ill people have difficulty sleeping many people jump to the conclusion that everyone who can't sleep must be ill. Memories of childhood scoldings also play a part with many people. They remember being told they were naughty for not being asleep, yet they probably didn't need that much sleep then and certainly don't now.

What causes it?

- Any illness, and especially a feverish one, or one that causes pain, will cause even the best sleeper to have difficulty sleeping.

- Drinking tea or coffee too close to retiring is a common cause. People forget just how potent a stimulant coffee is. Some people cannot sleep until 4 a.m. after one cup of coffee at 7 o'clock the previous evening.

- Deficiencies of vitamins B_1 and B_6 can cause insomnia, as can deficiencies of zinc, manganese, calcium and magnesium.

- Too big a meal just before retiring.

- In children sleep may be broken by night terrors, nightmares or sleepwalking—and, of course, some adults suffer from these too.

- Going to bed too soon after extreme mental or physical effort is a sure recipe for sleeplessness because the body is keyed up for action.

- Jetlag and time-zone changes.

- A bad bed.

- Depression. This is probably the most common cause of insomnia in adults. There is usually a depressed mood, a loss of weight and appetite, poor sex drive, irritability, tearfulness, poor concentration, poor memory, an inability to make decisions, and a general lack of vitality. Such people have difficulty falling asleep and then wake in the early hours (around 4 or 5 a.m.) and don't go back to sleep.

- In some neurotic states the sufferer has difficulty getting off to sleep or wakes frequently with bad dreams and nightmares. Some people are in a perfectly normal psychological state yet are woken by bad dreams and nightmares as a result of eating certain foods. Red wine and cheese seem to be particularly potent in this respect, which is hardly surprising as they contain a vaso-active amine called tyramine.

- Sexual frustration is a not uncommon cause of insomnia. Most people say that they sleep better after intercourse or masturbation.

- Schizophrenics, especially young ones, often spend hours tramping round the house at night.

- Senile dementia can cause a reversal of the normal sleep pattern, with the old person sleeping all day and lying awake at night.

- Manic people are so active that they can't find time to go to bed.

- Alcohol and drugs are important causes. The drinker who slumbers under the influence of drink may wake up with a full bladder, which, having been relieved, leaves him or her sleepless. Some alcoholics can't sleep because of the direct toxic effect of the alcohol. A little alcohol helps induce sleep but large amounts can have the opposite effect. This is also true of barbiturates.

- Many people with severe heart disease don't sleep well because they are breathless unless propped up with lots of pillows.

- Worry about day-to-day events and problems keeps many people awake but eventually they fall asleep and wake refreshed.

Prevention

- Any painful condition should be properly treated, and the cause cured if at all possible. If it can't be adequately treated pain-killers should be taken before retiring, to ensure that you get adequate rest and sleep. All pains seem to be worse if you are tired so getting good sleep helps reduce the pain the following day.

    Acute, feverish illnesses can usually be coped with fairly successfully. Drink plenty of fluids and take an aspirin to reduce the fever if it is keeping you awake. This kind of insomnia is usually very shortlived (only a night or two) and does not often cause much of a problem.

- Never drink tea, coffee, cocoa or cola drinks in the three or four hours before you go to bed.

- Take 100 mg of vitamin B complex. Some people need extra vitamin B_1 to cure their sleeplessness. Taking B vitamins (and especially vitamin B_3) too late in the day can have a stimulant effect and keep you awake. Take the B complex at 4.00 p.m. at the latest.

    Zinc should be taken at a dose of 25–50 mg daily; and a combination of calcium 1–2000 mg and magnesium 500–1000 mg last thing at night. The essential amino-acid tryptophan 1000 mg

can also be a useful dietary supplement, especially if depression is the cause of insomnia.

- Never go to bed on a full stomach. Allow an hour or two to pass before retiring after a large meal. Wind, nausea and indigestion prevent millions of people from getting off to sleep and only a proportion can be helped with antacids. For many people the combination of alcohol and a large meal is the problem–try leaving out alcohol when you go out late in the evening. On the other side of the coin are those who lie awake hungry with their stomach rumbling. Have a snack of cereal or biscuits, perhaps a hot milk drink, just before retiring.

- Apart from dietary restrictions on those foods which can be found by trial and error to cause nightmares and night terrors in children, there is little that can be done to prevent these events. Sometimes the child is obviously disturbed when awake and may well benefit from professional psychological help. Many children of troubled (for example, divorcing or separated) families sleep poorly and have frequent dreams and night terrors. Prevention starts with looking carefully at the child's waking day. A few children are terrified by science-fiction characters and things they have seen on TV–common sense can sort out most of these problems.

- It is helpful to relax before going to bed rather than expecting to sleep immediately, after a hectic physical, emotional or mental event. A hot bath can stimulate rather than relax – a tepid shower is probably better. Sitting down and listening to the radio, watching TV or reading a book are good ways of switching off from the demands of the day.

  I have mentioned that excessive exercise before going to bed is detrimental to sleep, so is exercise a promoter of sleep at all? The answer is definitely yes, but it has to be the right type of exercise and taken at the right time. Regular exercise is essential for vibrant health and most people sleep better if they have had at least some exercise during the day. The best exercise before bed is a brief walk. Certain yoga postures are said to encourage sleep and some people find that a period of relaxation (see page 87), including deep breathing exercises, helps relax them too.

- Jetlag and shift work are well-known promoters of insomnia. Both alter the body's time clock and as a result sleep suffers. The effects of jetlag are worst when crossing several time zones and get much worse if the time changes 8 hours or more. It is possible to overcome the pattern by keeping to your home time but if you are going somewhere on business or for more than a day then this won't work because you will have to fit in with the clock in the country you have travelled to. You can prepare yourself in advance, at least to some extent, by gradually altering your sleeping times in the week before you go – change them by an hour a day.

  When it comes to shift work the most disruptive pattern is the combination of day and night work. Most people eventually come to terms with night work if they do it all the time – the natural body clock simply resets – but with a mixture of day and night shifts you are fighting nature all the time. Avoid such work if you possibly can.

- Bad beds are a very common, yet preventable, cause of insomnia. Many people have a bed which is too small. Since 1920 the average height of young men has increased by 2 in and the proportion of men who are 6 ft 3 in or more has gone up from one in 250 to one in 40 today. So the old 'standard' bed is too small for many people, especially as the metric equivalent is even smaller than the old imperial standard size. A bed should always be at least 6 in longer than your body.

  Your bed may also be too narrow. Lie down with your hands behind your head. If your elbows overlap the edges of the bed, it is too narrow. Anyone over 6 ft tall probably needs a king-size bed.

  Until very recently in historical terms people slept on wooden boards or on the floor or a mat. This does not mean that all mattresses are unhealthy, but many are too soft. As we pass through periods of REM sleep most muscles of the body are paralysed. They give our bodies little or no support and a very soft bed will not support us either. Young people are not too badly affected by this but middle-aged and older people certainly are and wake up with backache and aching limbs. If in doubt err on the side of a harder bed. Replace your mattress at least every ten years.

A double bed is usually more spacious, even for two people, than two singles, but when two people share a bed there is a potential for sleeplessness. One of them may snore, toss and turn, sleepwalk, have nightmares, or get up to go to the bathroom. On the plus side cuddling someone else gives a sense of warmth and security that helps promote sleep. But sharing a bed does not mean that both have to have the same mattress. Today there are excellent zip-and-link mattresses available that enable one half of the bed to be softer and the other firmer, according to individual taste.

- Some people sleep badly because they are too hot or too cold. Old blankets become thick and matted, so that they hold the heat less well than when they were soft and fluffy. It is better to replace old blankets rather than pile more on top because the weight can be uncomfortable, especially for older people. A duvet is the perfect answer because it is light and makes bedmaking so easy. Room temperature and ventilation can make a real difference to insomnia, especially at the extremes of temperature – a hot, stuffy room and a cold draughty room both make insomnia more likely.

- If your room has thin curtains, you may be woken too early on light, summer mornings. Fit heavier ones, line existing ones or fit a blind inside the curtains. This could give you two hours' more sleep.

- Noise can be a real nuisance, especially on busy roads, and electroencephalograms done on people asleep in such situations show that they are registering the noise even though they are asleep. (Some people, used to the noise of a city, become insomniacs when they move to the peace of the country – they 'can't stand the silence'.) If you are super-sensitive to noise ear plugs are an answer, and if light rooms are a problem you can buy a mask or an eye-shade.

- Depression must first be recognised and then treated to prevent this common cause of sleep loss. See your doctor if you have any of the symptoms listed on page 189.

- Watch out for foods and drinks that give you nightmares or simply disturbed sleep.

- Although millions of people sleep perfectly well without ever having sex there is little doubt that intercourse and/or masturbation help the average person to drop off. Unsatisfactory sex on the other hand can prevent sleep. This is especially true in women who are left unsatisfied by their partners. Such a woman can always masturbate if she is left 'high and dry'. If she can't masturbate, for whatever reason, she may well be able to sleep better if she doesn't have sex.

  Sex is part of a pre-sleep ritual for many. Most of us use some form of pre-sleep ritual, often without even realising it. At roughly the same time each night we turn off the TV, put down our book or newspaper, make a hot drink, have a bath or shower, cuddle our partner, perhaps make love, and then go to sleep. Some people listen to music in bed, others pray – it doesn't matter what it is as long as it's a relaxing, predictable and unwinding process that prepares us for sleep. The best schedules are regular without being rigid.

- Stop worrying. If we have effective sleep rituals, the worries of the day slip away and we don't lie there thinking about them. Sex, or indeed any other activity that absorbs our attention, is a good antidote to worry. But often the worry is best confronted and discussed with your partner, if you have one. Try to think around the problem and then go to sleep at least having made some effort to solve it rather than trying to sleep on an unsolved problem. Serious problems can be solved at night when you are alone and peaceful and able to think. Don't lie there worrying about not sleeping – work through the problem and see what can be done. Some people find deep breathing or forms of meditation help them let go of their insoluble problems.

  Don't worry about insomnia. No one ever died of it and it will probably have very little effect on your performance. Keep a pad of paper and a pen by your bedside and make notes of what you decide to do to sort out the problem that's worrying you. Next day go through it rationally and implement whatever you can.

IRRITABLE BOWEL SYNDROME (IBS)

What is it?

A very common syndrome in which there is pain from the colon (large bowel) and an alteration in bowel habits. It is a leading cause of lost days of work and, apart from peptic ulcers, is the condition of the digestive tract most frequently seen by gastroenterologists.

The symptoms are abdominal aching or pain, diarrhoea, alternating diarrhoea and constipation, wind, and abdominal bloating.

What causes it?

The whole syndrome appears to be caused by increased bowel motility. This in turn can be caused by several things:

- Certain foods.

- Tea, coffee and alcohol.

- An infection with candida yeast.

- Stress.

- Certain drugs.

- Bowel infections.

- A digestive-enzyme deficiency.

- A low-fibre diet.

Prevention

- Many people with IBS can identify one or more foods that make their symptoms worse, and a study from Cambridge found food intolerance to be a major causative factor. The most common offending foods were wheat, corn, dairy products, coffee, tea, and citrus fruits. It is certainly worth going on to an elimination diet for a few weeks to see if the symptoms disappear. To do this you need to eat only a very few foods and to exclude all the foods listed above–and anything containing them. This usually means eating a diet composed of one

meat (lamb is good), fresh vegetables and water for 2–3 weeks. If your symptoms go you can try adding in the foods listed, one by one starting from the end of the list (citrus fruits). If you get any of your symptoms back cut out that food entirely for good and go back to the simpler diet for a few days until you are normal again. Repeat the process, trying each of the foods on the list, one at a time, for a few days until you have eliminated the culprit(s), which you should then cut out from your diet permanently.

- Cut out tea, coffee and alcohol and see if this produces a reduction in or elimination of your symptoms. Add each back in, one at a time, to identify the reaction-producing substance, as above.

- *Candida albicans*, the yeast that causes thrush, can be found in about half of the whole population's bowels. The consumption of antibiotics, any disruption of the digestive process, the consumption of a diet high in refined foods, and the use of steroid hormones, all make the growth of this yeast more likely. UK researchers have found that this overgrowth can produce symptoms exactly like IBS and that the 'IBS' can be cured by killing off the yeast.

- Most studies of IBS put stress high on the list of causes. (Some doctors even think it is a purely psychosomatic disorder but this is almost certainly not so). A study of 130 patients with IBS found that one or more psychological factors played an important part in causing the condition in the first place, or in causing relapses of it, in four out of five of those studied. For men business and career worries came high on the list, and with women family problems were the main culprits.

Psychotherapy can undoubtedly prevent IBS, and some people find taking regular exercise helps. Yoga or hypnosis may be of benefit–by helping you relax. A recent Swedish trial of preventive psychotherapy found that those receiving the psychotherapy fared much better than those who were treated with medical methods alone. Ways of preventing stress are considered on page 87.

- Treatment with antibiotics can *produce* IBS-like symptoms, usually because they profoundly alter the large bowel's normal bacterial and yeast population. The reactions may not occur until several weeks after the course of antibiotics has ended, hence the link between the two is difficult to make unless you know about it. People on long-term antibiotics (such as those on long-term tetracyclines for acne) are especially at risk.

- Acute infective diarrhoea, such as occurs in food poisoning (see page 220), can trigger the symptoms of IBS and they can persist long after the infection has gone.

- Certain people have a shortage or absence of the specific enzymes that digest lactose in milk. Such people get symptoms of IBS when they consume milk or milk products. If milk makes your symptoms worse, prevention is easy–stop drinking and eating milk and milk products.

- Whilst there is no doubt that a high-fibre diet seems to have a beneficial effect on many people with IBS, a few people actually only start getting IBS symptoms when they go on to a high-fibre diet. These people are wheat-sensitive and allergic to bran. Soya bran or rice bran are alternatives and are available from health-food stores.

KIDNEY STONES

What are they?

Stones made of calcium salts that are produced by and lodge in the kidney. Some stay there and produce no symptoms for years and others pass down the tube (the ureter) that leads from the kidney to the bladder, causing great pain as they do so. Such stones hospitalise more than a million North Americans each year. Many millions of others have small stones which pass without being noticed or with only a small amount of abdominal or loin pain.

What causes them?

The fluids that pass through the kidneys contain many different chemicals and minerals. Two of the more plentiful of these are calcium and oxalate, which combine to form calcium oxalate. If there is too little fluid or too much of these salts they begin to settle out and crystallise. More crystals are attracted until, like a snowball, the deposit increases in size and becomes a small, hard stone. This in turn can grow in size to almost fill the cavity of the kidney.

Just what starts off this crystallisation process is not known but it is thought that a tiny piece of organic matter such as a bacterium could do so.

The population appears to be divided into two broad categories – stone-formers and non-stone-formers. An analysis of 24-hour urine collections from stone-formers shows that between 40 and 60 per cent have too much calcium in their urine. One study found that stone-formers ate more purine-containing foods and another found that they consumed more meat, fish and poultry and less bread, grains and starch. Research shows that both protein and glucose increase the rate of calcium excretion in the urine and that the glucose effect is exaggerated in stone-formers. This led one researcher to claim that kidney stones are a disorder of

carbohydrate metabolism. Adding sugar to the diet increases the amount of calcium put out in the urine.

Another feature of the diet of the countries in which kidney stones are common is the amount of animal protein they eat. Research has found that the more animal protein we eat the more oxalate and calcium we excrete into our urine.

Dietary fibre traps and reduces the absorption of sugars, and wheat bran definitely produces beneficial effects on carbohydrate metabolism and the control of blood sugar. One study found that wheat bran reduced the absorption of calcium from the diet by as much as 50 per cent and that the increased absorption of calcium normally produced by sugar was reduced in those taking bran.

A study in Ireland, where 8 per cent of the population have a kidney stone at some time in their lives, found that the diet of fifty-one stone-formers was different from those who never formed stones. The stone-producers ate less fibre, got fewer carbohydrates from fruit, vegetables and grains and ate more fat and red meats.

An Australian study compared thirty meat-eaters with thirty vegetarians and found that the animal proteins caused an abundance of calcium to be excreted into the urine. They also found that the lower the calcium intake, the higher the oxalate excretion, so clearly reducing calcium intake alone is no good if you have kidney stones – you need to reduce your oxalate level as well.

Prevention

- Eat a diet rich in fibre, low in animal protein and low in sugar. Sucrose (table sugar) can increase the rate of absorption of calcium from the gut and also its level in the urine of some people. Lactose (milk sugar) also enhances calcium absorption by the body.

- Drink plenty of water or other watery drinks. Try to drink a glass of water in between the normal drinks you would have. This keeps the urine dilute and flushes out any tiny crystals that are about to form. Those who already have stones should aim at drinking enough fluids to produce 2–3 quarts of pale urine a day and should set their alarm clock to wake them at night to drink a glass or two. Most don't produce another stone if they take this action.

- Magnesium supplements appear to inhibit stone formation, a fact first documented as far back as 1697! A recent Swedish experiment gave 200 mg magnesium a day to a group of forty-one men and fourteen women who individually averaged about one stone a year and who as a group had formed 460 stones during the ten years before the experiment. After 2–4 years on magnesium only eight of the patients reported new stones. As a group their average rate of new-stone formation fell by 90 per cent. A control group was kept as a comparison and not given magnesium. After four years 59 per cent had developed new stones.

- Vitamin B_6 could be a valuable preventive too because of its oxalate-lowering effects. You can reduce your oxalate intake by avoiding spinach, rhubarb, tea, chocolate, parsley and peanuts, all of which are rich in oxalates. But you can also improve things with vitamin B_6. This vitamin seems to be especially valuable in lowering the oxalate level of the urine of stone-formers. Indian researchers recently found that only 10 mg of vitamin B_6 a day significantly lowered the oxalate levels in the urine of twelve stone-prone people all of whom had developed at least one stone a year in recent years.

  This relatively small dose of the vitamin produced better results than a group of drugs called the thiazides which doctors use to increase urine output and so wash out any stones. Unfortunately, thiazides have certain unpleasant side-effects: they produce light-headedness, elevate the amount of sugar and uric acid in the blood (promoting diabetes and gout), and can also reduce the level of potassium in the blood, which produces muscle weakness and cramps.

- It seems that certain individuals are sensitive to an increased dietary calcium which, in turn, results in high levels of calcium in their urine. It makes sense to limit your dairy produce intake if you are a stone-former. Having said this, be very careful not to so limit your calcium intake that you lay yourself open to osteoporosis (see page 292).

- It appears that in some people salt produces an increase in calcium in the urine. If you or your family are stone-formers it makes sense to cut out added salt altogether.

- Alcohol increases the excretion of uric acid, calcium and phosphate and has an adverse effect on vitamin B_6 and magnesium metabolism, both of which are useful in protecting against stone formation. Avoid alcohol or drink only in moderation.

- Vitamin C is metabolised to oxalic acid, so don't take high doses of the vitamin if you are at risk of forming kidney stones.

- If you have ever had an oxalate-containing stone (the commonest kind), avoid tea, coffee, chocolate, peanuts, spinach, rhubarb and beetroot because they are rich in oxalic acid.

LONELINESS

What is it?

A feeling of being alone in the world, together with all the negative emotions that accompany this feeling. It is different from solitude which is self-imposed and as a result can have much more serious effects. About one in five of all US households are single occupants (though not all of these will be lonely of course) and many other individuals are lonely even if they are surrounded by people. In this context loneliness could be said to be a combination of an individual's environment and personal expectations. Young people living at home are often lonely, especially if they have no boyfriend or girlfriend at a time when most of their friends have one. Older people are much better at being alone than are younger ones and it appears that loneliness is something we learn to cope with as we get older.

What causes it?

The most obvious cause of loneliness is literally being alone, but it doesn't have to be physical—it can be emotional or psychological aloneness. We can all be lonely from time to time, even within a family. Many married couples who appear happy to the outside world live lonely lives side by side under the same roof. Their bodies are physically close to one another but their hearts and minds are miles apart.

There are at least two main types of loneliness. In the first, the individual feels alone and passive, and sleeps, eats and cries most of the time. People suffering from this often see themselves as unlovable and unable to alter their lives. The second category contains the large group of adults who feel lonely for some reason and then read, listen to music, disappear to the greenhouse, study or whatever to fill their lonely hours. This then becomes a vicious circle because those around them imagine they don't want company, and their feeling of isolation and loneliness increases. Of course, not all pursuits such as these are signs of loneliness – they can be an oasis in a busy life – but if someone spends most of his or her time alone this should alert friends and family that all may not be well.

But it is not just adults who get lonely. Babies and young children are often very lonely – right from the day they are born. Many a baby is left in its cot awake for hours staring at the ceiling, but however many toys there are to play with the average baby craves human company and input. By and large it is probably fair to say that we leave our children too much in our culture, when they really want to be around their parents and particularly their mother when they are very young. I believe that babies should be with their mothers (or whoever is their primary care-giver) most of the time in the first year of life so as to prevent the learning of loneliness. Babies can be carried around in a sling or put in a carrycot in the kitchen or living room so that they can observe family life and be part of it.

Loneliness also paves the way for fear and other negative emotions. A busy mind wards off worries, especially unnecessary ones.

Grieving, for example after the death of a spouse or a parent, often involves a feeling of loneliness among the other emotions – all perfectly normal – and it can take up to two years to fully recover. Similarly, after a divorce many people feel desperately alone, possibly for the first time in their lives. This is especially true of the person who is left without the children (usually the man). This is a time when loneliness can lead to true depression, and even to suicide as the world seems hardly worth living in.

The 'normal', healthy person can be alone without being lonely and can balance a need for and enjoyment of others with a need for and enjoyment of solitude, if only from time to time. Such people don't feel the world is a bad place, or inferior or vulnerable, when they are 'alone' – simply that they can't and don't want to be with others all of the time. Many people need to reach their forties or even older before they can claim that they have achieved this delicate balance.

Prevention

- As we saw above, the prevention of loneliness begins in the cradle by encouraging babies to be part of everything going on in the home. In this way a baby learns that life is full of interesting inputs and that boredom is unnecessary.

- Older children should be brought up to understand that they can't always have parents or other adults around to play with them –

sometimes they must be able to entertain themselves for short periods. In this way children are brought up with reasonable expectations of the reality of adult life in which there will be periods of being alone which have to be coped with.

- Make a virtue of loneliness. Many people say that once they have come to terms with loneliness they can also enjoy it – if only for the freedom it gives them. The secret of managing loneliness in adulthood is to cultivate the right attitude of mind to it. There are positive benefits to being alone and there are ways of reducing the amount of time you have to be alone if you don't want to be.

- Take the opportunity to get to know yourself better. If necessary get professional help from a doctor or counsellor. By understanding yourself better you will be in a position to do something about your loneliness.

- Many lonely people are shy or have poorly-developed social skills. There are good books about these subjects and social-skills training groups are now widely available. At one extreme end of the spectrum are those who say that they prefer their pets to human beings. Such individuals probably need professional help. Pets are undoubtedly a boon to the lonely but to want to be with them to the exclusion of humans, as some seem to, is

not normal and could point to underlying personality or psychological problems – which could benefit from treatment.

- One US expert on loneliness finds that talking to oneself is helpful. Saying things aloud is a form of tension release, he claims. Other experts find that a diary is a good form of self-communication. In it you should record not only what happened that day but your daydreams and fantasies.

- Once you have insights into what you are like and what you want from life you can start to look outwards for things to do that will combat your loneliness. For many doing something for someone else works best. Helping an elderly or handicapped person or running something in the community such as a toddler group, or doing voluntary work at the local hospital, can work wonders for the unhappy, lonely person. If you want company yet find it difficult to meet people you get on with, try an evening class. At least all the people there will have one thing in common with you – the subject matter of the class.

- Be grateful for what you've got – think of those who have far less and then try to relax and enjoy what you have.

- If you are lonely within a marriage or other close relationship and are unhappy about it seek professional help.

MEMORY LOSS

What is it?

After the age of 50 or so we all lose the ability to remember things as well as we used to and memory loss is to some extent normal and inevitable. It is also rather annoying. There should be little deterioration in memory before the age of 70 or so, but after 80 most people have increasing memory loss.

But loss of memory in old people does not mean that they have difficulty remembering everything. They often lose the ability to remember things that happened recently, but do not have the same problems with things that happened a long time ago – they can regale you with all the details of what they did during World War I but can't remember whether yesterday was Tuesday or Wednesday or whether they had lunch today. It is as though their long-term memory with all its repetitions and reinforcements is locked into the brain more securely than the transient events that could have happened at any time. Without repetition a short-term memory lasts for about 30 seconds and then is gone. Lots of memories don't even last that long – they never get sorted into the memory bank at all. Concentration plays a big part in memory at any age and if we don't concentrate in the first place it doesn't register in our memories.

We can't possibly remember everything we experience in life, at least not consciously – though our experiences may be held in our unconscious minds and then dredged up by some method. Often, such memories come out in daydreams, fantasies, or while we are asleep.

What causes it?

- Normal ageing.
- Too little choline in the diet.
- Too much to remember.
- Smoking, drinking and drugs.
- Tiredness.
- Wrong mood.

Prevention

- There is nothing we can do about ageing but we see on page 126 how to prevent the effects of ageing, and some of these measures (and those outlined below) will undoubtedly help keep memory alive longer. A lively mind in a healthy body definitely helps.

- There is a lot of interest at the moment in choline in the diet. Lecithin is a major dietary source of choline and is especially plentiful in egg yolk. Doctors first became interested in choline because it is the precursor of acetylcholine which is essential for the flow of nerve impulses in the body. Studies have found that extra choline in the diet increases levels of acetylcholine in the brain and may help memory. In one study a 10 g dose of choline significantly improved memory and recall in normal, healthy people. Those whose memories were poorest at the start of the experiment were helped most. Lecithin can be bought in health-food shops, as can choline.

A study in Texas gave lecithin to people suffering from Alzheimer's disease (a form of mental deterioration that includes memory loss) and then re-tested their memories. Although their memories did not return to normal there was a definite improvement which lasted for 6–18 months. Choline and lecithin are totally safe to use–in one study there were no side-effects even when the subjects took 20–25 g a day.

- If you have too much to remember you will have to accept the fact that you will need to rely on tricks and devices if you don't want to forget things. Learn to improve your level of concentration and to make a positive effort to link the new thing to be remembered to something else you already know. Make lists. Write notes for yourself. Use other people to remember things for you and then enlist their help. Use modern technology to store information you don't have to carry in your head. Research has found that it is easier to remember pictures than words, so it can be helpful to create an image in your mind with which to link the new thought you want to memorise.

For example, if you want to remember to fill up the car with petrol and to buy some eggs think of the eggs floating in petrol. Similarly, when trying to remember names, link the person's name to what he or she does. So Mrs Garden who is a nurse would be remembered by a visual image of her with patients in beds in her garden, and so on.

- Cut down on or stop smoking, drinking and taking drugs. A study in Los Angeles divided twenty-three habitual smokers into two groups. One group was asked to smoke a non-nicotine cigarette, while the others smoked normal cigarettes. Both were then tested on their ability to recall a list of seventy-five items. The non-nicotine group recalled an average 24 per cent more words than did the ordinary smokers. In another study smokers and non-smokers were given a dozen colour photographs of people and told their names. After 10 minutes the non-smokers fared better at matching the names and the faces than did the other group.

- A study in Oklahoma tested the memory of young and middle-aged people before and after drinking alcohol. The results showed that even moderate drinking produced memory impairment. Certain medications, even some obtainable without a prescription, cause memory loss.

Some tranquillisers, and tablets for high blood pressure, cause memory problems, so if you think your tablets could be the cause, talk to your doctor. Don't just stop them to find out.

- Tiredness can seriously affect short-term memory. Most people find that their memory is best early in the day and gets less good as the day wears on. This is only true for short-term memory, though–the reverse is true for long-term memory.

- Getting in the right mood can help memory. It has been found that happy events are better recalled in happy situations and moods, and vice versa. In one study, subjects were asked to remember two lists of words, one while they were happy and one while they were sad. People who were sad during recall remembered about 80 per cent of the word lists they had learned when they were sad, compared with only 45 per cent of the words learned when they were happy. On a practical level it can be very helpful to re-create the mood of the event you are trying to remember.

MENOPAUSE PROBLEMS

What are they?

Troublesome symptoms of varying severity that affect most women at least to some extent around the time of the menopause (about the age of 50 in most women today). Throughout a woman's reproductive life she produces female sex hormones, but from the menopause onwards these are produced in reduced amounts. The first sign of the onset of the menopause is usually irregular periods. Although a woman's female sex-hormone levels may fall to below those found in most men, her male sex-hormone level can remain high and could account for the facial hairiness seen in some women at this time.

The most common symptoms around the menopause are hot flushes, vaginal dryness, pain on intercourse, headaches, night sweats, weight gain, light-headedness, muscle and joint aches and pains, dry skin, depression, excitability and a loss of confidence. There are, of course, many others too. The vast majority of these signs and symptoms can be reversed by giving female sex hormones, so clearly they are hormone-linked. However, such replacement therapy has fallen under a cloud since research has found an increased level of breast cancers in women taking oestrogens in this way. It also increases the risk of gall-stones and high blood pressure.

Once over the age of 50 or so ischaemic heart disease (which leads to heart attacks) becomes more common in women than before, and a few women lose their pubic hair and armpit hair and have degeneration of their vulva and vagina. Women also start to lose calcium from their bones and are more liable to fractures when they fall than are men. Some women welcome the onset of the menopause because it means they can now enjoy sex without worrying about contraception, but others mourn the passing of their fertile years and are miserable.

The menopause also often coincides with the departure of children from the home and the woman's husband may be at the stage of life in which he is becoming interested in younger women, perhaps to sow the oats he never did when he was young. This is now the second peak time for divorces (the first is during the first five years of marriage).

Having said this, the menopause is used somewhat as a catch-all and any problems a woman encounters at around this time of life tend to be attributed to it – often erroneously. About 10–20 per cent of women suffer no symptoms at all at the menopause.

What causes them?

- The fall in oestrogen (and to some extent testosterone) levels in the blood.

- Psychological changes that occur quite independently of the purely physiological ones. Few women are totally unmoved by what the menopause means for them as women and many have fears, both rational and irrational, about the future both of themselves and their relationship. It is under-

standable that a woman who sees herself as 'washed up' after the menopause, or 'not a real woman' – because she can't any longer have children – is open to all kinds of emotional and psychological ills.

- A vitamin E shortage.

Prevention

- Bring up children (and girls especially) to have a more realistic view of female sexuality which puts less emphasis on child-production as the sole validity for being a woman. Most women don't consciously think that sex is only for procreation but clinical experience shows that *uncon*sciously this is seldom far from their minds. Today's teenage girl will probably live for as long after the menopause as a non-reproducing female as she did before it and some of this time will probably be spent celibate, or nearly so, as her partner is likely to die some years before her. These are the realities that need to be taught to youngsters so that they can prepare for them realistically.

- Use an oestrogen-containing cream in the vagina to reduce dryness and soreness. This can prevent many of the genital symptoms associated with the menopause. Also, frequent sex and orgasms tend to reduce the speed at which the vagina degenerates. A study of post-menopausal women and their sex lives found that those who had sex rarely or not at all had more vaginal problems and pain when they did have sex than those who enjoyed regular sexual activity.

- Take vitamin E. Many women report relief from hot flushes within two days of starting vitamin E (800 IU daily). If the vitamin is taken with vitamin C it seems to work even better, according to one expert in the field. Once the flushes have been reduced for a week or so the dose of vitamin E can be gradually cut down to 400 IU daily.

- Taking the essential amino-acid tryptophan can help prevent the depression seen around this time.

- Calcium and magnesium have been found to prevent post-menopausal 'blues'. These also help the bones of the menopausal woman to remain stronger. After the menopause the body both puts out more calcium in the urine and absorbs less from the intestine. Taking more helps redress this balance.

- After the menopause there is a big jump in the low density lipoproteins (LDLs) in the blood. This type of cholesterol is especially associated with heart disease. This makes good nutrition even more important after the menopause. Lecithin, a substance found in eggs, soya beans and liver, has been shown to be effective in lowering blood triglycerides and LDLs in the blood, and vitamin C also has a cholesterol-lowering effect. The vitamin C you will be taking will also reduce blood stickiness and so cut down the chances of a clot forming in the heart and leading to a heart attack.

- Ginseng binds to oestrogen receptors and has an intrinsic oestrogenic activity of its own. Some women find it a good preventive and curative herb for menopausal symptoms.

- Uncommonly, the menopause unmasks a food allergy which has, in retrospect, been present for years. Sorting out this allergy (see page 216) can resolve and prevent some of the unpleasant symptoms associated with the menopause.

- Cold-pressed linseed oil (kept in the fridge) or evening primrose oil – 500 mg, eight capsules a day – can also be a useful preventive.

- Calcium at a dose of 400-600 mg twice a day has also been reported to have beneficial effects.

- Perhaps the best preventive measure for a woman's self-esteem and general well-being after the menopause is to try to get the best out of her sex life with her partner. Ideally, the seeds of such a life together should be sown well before the onset of the menopause, but if this hasn't been done, the menopause can be a good time to rethink your romantic and sexual life together.

Try to keep up an active sex life whatever happens in life to make things difficult. Be resourceful and inventive about overcoming problems. Keep physically and mentally active both as an individual and as a couple. Indulge in lots of mutual genital stimulation, even if you don't have much actual intercourse. Perhaps try sex aids for the first time in your relationship. Expect a few failures but don't be demoralised by them. Get medical help for any condition that makes intercourse painful or difficult. Ignore what anyone says about sex being only for the young.

MISCARRIAGE

What is it?

The loss of a baby before it is old enough to support itself–around 28 weeks of fetal life. After this time the death is called a still-birth. The spontaneous loss of a fetus is very common indeed. About eight out of ten of all conceptions abort spontaneously, though no one knows why this is so common. Perhaps the mother's natural monitoring systems detect an abnormality and reject the imperfect fertilised egg very early on. Whatever the reason, human embryos have a very poor survival rate compared

with almost any other animal.

When it comes to confirmed pregnancies, about 20 per cent result in a miscarriage, usually in the first twelve weeks. Some women miscarry repeatedly. After one miscarriage the chances of doing so again are 20 per cent; after three miscarriages, 30 per cent.

A miscarriage is like a mini-labour. There is pain and bleeding from the vagina. If you are pregnant any vaginal bleeding should be reported to your doctor at once.

What causes it?

In most cases no one knows. In women who habitually abort the reason is found in only about a third.

- Blighted ovum. The pregnancy starts to develop normally but the mass of cells never becomes a baby. No one knows why such eggs are blighted but it is thought that it happens when an abnormal sperm fertilises a normal egg. This has been found by looking at the sperms of the partners of women who seem to have repeated blighted ova–often the sperms are abnormal.

- About one in five miscarriages arise because of trouble with the cervix. This is the most common cause of miscarriage in the second and third trimesters of pregnancy. A loose or 'incompetent' cervix lets the growing fetus out too early and so the woman aborts. This usually occurs around fourteen weeks of pregnancy. An incompetent cervix can be caused by: an overdiligent D&C (at which the gynaecologist has stretched the cervix too much); a therapeutic abortion; or a difficult or rapid labour during which the cervix has been damaged.

- Hormone deficiencies probably play a large part in miscarriage. An egg, once fertilised, needs hormones from the corpus luteum in the ovary until the placenta is sufficiently well developed (at about 14 weeks) to take over. Some miscarriages occur at this take-over point.

- Uterine abnormalities are uncommon but often produce miscarriages. A uterus with a division down the middle may not provide enough room for the fetus to develop normally.

- Chromosomal abnormalities are not an uncommon cause. This can be a special problem for infertile men. Normal men have an average of 107 million sperms per millilitre of semen but men with chromosomal abnormalities may have only 31 million. In men with sperm counts under 20 million per millilitre 8.2 per cent had chromosomal abnormalities, according to one study.

- Psychological causes have been put forward as a possibility and this is not as unlikely a suggestion as it might at first appear. The higher centres of the brain have a powerful influence over a structure called the hypothalamus which in turn influences hormone production in the body via the pituitary gland. There is little doubt that a woman's hormone cycle can be profoundly affected by her psyche, as any woman who has ever missed a period – or had it brought on – as a result of stress will confirm. In one study researchers took two groups of habitual aborters, and gave supportive psychotherapy to one group and not the other. Three times as many women receiving the psychotherapy gave birth to babies compared with the other group. Another study found that simple psychotherapy increased the women's chances of actually going through the pregnancy fourfold.

- Congenital abnormalities of the baby are relatively common and are undoubtedly a cause of miscarriage. This is nature's way of weeding out fetuses that would not survive or which would do badly. About 5 per cent of early miscarriages have neural-tube defects (spina bifida or anencephaly). The success of this natural 'selection' process is indicated by the fact that only about 2–3 per cent of babies are born with serious abnormalities.

- Trauma to the cervix can cause a miscarriage in susceptible women. This means that intercourse should be undertaken very cautiously or even avoided completely around the 10–14 week time in a woman who has ever had a miscarriage or bleeding at this time.

Prevention

- The blighted-ovum problem can be prevented, at least to some extent, by freezing the man's semen in a deep-freeze in a laboratory. When unfrozen, most of the poor-quality sperms will have been killed off and the couple's chances of a successful pregnancy greatly increased.

- Cervical problems can almost all be prevented. Gynaecologists should be very cautious and gentle when dilating the cervix to do an abortion or a D&C, using only the smallest dilator they need to. Better management of labour, with the woman in an upright position (sitting, squatting, kneeling or standing) will greatly help reduce cervical trauma during birth.

- Perhaps the greatest single preventive for cervical problems is the use of a special stitch put in by a gynaecologist at about 14 weeks. This holds the cervical canal closed and keeps the baby safely inside. The stitch is removed at about 38 weeks, or earlier if the woman goes into labour before this.

- Hormone treatments can be given to prevent hormone-deficiency states that cause miscarriages.

- The surgical correction of uterine abnormalities and the removal of fibroids can prevent miscarriages in some of the women in whom these are a problem.

- Supportive psychotherapy should be more widely offered to any woman who has had more than one miscarriage because it works in a significant proportion of women.

- We look in some detail at how to prevent congenital abnormalities in babies on page 294.

- If any woman has a history of miscarriage or premature labour it makes sense not to have intercourse (or even, probably, orgasms) around the time at which she previously had the miscarriage. If you are worried about a miscarriage, don't have sex or an orgasm in weeks 10–14 of the pregnancy. There is no evidence that using a vibrator inside the vagina causes miscarriages, but it is probably sensible to steer clear of them around this vulnerable time.

MUSCLE CRAMPS

What are they?

Involuntary contractions of muscle groups (usually in the legs, neck or back) which make the area painful and tender. Some people get them in bed at night. A particularly unpleasant form occurs in some people in the muscles between the ribs when making certain movements – for example when turning round to look behind them when reversing the car.

What causes them?

Often the cause is unknown but several are recognised:

- Tired or stressed muscles, in swimmers or footballers, for example.

- Certain occupational cramps are well recognised. An example is writer's cramp, which affects typists, musicians and type compositors, as well as writers.

- Very hot working conditions leading to profuse sweating. Many of those who work in blast furnaces or ships' boiler rooms know all about this type of cramp. It is caused by a loss of sweat together with its salt, and the cramps are really the result of sodium shortage. In a similar way dehydration during serious illnesses involving a fever can cause cramps.

- Chronic alcoholism causes cramps in the legs and feet.

- An elusive but common form of cramp is the 'stitch' in the side – experienced, for example, by long-distance runners. It is thought to be caused by a cramp in the diaphragm muscle.

- A shortage of calcium.

- A lack of vitamin E.

- Uterine cramps occur in some women on the first couple of days of their period. These period pains are the biggest cause of lost work and school days in females. There are many 'cures' for these cramps, the best of which is a drug which prevents the release of prostaglandins in the uterus – now known to be the cause of the pains – but there is as yet no fully proven way of preventing period pains.

Prevention

- The prevention of sports-induced cramps is usually straightforward and involves doing proper warming-up exercises before embarking on any strenuous sporting activity. Avoiding chilling the muscles helps too, and some sportsmen and women find that binding up the area helps. As soon as you get any form of cramp it is best to stop what you are doing until the symptoms go. The best treatment for cramps is to put the muscles involved under tension (stretch them). Someone else will almost certainly have to do this for a cramped sportsman or woman.

- The prevention of occupational cramps is usually fairly obvious. Special attention should be paid to posture, seating, lighting, desk height, and so on.

- Those who work in very hot conditions should take salt tablets regularly.

- Calcium is vital for adequate muscle function. *Prevention Magazine* in the US carried out a survey in 1977 of 3,000 readers to find out how calcium had improved their health. Over half wrote to say that it had relieved their muscle cramps. Probably the best way to increase calcium intake is to take Dolomite tablets before each meal and one at bedtime.

- Vitamin E also seems to play a part in cramps. When a team of Los Angeles doctors gave the vitamin to 125 patients with night-time leg and foot cramps, 103 had complete or near-complete relief. Some of these people had had their cramps for thirty years. Almost half the patients got better on 300 IU units or less of vitamin E a day. The other half needed 400 IU or more, and many had to stay on the vitamin if they were to remain cramp-free.

  Vitamin E has also been used to treat a cramp-like condition in the legs known as intermittent claudication. In a study of forty-seven men with severe intermittent claudication, thirty-two were given vitamin E and the rest drugs to prevent and cure the cramps such men experience on walking. After three months the men were tested to see how far they could walk. In the vitamin group 54 per cent could walk the maximum distance set by the tester (just over ½ mile) but only 23 per cent of the drug group

could do so. It appears that the vitamin E improved the circulation in the legs. After eighteen months of taking the vitamin twenty-nine of the thirty-two men showed an increase in the blood flow to their legs whereas most of the men in the drug group had a decreased blood flow.

NAIL BRITTLENESS

What is it?

Nails so soft that they split into layers or split very easily once they grow beyond the fingertips.

What causes it?

No one knows for certain. Possibilities are:

- Circulatory disturbances causing poor nutrition to the nail bed, but there are usually other signs of this and it is not common in the fingers.

- An inherited tendency.

- Psoriasis. Usually the nails are also pitted.

- Iron-deficiency – the nails are usually spoon-shaped.

- Zinc-deficiency.

Prevention

- See a doctor for the treatment of

any circulatory disorder you have.

- Get psoriasis treated.

- Take iron supplements or eat more iron-containing foods.

- Use nail hardeners or nail polish to prevent the ends from splitting.

- Increase the wholefoods you eat and cut down on refined foods.

- Take a zinc supplement (up to 20 mg daily).

NAPPY RASH

What is it?

A reddened area of skin in the nappy area of a baby. This can develop into tight, papery skin with some peeling. The common rash tends to spare the folds and creases, but babies with sensitive skins and those prone to seborrhoea (cradle cap) may get a rash that extends into the folds and creases. A monilial rash (caused by thrush) has features of both and also has some spots elsewhere. It is also possible to have a rash that is purely monilial and consists just of isolated spots.

If a nappy rash is very severe there may be raised, red pustules which turn into raw, ulcerated areas. Undoubtedly a baby with this severity of rash will be irritable and will cry a lot.

What causes it?

- Common nappy rash is caused by urine irritating the skin in places where the nappy chafes. Plastic pants increase the humidity by preventing evaporation and so make this kind of nappy rash worse. It is thought that ammonia released from the urine is not the *cause* of this kind of rash but it can make the rash worse if the skin is already damaged.

- Diarrhoea of any cause can make a nappy rash worse.

- Allergies are rarely a cause but some babies appear to be allergic to certain chemicals used in the manufacture of paper nappy liners.

- Airtight and watertight plasticised disposable nappies provide little or no ventilation and may promote nappy rashes.

- Occasionally a nappy rash is the earliest sign of atopic eczema.

- One in two nappy rashes is caused by monilia (thrush). Any rash that has been present for three days or more is likely to have monilia in it.

Prevention

Preventing the common kind of nappy rash is simple:

- Change your baby's nappies frequently, never allowing him or her to stay for long in a wet or soiled nappy.

- Leave your baby without a nappy for as much of the time as possible – this is easier in the summer.

- Wash the bottom well and dry it thoroughly, and only then apply a barrier cream. Do this every time you change the nappy.

- Soak nappies in a sterilising solution before washing.

- Ensure that nappies are thoroughly rinsed to remove all the soap and detergent.

- A one-way fabric nappy liner works wonders but paper ones can actually make rashes worse.

- Ideally, avoid using plastic pants, though this is the counsel of perfection because it often means soaked clothing, bedding, etc.

- If you think a particular brand of disposable nappy is the cause of your baby's problem it could be the plastic or the deodoriser used. Try the baby in terry nappies for a few days to see if this will cure the condition. Once a culprit has been found, avoid it in the future.

OBESITY
(see also page 92)

What is it?

A condition characterised by excessive weight. It is generally accepted that the term obesity applies to people who are 30 per cent or more above their ideal weight – allowing for their frame size. About 15 per cent of 16–19-year-olds, and 54 per cent of men and 50 per cent of women aged 60–65, are thought to be overweight. Forty per cent of adult men overall and 32 per cent of adult women overall are overweight, with 6 per cent of men and 8 per cent of women truly obese.

Recent research has found that even being mildly overweight matters – it is not just the truly obese who are at risk. Weight is especially important to those with a family history of diabetes and heart disease and in those who already have high blood pressure. If you or your family have diabetes, heart disease or high blood pressure, it is especially important to watch your weight and that of your family.

Smoking is linked to weight too. Smokers tend to be less heavy than non-smokers *but* they are at greater health risk. Many people give up smoking and promptly put on weight but the hazards of smoking are greater than those of being overweight.

What causes it?

- Eating the wrong foods.

- Bad nutritional habits from the cradle.

- Too little exercise.

- Too much alcohol.

Prevention

- There is little doubt that most westerners are fat because they eat the wrong foods rather than simply because they eat too much. By consuming too large a proportion of one's calories as fat, sugar and refined carbohydrates, we absorb too much of the food we eat and end up fat. Guidelines for a healthy diet can be found on page 70. The answer is to eat much less fat, little or no sugar, and much more unrefined carbohydrate in the form of cereals, wholemeal-flour products, fruit and vegetables. Such foods are naturally slimming because they are so bulky that it is difficult to overeat them.

Eating such bulky foods may mean eating six smaller meals a day rather than two or three big ones, especially in the early days as you get used to large, bulky meals instead of fatty, sugary, condensed ones.

• Trouble with obesity often starts in the cradle when mothers give their babies cows' milk formula instead of breast milk. Studies of the arteries of young children killed accidentally have found that breast-fed children have much less atheroma (the sticky material that blocks up arteries and causes heart attacks in later life) than do bottle-feds. Also, many mothers add sugar to the formula and so accustom a baby to expect sweetness from early on. Bottle-fed babies on average grow up to be fatter than do breast-feds but the reasons for this are obscure. Perhaps it has to

do with the lack of oral satisfaction compared with the 'comfort sucking' a breast-fed baby enjoys–which makes the baby bottle-fed to a schedule more likely to turn to food for solace later in life. Breastfeeding exclusively for at least 4–6 months is undoubtedly the best start in life when it comes to obesity. And don't be put off by the podgy breast-fed babies you see. They lose their baby fat as they are weaned but the bottle-fed baby often does not.

• Exercise is thought to play a part in controlling the body's metabolism though no one is quite sure how. Fairly vigorous exercise is known to stimulate the metabolism (so that you consume more calories doing the same things) and evidence suggests that this raised metabolic rate continues for a day or two after the exercise stops. Many slimmers find that exercising fairly vigorously two or three times a week helps keep their appetite down.

Several studies have shown that fat people tend to eat less than do thin ones. Obese people, and men in particular, are likely to consume a lot of alcohol, though, and this is very fattening. The real problem for most fat people is inactivity. One Dutch study found that fat people ate less because they were physically less active and therefore used less fuel. Yet they still continued to eat more than they burned off: re-sult–obesity. This research group concluded that the main preventive against obesity is to take regular exercise.

- However you decide to lose weight make your principle 'slow but sure'. Short-term, rapid weight loss on fancy diets usually depends on losing water rather than body fat. It has taken you years to get fat and it will take many months to get slim. Aim at a 2lb loss every week after the rapid loss of the first week or two. Remember that the idea is not to eat less of the same foods but to eat more of bulkier foods, and to take more exercise.

OSTEOPOROSIS

What is it?

A condition in which the bones of the body become less strong–usually as a result of the loss of calcium. As we age our bones become weaker, partly because we put out more calcium in our urine and partly because we absorb less from our diet. Also there is little doubt that old people who eat poorly get too little of both calcium and the vitamin D that is needed for its metabolism in the body. After the menopause women, especially, lose bone strength. This comes about as a result of the reduction in their oestrogen levels after the ovaries cease to provide them.

The problem of oesteoporosis is a very real one. The number of hip fractures in elderly women is doubling every ten years and–as well as the suffering involved for the women themselves–the workload for the medical services that this represents is massive. One in four of all women over the age of 60, and half of all those over the age of 70, have osteoporosis severe enough to produce pain, a loss of height and a spinal deformity. One in ten women will break a leg by the age of 80 and a third of these will die of the complications. Half of those who could walk before the fracture will be permanently crippled. On top of all this there will be one third more women over the age of 65 in fifteen years' time–so it amounts to quite a problem.

Unfortunately, osteoporosis is often diagnosed very late, usually *after* a fracture has occurred.

What causes it?

- Genetic factors. These undoubtedly play a part, but there is little one can do to prevent them.

- An inadequate diet. As mentioned above, many elderly people simply eat too little of everything and along with this become short of calcium, among other things. Studies in the US have found that the average middle-aged woman takes in only about 500 mg calcium a day. The recommended daily intake is about 800 mg, and many osteoporosis experts think this should be 1,300 mg for such women. Given that women around the menopause lose 3 per cent of their bone mass each year (and in some bones the figure is up to 8 per cent) it is easy to see how vital a plentiful calcium intake is. One cup of milk supplies 300 mg calcium and small, bony fish are good sources too.

- Inadequate vitamin D. As this vitamin is essential for the utilisation of calcium in the body it makes sense to supplement the diet with it as well as calcium. Old people are often housebound and so get low on vitamin D which is naturally formed in the skin by the action of sunlight.

- Too little exercise. A four-year study of women aged 37–67 (average age 51) found that vigorous exercise stops bone loss in middle age. A non-exercise control group lost 2.4 per cent of their bone per year over the four-year period. In another study the same researcher was able to increase the bone weight of nursing-home residents (average age 81) by 2.3 per cent just by getting them to do exercises in a chair. A similar group who did not exercise *lost* 3.3 per cent of their bone mass. Walking on the spot also

works wonders – you don't even have to go out.

Prevention

- Calcium supplementation should probably be started around the age of 30, according to experts in the field. Dolomite is a good calcium supplement available from health-food shops and chemists, and vitamin D is widely available too. An effervescent calcium drink is also available (Sandocal).

  In a study at Kentucky State University, dicalcium phosphate (rather like bone meal) was given together with vitamin D to elderly women for about six months. After this time the bone density of more than half the women had gone up by 25 per cent. To be safe it makes sense to take 1 g of supplemental calcium a day. There is no truth in the myth that you will get kidney stones, especially in the elderly, if you eat this much calcium.

  Dietary sources of calcium include: dairy produce (but don't overdo it because most dairy produce is rich in saturated fat); green vegetables; small fish (provided you eat the bones); watercress; and bread and other flour products. Dried skimmed milk is exceptionally high in calcium and low in fat.

- Take more exercise. Even doing arm- and leg-raising exercises three or four times a day for a few minutes in your chair or bed will help. If you are really keen you can attach weights to your ankles and wrists before exercising – use any sensible household object to hold or alternatively strap a can of food to each foot.

- Take sensible precautions generally. Most falls in the elderly occur at home from standing height, often getting in or out of bed or a chair. Half of all such falls occur as a result of the effects of ageing – poor muscle strength, weakness, poor posture, instability when standing, slow reflexes and poor vision. Many old people feel faint when they stand up (because their blood pressure falls quite dramatically) so the answer is to stand up slowly, especially when getting out of a bath or a warm bed. These effects are particularly obvious in diabetics and in those taking tablets for high blood pressure.

There are many hazards to old people around the house that increase the likelihood of their falling over and coming to grief. Many of these can easily be overcome with a little thought. Obviously it makes sense to plan your home so that you don't fall over rugs, wires, telephone leads, slippery floors or difficult steps. Wear sensible, flat shoes, remove clutter from around the home, and have safety rails installed by the bath, the lavatory and the bed.

PERINATAL DAMAGE AND DEATH

What is it?

Until a few decades ago childbirth was dangerous for the mother and her baby. As recently as 1930 between forty and forty-five women in every 10,000 having babies died. Today this figure is one in 10,000. Great progress has been made in saving mothers' lives and in the 1950s attention turned to improving the lot of the baby. Considerable progress has been made in this direction but there is no room for complacency. Infant mortality today is still a real cause for concern – as many babies die in the first year of life as children and young adults die in the following twenty-four years!

Although a few of these deaths are totally unavoidable most are part of a much bigger problem. Some babies are born dead (still-born); some are born alive but too early and so stand a poor chance; others die in the first weeks of life; and yet others live but are handicapped – often for life.

The problem is not a small one in terms of numbers. In 1984 there were 3,640 still-births in England and Wales (who died between the twenty-eighth week of pregnancy and the end of the first week of life). French estimates have suggested that for every one 'perinatal' death 2.5 babies survive damaged. There are today about 16,000 damaged babies surviving in England and Wales each year. Some are very little affected and others are grossly handicapped and will live in an institution for all their lives. There are probably a quarter of a million children in the UK in special schools and attending normal schools who are mentally and physically handicapped, and 5,000 children live in long-stay hospitals from which they are unlikely to emerge.

What causes it?

- Poor preconceptual care.

- Poor diet in pregnancy.

- Medicines, drugs, X-rays or the Pill.

- Infections during pregnancy.

- Alcohol in pregnancy.

- Smoking before conception and during pregnancy.

- Environmental hazards.

- Genetic problems.

- Poor ante-natal care.

- Birth problems.

- Congenital abnormalities.

Prevention

- As soon as you think you want to start a baby it is good sense to make sure that all the conditions are right for your baby to get off to a good start. First, start eating properly. Make sure that you eat enough, especially if you are thin. If you are underweight your baby may grow slowly. Ensure that your diet is rich in protein, vitamins and minerals and complex carbohydrates. These latter should be in the form of high-fibre, unrefined carbohydrates. These also have the advantage of ensuring that you don't get constipated during pregnancy – a common problem.

  Drink plenty of fluids – keep off or cut down on tea, coffee, cocoa and cola drinks. Drink more water or dilute pure fruit juices (not squash). Aim to gain between 17 and 25 lbs in weight over the whole pregnancy. Any more could be disadvantageous. Come off the contraceptive pill at least three months before you plan to conceive. Use a barrier or other method until your body resumes its natural cycle and then try to conceive. Remember that it takes an average of 5.3 months for a normal, healthy couple to conceive if they are having unlimited sex. After taking the Pill a small percentage of women take many months to conceive but eventually almost all of them do so. If you have a coil don't remove it until you actually want to conceive. Come off all drugs but don't stop any prescribed drugs or medications until you have discussed it with your doctor. Stop or seriously cut down on your smoking and alcohol intake. Both can be hazardous in pregnancy and their effects on the health of eggs and sperms are not yet fully understood. Play safe.

- Keep away from infections, including childhood infections, 'flu and so on. By doing all these things for 3–6 months prior to conceiving you will stand a better chance of conceiving a healthy, normal baby.

- Obviously you can't choose your parents and there may well be diseases or conditions that run through your family or that of your partner. If you are worried about anything like this tell the doctor. He or she can arrange for you to attend a specialist, if necessary, to put your mind at rest or to establish whether or not the risk of a particular condition occurring is worth taking.

- During pregnancy eat well and don't put on too much weight. The ideal to aim for is 17–25 lb, but if you are very skinny at the outset you could add a little more. Eat as outlined above. Don't take any food to excess because it is now thought that large slugs of certain foods (see Food Allergies, page 216) can sensitise a baby in the mother's womb. Be moderate in all you eat. Be sure to have plenty of dietary fibre and lots of fruit and vegetables eaten raw or very lightly cooked to preserve the minerals and vitamins.

  There is a good case to be made for taking additional vitamin and mineral supplements during pregnancy, especially as so many foods are so poor in these valuable nutrients today. Do not drink pints of milk a day. This can sensitise your baby *in utero* to cows' milk protein. Also milk is very fattening and rich in fat. If you really want to drink milk make sure it is skimmed milk. Carry on drinking plenty of bland fluids and avoiding tea, coffee, cocoa and cola drinks, as before conception.

- Don't take any drugs at all and see your doctor to ask if you can come off any of the prescribed drugs you are on. This should already have been discussed before conception but now he or she may be prepared to reconsider the whole subject with more urgency. Almost all drugs cross the placenta and affect the unborn baby somehow, so you are better off without them unless they are life-saving. Morning sickness, constipation and other minor ailments, should be coped with by using dietary and natural remedies rather than drugs and medications. A high-fibre diet will prevent constipation, and dry toast and biscuits are good if you feel sick. Moderate doses of antacids for heartburn are probably safe.

  Keep away from X-ray machines and other X-ray hazards. If a child has to be X-rayed get someone else to hold him or her if there is even a remote chance that you are pregnant.

- Research on the adverse effects of alcohol on the fetus is now voluminous, and there is no doubt that even very small amounts of alcohol (a few drinks a week) can be harmful. You may find that during pregnancy you go off alcohol altogether (in which case you are lucky). If you really can't do without it keep it down to one or two drinks a week at most.

- Smoking is also well known to be dangerous to the baby. Women who smoke during pregnancy tend to have small or premature babies. Smoke affects the placenta and increases the risk of bleeding in the weeks shortly before the birth. Try to get your partner to stop smoking too because the baby will get the smoke you inhale from the air around you. Giving up smoking is the single most important thing you can do to increase your chances of having a healthy baby.

- Try to avoid people who have infections if you are pregnant. The most dramatic of the illnesses that harm babies is German measles. It is best to have a blood test to ensure that you have antibodies to the disease at least three months before you plan to conceive. If you suffer from German measles during early pregnancy your baby could be born deaf, blind or with heart disease. Having had measles does not make you immune to German measles – they are different diseases. It is advisable to have a test to check whether you are immune, and then to get immunised if your blood test shows that you need to.

- If you are continuing to work be sure that you are not exposed to chemicals, radiation or other environmental hazards. If you are at all worried talk to your employer, union representative, occupational health nurse or your doctor. Look into your benefits and allowances so that you claim for all you are entitled to. This could make all the difference in your efforts to eat well and look after your baby properly, especially if you are not well off.

- Numerous studies have shown that attending ante-natal clinic is of great importance in producing live, healthy babies. Several conditions such as spina bifida and Down's syndrome can be diagnosed early and an abortion offered. Ante-natal care generally aims to detect problems early and prevent conditions that predispose to handicap. The perinatal death rate of babies of mothers who go late for their first ante-natal visit is five times higher than for babies of mothers who attend early. As soon as you miss a period, tell your doctor and get a pregnancy test done at once – the doctor can tell if you are pregnant twelve days after the first day of your missed period. He or she will then arrange for you to be 'booked in' for your ante-natal appointments.

- Ante-natal care is more important for the poorer mother who lives in bad housing than for her more advantaged sister but, unfortunately, as with so many preventive measures, those who would most benefit often do not receive the help. An answer here would be to make ante-natal clinics more easily accessible, perhaps as drop-in centres in shopping precincts.

- The way that your labour is handled greatly depends on the obstetrician at your local hospital. There is no evidence that hospital is a safer place to have a baby (unless you are at high risk for some reason)–a home birth can be just as safe or even safer. Make a birth plan and discuss it with your obstetrician early on in pregnancy. If you want to avoid having an episiotomy, (see page 209), an epidural, and so on, say so and put it all in writing to the hospital. Surgical and other interventions can save babies' lives but can produce problems too. The best way of ensuring that you have as trouble-free a birth as possible is to go to ante-natal classes to learn about birth and to prepare you for what is to come.

  During the labour keep upright and walking around as long as possible and then give birth standing, squatting, kneeling or indeed in any position that keeps your body upright. This provably helps improve the blood supply to the baby, and makes labour shorter and less painful. Most women who give birth in this position are very loath or even refuse to deliver on their backs in

subsequent labours. Because labour is quicker the baby is less likely to suffer from a shortage of oxygen. All of these factors contribute to a greater chance of having a normal, healthy baby.

  Asphyxia (a shortage of oxygen) is the commonest cause of preventable death or handicap occurring at the time of delivery, but much of the danger can be avoided by giving birth in an upright position and by having trained staff with oxygen available in case a baby is born with asphyxia. Permanent brain damage can occur after a remarkably short period of time with an insufficient supply of oxygen to the brain.

- After low birthweight, congenital malformations are the next most common cause of infant death. In the UK 18 per cent of first-week deaths and 20 per cent of perinatal deaths are caused by congenital malformations. Some of these can be prevented by taking proper care before conception and during pregnancy.

- Treating neonatal jaundice is a way of preventing cerebral palsy (a diffuse group of neurological conditions that produce a 'spastic'). There are six spastic babies born every day in the UK–over 2,000 a year. In some cases the recognition of a failing placenta, followed by appropriate action, is another way of preventing this heartrending handicap: babies who are suffering from poor placental blood supply can be delivered with the minimum of trauma and have their asphyxia (if any) treated so as to be born healthy and normal. The prevention of premature babies and their care in intensive nursing facilities can dramatically reduce the numbers of spastic babies born from this cause.

PET-RELATED DISEASES

What are they?

The vast majority of pets do not produce any illnesses in children, or indeed in the rest of the family. Fleas are fairly common in cats and dogs but can be controlled by regular de-fleaing. If your pet scratches a lot, take it to the vet.

Worms can be passed to children via the bowel motions of cats or dogs. Almost all puppies are born with roundworms (toxocara) and by 6 months about half still have worms. The worm eggs can live in dust for months, so worming is essential. Kittens and adult cats need worming too.

Some children are allergic to certain animals, often in fact to the mites in their coats. This can be overcome by washing the animal regularly in special solutions to get rid of the mites.

Toxoplasmosis is an infection with a small, single-celled micro-organism that can produce congenital abnormalities in a baby born to a mother who has the illness during pregnancy. It is spread by cats and poorly cooked meat.

What causes them?

- Poor hygiene.

- Fleas and mites

- Allergies to certain animals.

- Worms and other diseases in the animals themselves that can be transferred to humans.

Prevention

- Never let animals lick your children's faces or mouths.

- Wash your hands–and see that your children do–after handling pets.

- Always wash hands before meals if there is a pet in the house.

- Train your dog to use a particular part of the garden to open its bowels.

- Make worming a routine–don't wait until you actually see worms. Ask your vet how often you should worm and what to use.

- Don't forget that kittens and puppies need worming too.

- Keep your pet's coat well groomed and free from fleas and mites.

- Never take your dog into food shops.

- Ensure that your dog and cat have their own beds and don't sleep on yours.

- Never let your dog or cat eat from your food dishes. Give them their own and wash these separately from yours with a separate dish-cloth or brush.

- Keep your dog well disciplined so that it comes when called and does not cause accidents on roads by running out uncontrolled.

- Don't feed your pet in between meals, especially from the table – it will not only become a nuisance and spoil mealtimes for you but could transfer infections to your hands and then to you.

- If a child is allergic to an animal see your doctor to discuss a course of desensitising injections. This often fails but can be worth a try.

- Never eat poorly cooked meat – you could get toxoplasmosis.

- If you are pregnant avoid handling cats' litter at all and even if you are not pregnant do so wearing rubber gloves.

PILES (Haemorrhoids)

What are they?

Engorgements and enlargements of 'cushions' of tissue that line the anus (opening of the back passage). They are very common in the West and were until recently thought to be a sort of varicose vein in the back passage. This theory is no longer tenable in the light of recent research which shows that we all have anal cushions of tissue that close off the back passage so as to keep stools in until we choose to release them.

What causes them?

Studies from around the world show that piles are mainly a disease of the western world. Monthy returns from seventy-seven rural hospitals in sub-Saharal Africa showed that fewer than three people with bleeding or prolapsed piles were found each year in each hospital. These figures are extremely low compared with the West where the disease is said to affect half the entire population over the age of 50!

It is now thought that as hard, sticky masses of stools are forced down the back passage, substantial shearing stresses are put on the anal cushions which, as a result, become pushed down as they part company with the underlying muscles. Both the straining and the hard faecal matter are caused by a low-fibre diet.

Prevention

- Drink more water. This tends to make the stools less hard and easier to pass.

- Eat more fibre in all its forms. This alone will make the stools easier to pass and so reduce the shearing stresses on the anal cushions.

- Lubricate the back passage before opening the bowels (with a little Vaseline or KY jelly).

POST-NATAL DEPRESSION

What is it?

A condition in which a woman becomes miserable or frankly depressed after having a baby. It is extremely common, with some surveys showing that eight out of ten women feel low, weepy and depressed, and are easily upset, in the first week or two after a birth. These emotions may or may not be accompanied by a feeling of anxiety around the time of taking the baby home from the hospital – a condition seen more commonly in first-time mothers.

Usually post-natal depression is not sufficiently serious to prevent the sufferer from functioning normally, but is very unpleasant for her. Such a woman typically cries at the slightest provocation, perhaps for no reason at all, feels she can't cope with the baby, is critical or openly aggressive towards her partner, feels guilty about not loving her baby enough, goes off sex, loses her appetite, can't sleep, has nightmares, and may have panic attacks.

A 1975 study found that of sixty-six women having their first babies 84 per cent experienced post-natal depression of some kind and 77 per cent were anxious. Twenty-four per cent were frankly depressed.

Post-natal depression starts at any time after the birth but the common 'baby blues' is experienced in the first few days and lasts only for a couple of days. More severe forms of depression start from 2–3 weeks post-natally, but can first appear as much as six months later.

What causes it?

No one knows for sure but there are several theories:

- Hormonal theories have always been popular because the levels of progesterone rise during pregnancy and then fall very suddenly immediately after the birth. Superficially this appears to be a plausible explanation but it is difficult to see how this sudden fall in hormone level could cause depression weeks or months later. Also, these very same hormones are deemed to be the cause of pregnancy depression in which progesterone levels are high – not low.

  It was noticed many years ago that there were certain similarities between premenstrual symptoms and post-natal depression. Dr Katherina Dalton, a pioneer in this field, wondered whether there might not be a connection – possibly a shortage of one of the circulating hormones. Unfortunately, it is not easy to measure hormones post-natally because the levels swing wildly until the menstrual cycle re-establishes itself. Whilst we still have a lot to learn about hormonal abnormalities, several researchers have meanwhile found other abnormalities. One of these is:

- Inadequate vitamin B_6. This vitamin now has a proven place in the management of premenstrual tension and it has also been tested in the post-natal situation. One researcher gave 100 mg of the vitamin for twenty-eight days to more than 100 women who had already had one baby (thus ruling out first-timers). The results showed that the B_6 group had much less depression than did those given a placebo and that the effects were particularly marked in those women who had premenstrual symptoms. Depression has been linked to a shortage of a neurotransmitter called serotonin and vitamin B_6 shortage can cause too little of this to be produced in the body. Research in Birmingham (England) has found that the substance from which serotonin is made fails to rise after birth in some women who later become depressed.

- Tiredness and sheer exhaustion are often cited as causes of post-natal blues but there is almost certainly more going on than this. Undoubtedly, physical and mental exhaustion are a *part* of the baby blues in some women but they are unlikely to be a major factor in true post-natal depression.

- The psychoanalytic approach to post-natal depression is based on the theory that women who become depressed after childbirth do so because of unconscious anger towards their baby and because of a rejection of the role of motherhood. This overlaps somewhat with a major category of causes of post-natal depression:

- Psychosocial reasons. There is little doubt that, whatever is going on hormonally and physiologically, for many if not most women psychosocial factors are involved. First-time mothers, those who have marital problems, those with money problems, the unemployed, and those who know little about babies, have all been found to be at greater risk of becoming depressed.

  The circumstances of the birth itself also play a part, with women who have had unpleasant or interventionist birth experiences faring worse. Many women whose babies are taken away from them to the hospital nursery feel very low and would rather have them with them. Could this be a reason why there are fewer cases of post-natal depression in home-delivered mothers? Women who breastfeed right from the start also have less depression than do bottle-feeders.

Perhaps as important as any of these factors is our society's attitude to childbearing and child-rearing. Many people have so little experience of babies before they have their own (modern families being so small) that first-time mothers are often shocked at the realities of life with a baby when they get it home, and four out of five say that their expectations are unrealistically romantic. It is this gap between fantasy and reality that is the greatest producer of post-natal depression in my opinion.

The vast majority of women get better from their post-natal depression without medical help, but what can be done to prevent it arising in the first place?

Prevention

- The education of all young people, right from the earliest years, to see babies and parenthood in a realistic light must be the starting point for prevention.

- Greater contact between young people, before they have babies, and older people with children could help get their ideas straight from early on.

- A birthing system in which women (and couples) feel that they have as much say and control as possible over what is happening will prevent a lot of depression.

- Fewer operative and medical interventions in the birthing process.

- A policy of 'breast is best' and good back-up support for it antenatally and post-natally is essential.

- Babies should normally be allowed to stay with their mothers in hospital. Putting babies into a hospital nursery should no longer be routine. Ideally, all mothers should have their babies with them all the time they are in hospital.

- Supportive staff in the post-natal ward should treat the women as adults and not little girls. This will prepare them for the reality of the world outside when they will be alone with their baby.

- Social workers and other professional helpers should be more readily available for women with real domestic or family problems. This would enable 'at risk' mothers to be identified and helped ahead of the birth to prevent depression occurring.

- Vitamin B_6 could be tried in any woman who usually has premenstrual symptoms.

PREMATURE EJACULATION

What is it?

A condition in which a man ejaculates

before his penis erects, at the moment of penetration or immediately afterwards. There have been many more lengthy and complex definitions but this is a workable one for all practical purposes.

What causes it?

There are probably about twenty reasons for premature ejaculation but the most common is that the otherwise normal man has not learned to recognise the sensations that immediately precede ejaculation. In most animals copulation is a very brief business but humans have developed skills in prolonging the whole process of arousal and delaying ejaculation so as to give both participants more sensations.

Just why some men can't recognise the 'almost there' sensations and go beyond the point of no return before they want to is a complex subject and involves both physical and psychological factors.

- Physical disorders of the man's genitals are rare causes – most men have no medical or anatomical reason for their premature ejaculation.

- Much more common, though, are the psychological causes, which include: a fear of women; a fear of being controlled by women; the view that women are really sexless and so don't want a man to ejaculate in them; the view that sex is an unwelcome assault on the woman; and a general anxiety about or fear of

sex. Such views are surprisingly common yet the man who holds them may not even realise that he does so – they are locked away in his unconscious mind. Previous bad experiences make many premature ejaculators worry that the same thing will happen again and they become so anxious that they ejaculate too soon once again.

- Poor masturbation training. Because of guilt a man may have masturbated only hastily and guiltily right from the beginning, with the result that as an adult he is programmed into speedy ejaculations.

- Furtive early intercourse, perhaps hastily in the back of a car or in the girl's home, can produce men who become locked into fast arousal and ejaculation cycles.

- Feeling unsafe and anxious for any reason can cause premature ejaculation.

- Not having had sex or masturbated for some time makes some men ready to ejaculate at a moment's notice.

- Some men with hostile feelings about their partner want (unconsciously) to punish her, so they withhold from her their ejaculation and the pleasure it gives her. Some men express their dissatisfaction or rage with their partner in this way rather than doing so outwardly. For a few men who cannot otherwise exert any power or control over their partner premature ejaculation is the only way they know.

- Fear of a particular sexual occasion–especially when it comes to extramarital sex–is a common cause of premature ejaculation, and many young men are so anxious at their first intercourse that they ejaculate too soon.

Prevention

Clearly, few of these causes can be readily prevented by any one man or his partner because they go back to his upbringing–or indeed hers. Often a professional can help cure such background misunderstandings or inhibitions and so help the man regain his control. For many such men their premature ejaculation is an unconscious way of avoiding sex yet neither they nor their partners realise this is so. The prevention of further trouble involves sorting out the root cause and this can be time-consuming and difficult.

However, many couples don't want to go down this path and would like to try something themselves. This is certainly worth doing, as it can produce good results and prevent premature ejaculation becoming a way of life. Here then are some basic preventive tips:

- If the man thinks the woman in any way contributes to the problem he should say so and the couple should talk it through. If he feels that he is trying to get back at her for some other dis-

satisfaction in life then they should talk it out and resolve the other problem in another way so that they don't carry it over into sex.

- If the couple are having sex too infrequently so that he becomes 'trigger-happy' the answer is usually obvious. If more regular intercourse is not possible the man should masturbate every few days or his partner could masturbate him.

- Open display of the woman's sexuality, including the sharing of her fantasies, helps many such men to start to see women as earthy sex-loving human beings instead of a sexless madonna who should not be defiled. This sort of revelation alone can make a lot of difference.

- A very good and well-proven preventive is for the man to masturbate or get the woman to masturbate him (to orgasm) before intercourse. This defuses the situation and the man can later have a controllable orgasm to the pleasure of them both.

- Using a sheath can so reduce the level of sensation that the man receives from his penis that he can sometimes be totally cured of his problem.

- Weak anaesthetic creams or ointments work in the same way.

- Contracting the anus tightly at the end of each thrust helps some men gain control, as does penetrating deeply with the penis.

- Stop–start intercourse can also produce good results. In this the man makes love, but as soon as things begin to get too excited he stops thrusting and concentrates on the pattern of the wallpaper or counts the rings on the curtain rail, for example. Many women enjoy this teasing intercourse and it can help the man learn how to control his progress to ejaculation.

- A little alcohol can be a good preventive. It reduces the man's anxiety about the act of intercourse (and he also has an excuse should things go badly).

- Here is an exercise for a woman to do with her partner, to help him learn to recognise the 'almost there' signs that his body produces and to be able to control them. This can be done by any caring couple who really want to succeed.

  Set some time aside one evening and take the phone off the hook. Read something sexy or get in the mood in whatever way you choose. The woman should stimulate the man's penis until it is fully erect. He then tells her when he feels he is about to climax, so that she can squeeze his penis very firmly (putting her finger and thumb on opposite sides of the rim at the base of the head), which will stop his erection in seconds.

Once he is limp she can start to re-stimulate him until he is erect again, whereupon she can squeeze him again. Continue this cycle until the woman can erect the man and collapse him at will for up to half an hour. At the end of this session she should masturbate him, or he should do so himself, so that he is not left 'high and dry'.

Once you have practised this for a few sessions you will be confident that he can control his ejaculations. In the next few sessions the woman can stimulate the man as before, but instead of squeezing his penis to stop the erection, she should leave his penis alone when he says he is about to climax, perhaps even getting him to do something else around the house. Repeat this procedure several times at one session. End with masturbating him as before.

The next stage involves the woman giving the man a really hard erection and then getting on top of him and gently putting his penis inside her. She should just sit on it without moving, getting him used to the feeling of being erect inside her and not 'coming off'. She should then move gently, and when he feels he is about to come off she either squeezes him with her fingers as before or lets him go down of his own accord.

Slowly, over several weeks the woman will be able to exert such control over the man's penis that he will never come unless they both want him to. After such training most men can take over their own ejaculatory control and remain erect for half an hour or more inside their partner's vagina, only coming when she is also ready.

PREMENSTRUAL TENSION (PMT – *premenstrual syndrome* – PMS)

What is it?

The premenstrual syndrome is a collection of symptoms and bodily and mental changes that occur, usually regularly, anything from a few days up to two weeks before the onset of a woman's monthly period. The problems stop with the onset of bleeding.

The syndrome has tended to appear a somewhat woolly collection of symptoms and signs (more than a hundred have been reported) and this has led many, mostly male, doctors to question its existence as a real entity. To the women who suffer from it, though, it is real enough, and although there is undoubtedly a psychological element to many cases it is by no means a problem that is 'all in the mind'.

The most common complaints are of anxiety, nervous tension, mood swings, irritability, weight gain, breast tenderness and headaches.

Between 30 and 35 per cent of women of childbearing age suffer from it. Almost 5 per cent of women are severe sufferers and become suicidal, accident-prone or very difficult to live with when they have PMT.

Recent research has shown that there are several fairly clear-cut sub-fractions of the condition which respond to different treatments:

PMT-A women complain mainly of nervous tension, anxiety, irritability and mood swings occurring as much as two weeks before the onset of their period. The symptoms get worse and are sometimes followed by mild to severe depression, improving with the onset of bleeding. These symptoms have been found to be caused by too much oestrogen – research indicates that oestrogens act as stressors to the nervous system. Progesterone, on the other hand, has a calming effect. Research shows that the liver is unable to de-activate these raised levels of oestrogens without adequate supplies of B vitamins.

PMT-C women find their appetite increases two weeks before a period and they crave sweet, sugary things. The craving is especially bad if the woman is under stress. An hour or two after eating the sugar-rich foods the woman feels low, tired and shaky. If you are under stress and eat a lot of refined sugar several things happen. Stress changes the levels of certain brain enzymes, which creates a relative deficiency of a substance called dopamine. The highly refined sugar eaten forces the amino-acid tryptophan into the brain cells where it is converted to serotonin. An excess of serotonin causes palpitation, nervous tension and drowsiness, among other things. The refined sugar triggers the release of too much insulin and this reduces blood-sugar levels. A deficiency of a hormone called prostaglandin E (PGE) may also be involved. PGE suppresses the insulin response to sugar and reduces the nervous system's responses to a decreased blood sugar. The following nutrients are needed for the formation of PGE from cis-linoleic acid, which is its dietary building block: magnesium, zinc, and vitamins B_3, B_6 and C. Perhaps the craving for chocolate so many PMT-C sufferers have is really for the magnesium and phenylethylamine (related to dopamine) that chocolate contains.

PMT-H women mainly complain of weight gain during the last few premenstrual days. Their body weight goes up, their breasts, hands, feet, faces and ankles swell. Rings become tight, shoes and skirts are tighter than normal, contact lenses feel less comfortable or even cannot be worn, and the breasts and lower abdomen are tender. Most women in this group gain only 3 lb or less in weight but it seems to be all in sensitive places. Some gain as much as a stone.

Such women often have normal oestrogen levels but have elevated levels of hormones produced by the adrenal glands that control salt and water retention by the kidneys. High brain levels of serotonin stimulate the release of ACTH–a brain hormone that makes the kidneys retain salt

and water. Excess carbohydrate consumption makes the body produce too much insulin, as we saw above, and insulin is known to make the kidneys retain more salt than they should. Stress also makes the kidneys retain salt and water.

PMT-D women have premenstrual depression, are withdrawn and confused, cry easily, can't sleep, are forgetful, and may even be suicidal. Many such women, if they have no other signs, are not diagnosed as PMT sufferers and end up with psychiatrists. Some of these women improve with oestrogen supplements.

What causes it?

No one knows precisely but there are several factors known to be implicated.

- Hormonal changes are a crucial feature of the menstrual cycle in all women. In the first two weeks of the cycle (i.e. the first two weeks after the start of a period) there is a substantial level of the hormone oestrogen, and in the second two weeks the level of another reproductive hormone, progesterone, rises. These sex hormones affect not only a woman's sex organs and her breasts but every organ of her body, and an imbalance can produce a wide range of symptoms.

Many experts now believe that low levels of progesterone are to blame for most, if not all, of the symptoms seen in PMT. Women with PMT have relatively lower levels of this hormone than do non-sufferers. It is the balance between oestrogen and progesterone in the blood that seems to be crucial. Oestrogen can antagonise progesterone so that even if you produce enough progesterone it can be wiped out by too much oestrogen. Normally progesterone acts as a natural diuretic, clearing fluid from the body. If a woman's progesterone levels are low she accumulates salt and water, feels bloated, has joint pains, gains weight, feels tense, gets tired easily and can even have visual disturbances. A few women become so bloated, that they are unable to wear their contact lenses.

But the most important action of progesterone in this context is on sugar metabolism. Without enough progesterone the body is unable to deal with sugar properly and the result is hypoglycaemia (low blood sugar – see page 248). It is this that produces so many of the mental symptoms seen in PMT. Hypoglycaemic signs include headaches, migraines, fainting, weakness, irritability, aggressiveness and panic attacks. Once menstruation begins, sugar metabolism returns to normal and the woman feels well again. Alcohol and caffeine can also play havoc with blood-sugar levels and are best avoided premenstrually.

- Childbirth seems to increase the chances of suffering from PMT. The more babies a woman bears (especially if she has toxaemia) the more likely she is to suffer from PMT.

- Age. PMT generally increases with age. Women in their thirties seem to suffer most.

- Stress. This definitely seems to make PMT worse and even to precipitate it. Married women complain of more severe PMT than do single women, which may be accounted for by marital stress.

- Lack of physical activity seems to play a part too.

Prevention

- Learn about PMT. Become aware of your body. Keep a diary of any symptoms you have at any time in the month for at least three or four months so that you understand what is related to your menstrual cycle and what is not.

- Find a PMT club or group to join – other women's experiences can be very reassuring and even curative.

- Keep a note on the family's calendar so that the rest of the family know why you are behaving strangely and can make allowances.

- Having learned by self-observation when to expect symptoms, do the following from ten days before their onset until the day you start bleeding:
  1. Stop eating added sugar, sweet foods, refined-flour products and between-meals sugary snacks.

2. Stop adding salt to your cooking or to your food at the table. This will help reduce the amount of fluid you retain and could make you feel a lot better.

3. Stop drinking coffee and cola drinks. Drink only weak tea or other non-caffeine-containing drinks.

4. Reduce or cut out alcohol and smoking.

5. Start eating six small, high-protein meals a day rather than two or three big meals–don't eat *more* over the day; simply spread it out evenly so you don't go for long periods without eating.

6. Increase your intake of foods rich in magnesium. These include millet, corn, brown rice, potato, cashew nuts, peanuts and tomatoes. Reduce your intake of dairy foods because, being rich in calcium, they interfere with magnesium absorption.

7. Take brewers' yeast tablets (two a day) to improve your sugar metabolism.

8. Take six capsules of evening primrose oil a day. This is especially useful for women whose main complaint is breast swelling.

9. Reduce your intake of fats, avoiding particularly animal fats and hydrogenated margarines. Consume only high quality margarines, high in polyunsaturates.

10. Take daily exercise, preferably out-of-doors. Walking and running are ideal, as are aerobic exercises and swimming.

11. If you are a PMT-H type restrict your fluid intake and beware of hidden salt in your diet as well as obvious salt. Pickled foods, preserved foods, cured meats, spinach and celery all contain large amounts of salt, so be careful. PMT-A women seem to improve with the addition of vitamin B_6.

12. If this preventive regime doesn't work then progesterone (a natural hormone made from inedible yams) can be given by a doctor. Progestogens, the synthetic versions of progesterones used in the contraceptive pill, tend to make PMT worse. Natural progesterone is best, given as a vaginal pessary or as a suppository. For some women even quite a short course of progesterone can stimulate their hormone production to normal levels.

•   Try to cut down on the stress in your life–this will help your PMT symptoms. (See page 87).

•   It is my own personal clinical experience, and that of several others who work in this field, that many women who suffer from PMT have emotional or marital problems that are the cause and not the result of their PMT. I find that there is often a substantial psychosexual element with many of these women and that they often give a history of troubled sexual or interpersonal relationships. I have cured many women of their PMT by psychotherapy alone and a lot of women have told me that they can date the onset of their PMT to a particular psychological, emotional or sexually-linked event in their lives. Prevention in these women involves sorting out their underlying psycho-sexual problems.

PROSTATE PROBLEMS

What are they?

The prostate gland is an organ the size of a walnut situated at the base of the bladder in males. The first part of the urinary passage flows through it on its way to the penis. Slightly above and behind the prostate are two sacs called the seminal vesicles. These store sperms ready to be ejaculated at orgasm. The prostate gland produces a fluid that nourishes the sperms on their journey to find an egg to fertilise in the female genital tract.

In a large number of men the prostate enlarges in old age. This produces a feeling of discomfort in the pubic area, and gradually the bladder becomes unable to empty fully, involving the man in frequent trips to urinate. The urine then takes some time to come and the stream is poor. Such men wake a lot at night to pass water. Eventually the bladder mouth can be totally shut off by the enlarged prostate and causes a complete inability to pass urine. If untreated this causes toxic symptoms because the body is unable to get rid of nitrogen-based waste matter in the urine.

A much rarer condition is prostatic cancer. Removal of the gland is mandatory in this condition and may become necessary in benign (non-cancerous) prostatic enlargement.

Lastly, the gland can become inflamed – a condition called prostatism or prostatitis.

If you ever have any of the following, see your doctor to have him or her check up on your prostate.

1. Difficulty in starting to pass water or a poor stream once you do.

2. A chronic sense of fullness of the bladder.

3. Impotence or premature ejaculation.

4. Pain on ejaculation.

5. Erections that occur without any special stimulation.

6. Blood in the urine or in semen.

7. Low back pain.

8. Needing to get up at night to pass water.

9. Pain in the testes.

What causes them?

- Irregular sexual function or prolonged abstinence from sex can cause prostatism and probably benign enlargement.

- Ageing.

- Vitamin E deficiency.

- A shortage of certain amino-acids.

- Faulty fatty-acid metabolism.

- Magnesium deficiency.

- Zinc deficiency.

- Coffee and sugar.

Prevention

- The prostate is part of the sexual apparatus of a man so it is only sensible to look at sexual activity as a cause of prostatic problems. Clearly a man's sexual habits must influence the workings of his prostate.

    The prostate produces fluid all the time which, having built up, needs to be discharged by ejaculation. The build-up appears to take approximately three days in the average young and middle-aged man and longer in the older man.

    Finding that younger men are experiencing prostate problems which in the past were confined to the elderly has led various experts in the field to suggest that prolonged sexual excitement without ejaculation is bad for the gland. This is rather akin to the pelvic congestion that occurs in women who are aroused re-peatedly but don't have an or-gasm – they too suffer from all kinds of pelvic and lower-back symptoms. Also, it is proposed that when such a man does ejaculate his prostatic contractions are poor and that he has a poor-quality orgasm with incomplete emptying of the gland.

Residual fluids degenerate in the gland and cause inflammation and need more muscle power to expel them next time.

No single type of sexual activity necessarily produces prostatic damage, but both excessive mas-turbation or intercourse and too little could do so. The answer must be to find your own sexual rhythm and be guided by how you feel. Certainly, long periods of abstinence from sex may pro-duce prostatic fullness, tender-ness and eventually infection which can be difficult to treat. Zinc supplements and regular emptying of the prostate both help.

- Many animal experiments show that vitamin E deficiency causes all kinds of abnormalities and problems in the sexual life and reproduction of animals. It there-fore makes sense to eat foods rich in the vitamin.

- Natural substances occurring in wheatgerm oil have proved valu-able in animal experiments. It is an old belief among the peasants of the Balkans of eastern Europe that pumpkin seeds are of value for prostatic well-being. Analysis of these seeds shows that they are rich in all the nutrients known to be of value to prostatic health. Other valuable seeds are those of the sunflower. These seeds con-tain the amino-acids glycine, alanine and glutamic acid. A study in the US of forty men with benign prostate troubles found that in 32 per cent of them their prostates shrank to normal size and there was some reduction in size in 92 per cent when they were given these amino-acids. The need to get up at night was reduced or eliminated in 72 per cent and urgent urination was relieved in 81 per cent. Men who received placebo capsules had no similar improvements. This study, rather than stimulating further research, has been largely ignored. Foods that are especially rich in these amino-acids are brewers' yeast, milk, eggs, beef, liver, lentils, nuts and corn.

- Unsaturated fatty acids have been shown to be of value in benign prostatic enlargement. In a study of nineteen men with this condition who were fed unsaturated fatty acids, all had less residual urine at the end of the treatment and twelve of them had none. For thirteen of the nineteen the dietary change meant they no longer wanted to get up at night to urinate. Cystitis cleared up. Dribbling was eliminated in eighteen of them and in nineteen the size of the prostate gland went down. Lecithin is a good source of unsaturated fatty acids.

- Magnesium deficiency has been studied in France in this connection – as long ago as 1930 a French specialist found that it was a valuable food supplement in men with prostatic problems. In one study twelve men with prostatic problems were given magnesium tablets. Ten of them were cured. Another French doctor found that magnesium reduced the swelling of benign enlarged prostates. Often, the reduction in size was small but the improvement in the man great. The specialist concluded that magnesium contributed to the battle against senility. Food sources of magnesium are Dolomite tablets, wheatgerm, honey, nuts, brown rice, seeds of various kinds and kohlrabi.

- Zinc is now the most researched of all the trace elements, with more than a thousand learned papers a year appearing on the subject in the western world alone. Zinc is especially plentiful in the prostate gland for reasons that are as yet unknown. There is a well-established link between a lack of zinc and prostate problems. A prostate gland that is abnormal due to infection contains less zinc than a healthy one. In benign enlargement zinc levels are the same as normal but in cancer of the gland zinc levels are low. Semen too is very rich in zinc but it is still not known why all this zinc is necessary in the male reproductive tract. Zinc appears to be related to spermatic physiology so perhaps prostatic fluid (which contributes substantially to the amount of fluid a man ejaculates) is rich in zinc to sustain sperms and to help them mature.

In a Canadian study, a 35 per cent fall in prostatic zinc levels resulted in mild enlargement of the gland. When the drop in zinc approached 40 per cent the men suffered from chronic infection of the gland. When it dropped by 66 per cent the men developed cancer. Foods rich in zinc are seafoods, brewer's yeast, onions, bran, eggs, nuts, rabbit, peas, beans, lentils, wheatgerm, gelatine and beef liver.

- Coffee and sugar have provable effects on the prostate gland. Every year thousands of men in the UK and US die from prostatic cancer or from the more severe effects of benign enlargement. In Japan cancer of the prostate is almost unknown and even benign enlargement is uncommon. Japanese researchers examined the differences between the diet of men with prostatic troubles in Japan and in the West. There were, of course, many differences but the most compelling was that the Japanese male drinks almost no coffee. The Japanese researchers then went to World Health Organisation statistics and found that in Sweden, where the death rate for prostatic cancer is the highest in the world, coffee consumption is also the highest in the world (8 kg per person per year). They then went through a list of twenty countries and found that for nearly all of them the correlation applied.

They next checked for research into cancer-causing agents in coffee. A US study had indeed found that benzo-pyrene and other cancer-producing hydrocarbons are present in lightly roasted coffees such as are drunk in the US and Europe. Very long roasting does not produce a coffee rich in these substances – such coffee is drunk in Italy where cancer of the prostate is half that of Sweden. So could it be that over thirty years of coffee drinking these tiny amounts of carcinogens can produce prostatic cancer? Sugar consumption is also statistically linked to prostatic cancer and whilst no correlation can be found between coffee consumption and other types of cancer in the body, this is not so with sugar. There is a higher incidence of cancer of the breast, ovary, intestine and rectum the more sugar a person consumes. This raises the question as to whether it could be the sugar in the coffee that could be causing the prostatic cancer and not the coffee itself. More research is needed.

PSORIASIS

What is it?

Psoriasis is a common skin condition affecting a million people in the UK and a further 7 million in the US. About 80 million people suffer from it worldwide. It appears as red, raised pustules covered with silvery scales and it can occur on any part of the body, though knees, elbows and the scalp are the most usual sites. The nails are involved in about one in three sufferers. Approximately one in seven people having suffered an attack of psoriasis then remain clear for more than a year, but to remain clear permanently is rare.

Psoriasis affects men and women equally, usually starts between the ages of 14 and 45 and is particularly common during adolescence, pregnancy and the menopause, though it can disappear at these times too. Certain races seem to be immune to the disease, notably the North American Indians.

What causes it?

The basic cause is not known. Heredity definitely plays a part though the actual pattern of inheritance is not yet understood. The genetic tendency can, however, be triggered by injury, a throat infection, certain drugs, and both physical and emotional stress.

Prevention

Apart from generally trying to avoid the triggers listed above, prevention for psoriasis amounts to minimising its effects by avoiding things that make it worse.

- As many as 50 per cent of all psoriatics are made worse by emotional stress and worry. The psoriasis then produces more stress, and so on. Relaxation exercises, meditation and hypnotherapy can help prevent such stresses.

- Some psoriatics (about one in five) are better in the summer. One in twelve is better in the winter. Some sufferers, especially those with fair skins or red hair, are made worse by the sun, and areas that are burned may progress to psoriasis.

- Drugs used to treat conditions other than psoriasis can produce a rash which turns into psoriasis. Steroids may provoke or worsen psoriasis. Certain tranquillisers, aspirin, and codeine-containing drugs and medications can aggravate psoriasis in some sufferers. There is no evidence that the Pill has any effect on psoriasis.

- Many diets have been tried and some helpful results are beginning to trickle through. Recent research suggests that there are subtle changes in the metabolism of certain derivatives of dietary oils in psoriasis. It could thus be possible to improve psoriasis by long-term changes in diet. This makes the following worth a try:

1. Reduce animal fat intake.

2. Eat plenty of fresh fruit and vegetables.

3. Take high doses of zinc (preferably under medical supervision).

RAPE

What is it?

A sexual assault, usually involving intercourse, on a woman against her will. It is an increasingly common crime in large cities everywhere and in the US it is at epidemic proportions. Any figures as to exactly how often it happens are purely speculative because experts in the field estimate that between 75 and 90 per cent of all rapes go unreported. Most rapes occur at the hands of someone known to the woman and the assault itself often occurs in circumstances which make establishing that the woman really was unwilling very difficult.For example, the claim of a woman that she was raped when hitchhiking alone may be countered by a claim by the car driver that she led him on. A woman may lead a man on sexually and then think better of it before intercourse has taken place – her change of heart does not always get through to the man.

Unfortunately, many rape victims have further unpleasant experiences after the rape itself in the hands of the police: intensive, often sceptical, questioning, disbelief, humiliating gynaecological examinations, and so on. For these,and many other reasons, most women do not choose to pursue the charge of rape to the bitter end.

What causes it?

- Most rapists are immature, often violent in other ways and dislike women in general. They have often been intimidated or humiliated by women. Some can only become sexually aroused if the sex act is violent and can't enjoy or even have sex with a compliant woman.

- Alcohol and rape often go together – partly because an immature man such as this may only be able to bring himself to do anything at all sexually when fortified with alcohol. A US study found that half of all convicted rapists had taken alcohol before committing the crime and that 35 per cent of them were actual alcoholics.

Prevention

- Keep away from lonely areas, especially at night. Go with someone else or wait until someone else comes by and walk a little behind them.

- Avoid areas where there are known to be street gangs.

- Take taxis late at night if at all possible.

- If you think someone is following you run into the middle of the road and stop a car.

- Never get into your parked car at night without first looking in the back seat.

- Park under a light at night.

- Put locks on your doors and

windows at home. Never open the front door without using a safety chain.

- Always ask to see the identity cards of workers who come to the house unless you know them.

- If attacked, scream–this can immediately put off many (but not all) rapists. If he does not desist, pull your knee up into his groin and dig him in the eyes with your fingers.

- If the rapist is armed take it quietly and don't do anything heroic–a combination of a weapon and a few drinks can be lethal. Once you have decided on this passive role talk to your attacker. Some rapists, once they have the realisation forced on them that their victim is a person, can't go any further and run away. Many women have talked a rapist out of the attack at this stage but it may be difficult to remain calm enough for this.

  Be careful not to fuel your attacker's ardour by mentioning the suffering he is causing you– this will usually make matters worse. Try to memorise things about him–his speech, clothes, appearance, and so on–so that you can describe him to the police. If he rapes you act as lifeless as possible and certainly don't show any emotions or this could make him more violent.

- If you feel that someone you know is likely to rape you contact a local rape crisis centre to discuss

it and get their advice. The address can be found in the telephone book. They are also very helpful when it comes to coping with the aftermath of a rape whether or not you report it to the police. If you are raped, contact a centre as soon as you possibly can after the rape occurs.

SEX DRIVE LOSS

What is it?

We all have a drive to have intercourse or some kind of sexual outlet and this drive varies in intensity throughout our lives. Younger people on balance have more drive and at every age what we actually end up doing is the result of the balance between our natural drives and our cultural inhibitions.

Any discussion about 'poor' sex drive is difficult because you have to be sure about what you are comparing yourself with.If you are making comparisons with a mythical 'norm' you imagine to be present in society, you could be in for trouble because the range of normality in sexual matters is so great. If you are comparing yourself with *yourself* that could be more sensible but even so is difficult because we all experience normal variations in how much we feel like sex.

Males are at the peak of their sex drive in the late teens and women probably in their thirties, but there are many variables that operate in quite normal, healthy people to alter their sex drive, even from day to day.

What causes it?

- Drugs. The most commonly suggested culprit is the contraceptive pill. Research with dummy tablets given to women who thought they were taking the Pill, however, shows that this has been somewhat overstated as a side-effect of the Pill. Having said this, some women feel depressed or sexless on one particular type and yet are perfectly happy on another brand. Sleeping tablets, high doses of steroids, some drugs taken to relieve high blood pressure, diuretics (water tablets) and some angina drugs can all cause a loss of sex drive. Tranquillisers, in even quite moderate doses, produce indifference in some women and as a result they lose interest in sex. Given that so many women are taking tranquillisers this is an important cause of a loss of sex drive.

- Depression is a potent cause of a poor sex drive and given that it is the commonest psychological illness should always be considered in anyone (especially a woman) who goes off sex.

- Serious physical illness such as arthritis, kidney disease, chronic anaemia and breast disease can all reduce a person's interest in sex.

- Physical and mental exhaustion can have a disastrous effect on one's sex drive. After having a baby, after an operation, or after many, even quite trivial, illnesses (such as 'flu) many people go off sex because they feel generally 'low' and run down.

- Stress is a common reason for a loss of sex drive. Any life crisis, from moving house to a bereavement, can kill one's sex drive for a while.

- Bad experiences are a less common cause but an understandable one. A rotten relationship, a bad love-making episode, an abortion, being jilted, and so on, can all make certain people say, 'To hell with sex—it's far too much trouble.' Such individuals go off sex for weeks or months but usually return to sexual activity eventually.

- Serious inhibitions produced in childhood and during growing up. Most of these reside in the person's unconscious mind yet they restrict the pleasure the individual is able to get out of sex. Often their pleasure is so limited that they end up having very little sex drive at all.

- Falling out of love. One in three marriages goes wrong and possibly at some stage in every marriage there is a time when the couple don't feel much for each other. At such times either one or both goes off sex.

- During an extramarital affair. This loss of sex drive occurs mainly because of the guilt involved. Some people go off sex with their regular partner during an affair partly out of fear that he or she will be able to detect some small difference in love-making which originated in their love-making with the lover. Sometimes a bad relationship outside the marriage can reflect on the marital one, and produce a loss of sex drive.

Prevention

Obviously factors such as the level of inhibitions one has about sex can't be prevented in the here-and-now because their seeds lie deep in childhood. However, much can be done with the help of an insightful professional to heal even some of these old wounds.

- Go through the list above and think out what you could do to prevent further loss of sex drive occurring. You will be surprised at the good results you get simply by revealing things between you as a couple. If you don't make much progress get professional help—it's well worth while. So treating the underlying cause should be the first preventive measure against any further or future loss of sex drive.

- Make your lives more erotic. Increase your level of sexual awareness by: reading erotic books; watching sexy videos or films; sharing sexy magazines; sharing your fantasies; increasing the erotic potential of your bedroom; learning to massage each other; going on a holiday together, however short, to be totally alone; and so on.

- Step up your masturbation rate. This almost always works wonders and gives you a chance to enrich and rehearse your fantasy life. This works especially well for women. Most such women find that if they step up their masturbation rate they want more intercourse.

- Get your confidence back in your genitals, by using sex aids if necessary, and by learning to please each other genitally without intercourse. Practise mutual masturbation until you can both give each other better orgasms than by self-masturbation.

- Return to courtship behaviour: send each other little notes; give one another small presents; take every opportunity to cuddle and kiss in everyday life without going on to have sex; spend more time together; go out with one another as if you were on an early date; and so on.

SEXUAL BOREDOM

What is it?

A feeling that after some time with the same partner things have become predictable and lost their spice and excitement. Most couples who have been married for more than ten years or so complain that sex is boring some, or even all, of the time. Sexual boredom is not inevitable, though, and can be prevented as we shall see. Having said this, many couples are apparently perfectly happy with sex lives that would be judged as very 'boring' by others. It is what suits any one couple that matters and not what other people think.

What causes it?

- Being bored with yourself. If you feel you are boring and don't get much joy out of life it is hardly surprising that sex seems boring too.

- As well as being bored some people are boring–they do the same things time after time, so that having them in bed is like making love with a robot. This is a common criticism of men by their women. Many such people are boring out of bed too.

- Just letting things slip. This is a common cause. Most couples are not bores–they've just stopped putting in much effort. This can happen in all departments of the relationship, of course–not just with regard to sex.

- Laziness. Most people settle for the least sexual activity they can get away with within their re-

lationship and then wonder why they get bored. We all expect to spend time and care shopping for and preparing a good meal, yet most people expect good sex simply to happen as if by magic. Of course, it rarely does and those whose sex lives are not boring spend time preparing and planning for sex.

- Being aware of what your partner wants. Quite often what your partner does to you is what they want to be done to them.

Prevention

- Start a new interest in life; take up a hobby; go to an evening class; do something that you have always wanted to do, and not necessarily with your partner. Examine your job and see if you could get more out of it or put more into it. If as a result of any of these things you become more interesting to yourself or your partner you are on the way to preventing sexual boredom.

- Try to be more spontaneous and, if necessary, get professional help to overcome any personality problems that are holding you back.

- Try something different. When did you last explore something new in your sexual relationship? You have probably, without consciously realising it, settled for less than the best. But in the search for novelty don't throw out or jeopardise your existing, if routine, pleasures. Our interest in new things has to be traded off against the security of the familiar and reliable. Too much hectic change is unsettling in sexual matters as elsewhere in life.

• Be yourself. Stop trying to be something your partner wants – exert your own needs and desires. Don't hide your feelings – it's more sexy to reveal them to your lover. You need to be selfish at least to some extent if you are to prevent boredom. Unfortunately, we are brought up to be reticent about what we would most like and often settle for far less.

• Share your fantasies. The most important sex organ is the mind! Be wary, though, about what and how you share. Be sensitive to your partner, especially if your fantasies involve someone of the opposite sex whom he or she knows. Many women especially fear that today's fantasy could become tomorrow's fact – though this rarely occurs.

• Go for the best at all times. Get away from stereotypes and make your love-making unique to you as a couple. This is true romance. It also makes it less likely that either of you will look outside for sexual pleasures – if only because the chances are that you will be

getting more fulfilling sex at home.

• Talk to each other about what is important to you – and not just regarding sex. Make time to share what really matters to each of you in life. As you explore each other more you will become genuinely more interested and interesting and will find sex less boring too.

• Improve your surroundings. Make your bedroom more cosy and more sexy. Perhaps get a TV or video for the bedroom. Ensure that the room can be warmed up quickly. Get some erotic literature, perhaps some sex toys, and so on.

• Forget about being 'in the mood'. Many people, women especially, believe that unless they feel 'romantic' they shouldn't have sex. This in itself leads to mounting boredom because there is no one mood in which enjoyable sex can or should take place. Try having sex when you are bored, miserable, angry, sad or quiet as well as when you feel happy or 'sexy'. This produces new emotions and can be a real eye-opener.

• Stop having sex for a while if it is boring you. Go back to courtship behaviour. Learn to enjoy each other in ways that don't end in intercourse. Once you have increased your repertoire in this way you will return to sex with a new vigour and certainly be less bored!

SIGHT PROBLEMS

What are they?

At one end of the spectrum there is complete blindness–a condition affecting some 16 million people around the world. There are several causes, including detachment of the retina, amblyopia, glaucoma, congenital blindness, trauma to the eye, diabetic retinopathy and various infections. The common conditions affecting the eyes (and sometimes leading to blindness) in western countries are considered under the headings glaucoma (page 222), diabetes (page 195) and cataract (page 173).

This section deals with the much more common, yet rarely sight-threatening, conditions: short sight, long sight and presbyopia (old sight). These conditions affect most of us to some degree, with more than half of all North Americans and British between the ages of 6 and 74 wearing glasses or contact lenses all or some of the time. Unfortunately, the problem seems to get worse with age. Fewer than 12 per cent of 6–11-year-olds need correction yet about 95 per cent of those aged 65–74 do. Whether or not such a deterioration in vision is inevitable is open to debate. Research over recent years suggests that much could be prevented.

What causes them?

- Poor nutrition.
- Poor lighting.
- Mental strain.
- Wearing spectacles.
- Too little exercise of the eyes.

Prevention

- The eye is an extremely sensitive barometer of diet. When the eye's diameter changes by even as little as a millimetre it makes a big difference to vision. At one end of the poor-nutrition scale, a quarter of a million Asian children go blind each year from malnutrition. Xerophthalmia, the main cause of such blindness, is a result of generally poor nutrition and in particular of a lack of vitamin A. Few westerners, however, are at risk of *losing* their sight due to a faulty diet. Many, though, have far worse sight than they should have.

  An early sign of vitamin A deficiency is poor vision in dim light. One study of 100 people taken at random found that twenty-six of them had at least some degree of night blindness. The prevention for this is to eat foods rich in vitamin A. Liver is the best source but fruits and green leafy vegetables are good sources. Zinc too has been found to be vital for night vision. Studies of people with the condition who did not respond to vitamin A supplements have found that adding zinc made the difference. Zinc is now known to play a vital role in the conversion of vitamin A to its active form, retinoldehyde, in the retina. Vitamin B and folate in particular are now being studied in the context of healthy vision.

It appears that green and yellow vegetables are vital if one is to maintain healthy vision. Some food additives, particularly monosodium glutamate (MSG), have a particularly bad effect on the eyes, according to one US researcher. When added to commercial foods in large amounts it damages the nerves. He feels that MSG should not be given to children, though he is less cautious about adults as they have a natural barrier to the toxic effects of the substance.

Although short-sightedness is not mainly caused by diet certain research seems to show that a poor diet worsens it. One study found that myopic people who ate too much sugar and protein, were deficient in chromium and didn't metabolise calcium properly. There are now numerous studies linking poor nutrition to eye problems and vitamin E is an exciting area of research. Highly vitamin E-deficient animals go blind in time. The human retina, it appears, is susceptible to oxidation–unless protected by an anti-oxidant such as vitamin E. Research in rats has found that a diet poor in vitamins E and A results in permanent damage to nearly half the animal's visual cells in eight months. There is little doubt that a wholefood, unrefined diet is the best starting point to improving poor sight.

- All eyes need good light if they are to work well and without strain. This particularly applies to older eyes. A recent study of visual acuity in fifty-six old people (average age 76), both in their homes and in a controlled clinical setting, found that general levels of lighting were often so poor in the homes of elderly people that the number of people functioning as 'blind' was twice what it needed to be. Simply increasing the wattage of the lighting, they found, improved the vision of 82 per cent of the people. Don't skimp on lighting. A 100-watt light bulb costs only pennies more a month to run than a 60-watt bulb.

As the eye ages, the lens becomes clouded and less pliable and the pupil decreases in size. Less light reaches the retina and near-focusing ability declines. Most people get glasses for their focusing problem but do little to increase the light that enters the eye. Research has found that the reduction of light reaching the retina is 50 per cent by the age of 50, and 66 per cent by age 60. Older eyes also react more slowly to changes in light levels, and because the cloudiness of the lens scatters light all around the inside of the eye, simply increasing the amount of light helps all this greatly. But this need for more light, especially at work, is not just confined to the old. Research shows that middle-aged workers need more light than do younger workers. An Ohio State University study found that 30–40-year-olds needed 17 per cent more contrast to see an object as clearly as 20–30-year-olds, and that those aged 60–70 needed two and a half times as much contrast to be able to see as well as the younger ones.

Older people, especially, are susceptible to glare and brightness. An older person facing a window all day at his or her desk is looking up at very bright light and then down at the work. This causes eye fatigue as the pupils enlarge and constrict. Also, when you look down with constricted pupils you will see very badly.

A way of seeing whether you are subjecting yourself to too much glare is to lay a mirror on your desk or table. If you can see a bright zone in the mirror when you are seated normally, it is a glare that could be causing you eye strain. Very highly-reflective surfaces can have the same effect too. Alter either the light or the furniture, whichever is easier, to overcome this problem.

When considering levels of illumination remember that intensity of light follows the inverse square law which means that moving a 25-watt bulb from 8 ft to 4 ft away is the equivalent of replacing it with a 100-watt bulb.

- Mental strain. Dr Bates, the man who became famous through his eye exercises to promote healthy vision, considered that most defective vision is caused by mental strain, and that a nervous temperament with a tendency to mental tension and rigidity of thought is the cause of most cases of serious visual deficiency. Whilst there is undoubtedly some truth in this it is too narrow a view, in my opinion. Having said this, relaxation exercises definitely do seem to improve vision. Three that are worth trying are:

Palming is done as follows. Sit in as comfortable a position as possible and relax. Close your eyes and cover them with the palms of your hands, crossing the fingers over the centre of the forehead but so that the right palm is on the right eye and the left on the left. Don't press on the eyes themselves. Allow your elbows to drop to your knees with your knees fairly close together. Close your eyes and keep them closed. Relax your mind too–don't think of things that upset you. Imagine the blackness you see getting blacker and blacker. Do this for 20–30 minutes twice a day and you will soon notice an improvement in vision.

Blinking. Normally the eye blinks at regular intervals all the time it is open. In people with defective vision the eye becomes more fixed and strained and blinking less frequent. It is often done sporadically and with effort. Try to get into the habit of blinking frequently and regularly. Consciously make yourself blink once every ten seconds or so no matter what you are doing and especially when reading or doing close work.

Swaying is another useful technique. It relaxes the mind and the body at the same time, and helps relieve eye strain. Stand with your feet about 12 inches apart with your hands hanging by your sides. Sway your whole body (not just your trunk) from side to side like a pendulum. Raise each heel alternately from the ground. Do this for 5–10 minutes twice a day. After swaying for a minute or so with the eyes open, close them and carry on swaying. Create a mental image of the object (a window, for example) that is in front of you and at which you were looking before you closed your eyes. Re-open your eyes and really look at the object for another minute, swaying all the time. Repeat this process with eyes open and eyes closed.

- Many experts in the natural treatment of eye problems claim that spectacles actually do more harm than good for many people. They claim that this can be clearly deduced from the fact that most people who wear spectacles continue to experience deteriorating sight over the years rather than being 'cured' of it. It is certainly true that wearing spectacles throws the whole process of seeing out of gear and that glasses make the eyes lazier rather than encouraging them to heal themselves.

    Few people could or would happily throw their glasses away when starting on a natural cure for their defective vision – although it is claimed that the best results occur in this way – but you can stop wearing them unless they are absolutely vital for the task in hand at the time. Even if they are left off for only a few hours a day the eyes begin to react naturally and after a couple of weeks of treatment most people are surprised at the improvement in their vision. Eventually, some such people can do without spectacles altogether and most will need weaker ones.

- Much of modern life makes our eyes lazy – eye exercises appear to help improve vision simply by re-educating the eyes. There are several exercises that are claimed to help. For example, memorise a small object with your eyes open, then after getting a clear mental picture, close your eyes and try to remember it as well as you possibly can. Open your eyes, look at the object again and repeat the cycle. Do this for five minutes every day without your glasses.

Reading without glasses is good eye training. The secret of this is to read without strain. Here's how to do it. Palm (see above) for a few minutes, then take a book or magazine and start to read at the distance at which you can best see the print. Read a few lines, or however much you can until you feel your eyes becoming tired. Stop. Close your eyes completely for a few seconds and then start again. Blink frequently and consciously as you read. Try this regularly and you will find that you can read more and more without eye strain. Ensure that these exercises are done in a good, non-glaring light.

Another useful exercise is to practise moving your eyes up and down, round and round, from side to side, and so on, rhythmically and systematically for a couple of minutes at odd times during the day (when standing in the queue at the supermarket, for example). Rest in between each exercise.

Yet another exercise involves holding up your index finger about 8–10 inches in front of your face and looking intently at it. Then look away from the finger to an object on the other side of the room. Look back and forth from one to the other ten times, rest for a few seconds and then repeat the sequence.

Some people find that doing simple neck exercises helps improve their vision. These should be done on rising in the morning.

Raise first one shoulder and then the other and rotate them so that the point of the shoulder describes circles in the air. Do this twenty or thirty times on each side.

Allow your chin to drop as far forward as possible into your chest, keeping your neck relaxed. Raise the head and allow it to fall backwards as far as possible. Repeat ten times. Now rotate your head so that your ears come close to your shoulders as you do so. Do this ten or twenty times slowly.

If done daily these exercises and diet changes should start to produce positive results in a very few weeks. You may need to see your optician to get weaker glasses over the first few months, or you may find that you can leave them off for longer periods during each day.

SKIN CANCER

What is it?

There are basically two important types of skin cancer. The non-malignant type is the more common and is seen in fair-skinned people who expose themselves excessively to sunlight. It is easily treated and does not kill. The malignant type is called a malignant melanoma and is a killer.

Skin cancers are most common on

the face and other areas where the skin is exposed to the sun. Any skin damage that does not heal properly should be seen by a doctor. Also, should a pigmented patch of skin you have had for years start to become more pigmented, be suspicious and seek advice. One type of skin cancer starts as a pale, pearly, raised, translucent nodule that slowly enlarges and then ulcerates. The next most common type is a small, raised area or patch that can be reddened or darkened and hard. A common site for this latter type is on the lower lip.

What causes it?

Researchers at the University of Arizona (a very sunny site) found that the incidence of the malignant form of skin cancer jumped 34 per cent over a ten-year period. Since 1960 until the present day the incidence of the non-malignant type has also risen by a startling 500 per cent. Nearly half of all the tumours were found in people aged between 50 and 69. Malignant melanoma is rising in incidence at a rate of 5 per cent per year in the US.

Other researchers have found that pale-skinned, easily burned people with an estimated lifetime sun exposure of more than 30,000 hours have a twenty times greater risk of developing skin cancer than a comparable group with less than 10,000 hours of sun exposure. More than 200,000 cases of skin cancer occur in the US annually though the incidence is much less in the UK because there is less sun. Northern climates have less sun and so less cancer of the skin. For every 265 miles you go closer to the equator the incidence of skin cancer doubles.

Another form of skin change caused by sunlight is the breakdown of the normal connective, elastic tissue called collagen. This produces premature ageing of the skin and is a reason why Californian women so envy the skin of English women.

Prevention

- Use a sunscreen preparation if you are in the sun a lot.

- Be guided by the general rules for preventing sunburn (see page 346).

SKIN DRYNESS

What is it?

Itchy, irritating, dry skin from any cause. The skin becomes prematurely wrinkled and often drives the person (especially a child) mad with itching.

What causes it?

- Extremes of temperature from freezing winds to direct sun.

- Ageing itself makes skin drier.

- Central heating without humidifiers.

- The use of detergents as bath foams (especially children's 'fun' bath products). This removes the natural oils from the skin.

- The misuse of cosmetics which block the oil glands that normally lubricate the skin.

Prevention

- Drink more water.

- Stay out of harsh sunlight unless you wear an effective sunscreen.

- Never use detergents in the bath and use soaps sparingly.

- Wear gloves if you use detergents for washing up dishes.

- Try to get a humidifier installed in your place of work or any other air-conditioned building where you spend a lot of time.

- Use only small amounts of skin lotions – the skin can absorb only so much, after which you block the natural ducts that bring oils to the surface. The best moisturiser for the skin is water – not oils. Use oils and creams, therefore, on slightly moistened skin. Many good moisturiser creams are mostly water for this reason.

- One skin expert uses a mixture of five vitamin A capsules to a 4 ounce jar of hand or body lotion to alleviate dry skin, with some success.

SMOKING DISEASES

What are they?

Diseases that are caused directly or indirectly by smoking tobacco. The best known is lung cancer but this is only the tip of the iceberg, as we shall see.

Smoking is the single greatest cause of death in the UK, and the World Health Organisation has said that the control of smoking would do more good than any other single action in preventive medicine. At least 100,000 deaths are attributable to smoking in Britain each year with an average loss of about ten years of life. It accounts for 90 per cent of deaths from lung cancer; 75 per cent of deaths from chronic bronchitis; and 25 per cent of deaths from coronary heart disease in men under 65. The risk of coronary heart disease attributable to smoking is greater in younger men so that a man under 45 who smokes twenty-five or more a day may have a fifteen times greater risk of dying from a heart attack than if he were a non-smoker. Here are some chilling facts:

- Early studies suggested that relative mortality risks among female smokers were less than those of male smokers, but it is now clear that these studies were comparing the death rates of a generation of lifelong male smokers with a generation of women who had taken up smoking much later in life. The smoking characteristics of the two sexes are now becoming more and more alike, and the rates of smoking-related diseases are drawing closer together.

- Women who take the contraceptive pill and who also smoke cigarettes are more likely to have a coronary attack, stroke, and blood clots in the leg veins which may shift to the lung (pulmonary embolus), than are non-smokers who are on the Pill. One study has shown that for women aged 25-34 on the Pill the relative risk of death from circulatory disease was 1.6 for non-smoking Pill takers but 3.4 for smokers; women aged 35–44 the risks were 3.3 and 4.2 respectively, and for women over 45, 4.6 and 7.4. There is also a considerable increased risk for women on the Pill who smoke and who have one or more known risk factors for coronary heart disease.

- The natural menopause occurs on average 2–3 years earlier in smokers.

- Fetal growth and birth weight. Babies born to women who smoke are on average 200 g lighter than babies born to comparable non-smoking mothers. The relationship between maternal smoking and low birth weight is independent of all other risk factors which influence birth weight including maternal size, race, socio-economic status and the sex of the child. Furthermore,

the more cigarettes a woman smokes during pregnancy, the greater the probable reduction in birth weight. However, if a woman stops smoking before the twentieth week of pregnancy, her risk of having a low-weight baby will be similar to that of a non-smoker.

- Children whose mothers smoke ten or more cigarettes after the fourth month of pregnancy tend to show poor progress at school, at least up to the age of 16. In both reading and mathematics tests they do less well than other children. This effect is found after allowing for other factors affecting educational level.

- Spontaneous abortion. Tobacco use during pregnancy causes a two-fold increase in the risk of spontaneous abortion (miscarriage).

- Complications of pregnancy. On average, smokers have more complications of pregnancy and labour, which can include bleeding during pregnancy, premature detachment of the placenta and premature rupture of the membranes.

- Perinatal mortality (defined as still-birth or death of an infant within the first week of life) increases in direct relation to the number of cigarettes smoked during pregnancy. In one large study, the perinatal mortality risk increased by 20 per cent for the infants of smokers of less than twenty cigarettes per day and by 35 per cent for smokers of twenty or more a day, compared with that of non-smokers.

- Breast feeding. Research has shown that smoking cigarettes may contribute to inadequate breast-milk production. Nicotine has also been found in the breast milk of mothers who smoke, although the effect on the baby is not yet fully understood.

- Long-term growth. Studies of long-term growth and development give evidence that children of mothers who smoked in pregnancy may have slight but measurable deficiencies in physical growth and intellectual development up to 11 years of age. Infants of parents who smoke are also more susceptible to chest infections, bronchitis and pneumonia than are the children of non-smokers.

- The act of breathing in other people's smoke has been labelled 'passive', 'involuntary' or 'second-hand' smoking. Many non-smokers experience nose, throat and eye irritation from passive smoking; and there is evidence that long-term exposure may be harmful even to normal,healthy adults. Non-smokers dislike the smell of tobacco smoke in their clothes and hair following exposure.

The smoke from the burning end and from the mouthpiece of the cigarette is more irritant than the smoke which is breathed out. Since pipe and cigar smokers tend to inhale less than cigarette smokers, the contribution of their smoke to atmospheric pollution may be greater than that of cigarette smokers.

- Non-smokers who report recent exposure to smoke have been found to have nicotine concentrations in their saliva and urine which overlapped those of smokers who had smoked up to three cigarettes before sampling.

- Carbon monoxide (CO) levels in air heavily contaminated by tobacco smoke can exceed those permitted in industry for an eight-hour exposure. The amount absorbed by the non-smoker increases with the period of exposure.

- Recent research found that non-smokers who worked for twenty years with smokers, but who were not exposed to cigarette smoke at home, had sustained measurable lung damage similar to that in smokers who did not inhale.

- A Japanese study has shown that the non-smoking wives of cigarette smokers developed lung cancer at higher rates than non-smoking wives of non-smoking husbands. The study followed up 91,540 non-smoking wives for fourteen years. The lung-cancer mortality rate of those married to men who smoked twenty or more cigarettes a day was twice as high as that of women who were married to non-smokers.

- In another study, in Greece, it was found that for non-smoking women the relative risk of lung cancer associated with having a husband who smokes was an estimated 2.4 for women whose husbands smoked less than twenty cigarettes a day and 3.4 for those whose husbands smoked more than this.

- Young children can be harmed by passive smoking. Infants under a year in age run twice the risk of developing a serious chest illness if both parents smoke. Also, children of parents who smoke have more upper respiratory infections than do children of non-smokers.

- Since the early 1970s the proportion of adult cigarette smokers (over 16) in Great Britain has been decreasing. Between 1972 and 1982 the proportion of adult male smokers fell by over a quarter and that of women by about one fifth. Smokers have been a minority in the adult population since 1976.

  It has been estimated that there are about 16–17 million adult smokers in the population of Great Britain, and nearly 10 million ex-smokers. Between 1980 and 1982 about one million people gave up smoking.

- Since 1978 men have been smoking on average fewer cigarettes per week, although they smoke slightly more now than in 1972.

- Cigarette sales in the UK have been declining steadily since 1974.

- There is a link between cigarette smoking and socio-economic group, showing a continuing trend for more smokers (men and women) in manual than in non-manual groups but in 1982 smokers were, for the first time, a minority in every socio-economic group.

- In England and Wales alone about 95,000 people are killed by smoking each year. It has been estimated that out of 1,000 young men who smoke in the UK, 1 will be murdered, 6 will die in road accidents and 250 will die prematurely as a result of their smoking. Most die from one of the three main diseases associated with cigarette smoking: lung cancer; chronic bronchitis/emphysema; and coronary heart disease. Lung cancer is caused almost entirely by smoking. In 1981 about a third of the total deaths from lung cancer were in people aged under 65. Although deaths from this disease are declining among men, they are rising among women.

- More than two-thirds of all smokers want to give up.

Why bother to give up?

- You will save money – about £10 a week if you smoke twenty cigarettes a day.

- You will have better-smelling breath and clothes.

- Your teeth and fingers won't be stained.

- You will feel fitter.

- You will lose your morning cough.

- You will be increasing your life expectancy considerably.

- You will have fewer colds.

- You will be nicer to be with – kissing a smoker is not much fun.

- You will be setting a good example to your children – and they will be less likely to smoke.

- Your children will have fewer colds and less risk of pneumonias.

- You won't be risking the health of others around you who inhale your second-hand smoke.

Prevention

The prevention of smoking can be tackled at three levels. *Primary prevention* tries to persuade young people not to take up smoking. *Secondary prevention* tries to persuade existing smokers that it is worth giving up before their health suffers. *Tertiary prevention* tries to help those who already have a health problem to give up, with the intention of halting that problem and prolonging their life.

Whatever stage you are at, once you are a smoker it is difficult to give up. Full understanding of the facts outlined above is generally not the total answer – you will probably need some kind of additional motivation. Many people stop smoking if advised to do so by their doctor. In one study, 62 per cent of those who had recently had a heart attack were persuaded to stop for at least a year, and in another study of heart-attack victims those who stopped smoking had half the number of relapses (fatal and non-fatal).

Here are some practical tips on how to stop:

- Make a firm decision to stop. Decide on a specific day, which should be a low-stress day.

- Tell other people around you at work and socially that you have stopped.

- Try to avoid smokers and smoky places.

- Get your family and friends to help you stop smoking by giving you moral support and being understanding when the going gets tough.

- Avoid situations in which you have found from experience smoking is most likely.

- Start on a healthy-lifestyle programme – including taking exercise and changing to a healthy diet (see page 70). Take up a new hobby or interest.

- Put aside the money you would have spent on cigarettes in a specific place and save for something you have always wanted but 'couldn't afford'.

- Ask others not to smoke in your presence. Make your house and your office 'non-smoking' areas.

- Throw away all your cigarette lighters, ashtrays, and so on.

- Join a local group that will help you. In the UK Action on Smoking and Health (ASH) will tell you how to find one of the twenty centres around the country.

- Try nicotine-containing chewing gum, hypnotherapy, acupuncture, aversion therapy and group therapy if they seem a good idea to you. It is never easy to stop smoking and any crutch that helps is useful.

- Find other things to do with your hands that will help you cope with tension. Knitting, 'worry beads', playing with a bunch of keys, or whatever, all work.

- Get your family and friends to sponsor you to stop smoking.

- Have a bet with someone as to how long they think you will give up for.

- In the early days of giving up, change your routine so that old trigger-points and situations don't get at you while your urge to smoke is great.

- Keep busy. Sitting around thinking about smoking and how much you miss it will soon have you longing to go back to it.

- Be prepared for the mood swings as your body gets used to doing without the 100–400 puffs a day it has been accustomed to.

- Don't kid yourself about how strong-willed you are–keep away from people and situations where you could be put to the test. One small slip and you will have undone all your previous efforts. One day in the distant future you might be able to enjoy the odd cigarette or cigar after a meal but in the early days this is too much to hope for. Complete abstinence is the only way.

- Give yourself a treat every day. Make sure that not all of them are in the form of foods, or you will soon get fat.

Obviously it is best never to start smoking in the first place. Here are some tips on 'primary' prevention:

- Breastfeed your children exclusively for at least six months and offer the breast after that whenever they need comforting. Psychiatrists and analysts have found that many smokers are 'frozen' at the oral stage of life during which a baby's main pleasure comes from his or her mouth. If breastfeeding (or bottle-feeding even) goes badly and the baby is left to cry, its oral needs unfulfilled, it is thought that later in life he or she will turn to other forms of oral gratification. Undoubtedly, smoking is the most common of these, though earlier on in life dummy- and thumb-sucking are also widespread. Most normally developed adults don't seek oral pleasure in this way and don't respond to stress and anxiety by putting something in their mouths. Some, of course, do and these can be found at any slimming clinic or club.

- Perhaps the best preventive measure adults can take for their children is to ensure that they themselves don't smoke. This will greatly reduce the likelihood that the children around them will want to smoke.

- Next, it's worth trying to bring up our children to be able to resist peer pressures to take up the habit. Most young children say they don't ever want to smoke yet obviously a percentage will be smoking by the age of 15. We should teach children that to take up smoking only because of pressure from their peers is to show that they cannot hold their own against their peers by doing only what they really want to do. They should be encouraged to think of smoking not as tough or glamorous but as an attempt to appear tough or glamorous by those who lack confidence. Such thinking has been shown in tests in California to protect children against drugs and alcohol too.

Another successful ruse is to use older young people to deliver the anti-smoking message in their own style. Play-acting helps in group work and can be fun too. Parents can also get across the message that:

1. You don't have to be conned by smoking advertising.

2. They wish they had never taken it up because they can't afford it.

3. They are glad they gave it up and how much better they feel.

4. It is possible to resist smoking just to go along with the crowd.

5. Smoking doesn't make you 'cool'.

6. By resisting smoking you will also be able to resist drugs and alcohol.

A study of 526 Californian students who were encouraged in this way found that those who were trained to be able to resist the pressures to start the habit began smoking at less than half the rate of those who did not have the training.

SQUINT (lazy eye)

What is it?

A condition in which the eyes don't look at an object in conjunction. The word 'squint' is also used to describe the condition in which children especially screw their eyes up to look at something. This is not really a squint at all but it makes sense to take your child for an eye test if he or she does this.

What causes it?

- In babies under the age of three

months a squint (of the cross-eyed type) can be normal but over this age you should tell your doctor about it.Such squints are more likely to occur if either parent squinted in childhood. If a squint is left it can cause blindness in the affected eye as the brain suppresses the image from that eye because it is out of line with the good eye's image.

- Short sight or long sight which is worse in one eye.

- Measles.

- Meningitis.

- Apparent squint. Sometimes a child appears to be squinting when in fact it is an illusion caused by folds of skin at the nasal side of the eye giving the appearance of a squint. These disappear as the child grows.

Prevention

Most squints cannot be prevented from occurring in the first place – prevention is a matter of recognising and treating the condition that causes them. If you take action as soon as your child starts to squint you can catch it early and prevent it from getting worse – and certainly prevent blindness.

Try covering the good eye so as to encourage the muscles controlling the movements of the squinting eye to work properly. This also encourages the re-education of the brain into perceiving the image from the squinting eye. If this doesn't work an operation may be needed.

STRESS

We looked at stress in some detail in Part One and we saw how relaxation, biofeedback and meditation could help prevent it. Let's look here at some everyday things that anyone can do to de-stress themselves. Some are preventive, in that they mean that the stress will not continue to plague the individual, and others are more curative.

- Have a good cry. According to one research biochemist crying at times of stress helps remove from the body potentially harmful chemicals produced during such times. To try to get evidence for this theory the researcher compared emotionally induced tears with tears that were the result of eye irritation (such as when peeling onions). He found that most people feel better after a cry. In one survey 85 per cent of women and 73 per cent of men said that they felt better after crying if the cause for their crying was emotional. On the opposite side of the coin, those who hold back their tears are more prone to stress-related diseases such as high blood pressure, colitis, and ulcers. A study of 100 men and women with stress-related disorders found that they were more likely than others to see crying as a sign of weakness or as a loss of control.

- Talk about it – don't bottle up your problems until you burst with stress. When faced with stress people either bottle it up, explode or resolve the conflict. One study found that people who refused to get angry when faced with conflict had lower blood pressures. One subject, for example, when attacked by his boss would say, 'Let's be cool, let's deal with the problem.' So explaining the problem in a detached manner is a good way of coping with stress. You acknowledge your anger but are not openly hostile or aggressive.

- Have more fun in life. Many people run their lives in ways that give them little or no fun. This means that they are always so close to their problems that everything seems overwhelming. Holidays can be of real value because the new events and the very fact of being 'away from it all' for a while enable or even compel you to forget your normal stresses. Hobbies can do this on a day-to-day basis but it is vital to have a hobby that does not stress you in the same way that your normal life does. Most people working in this field suggest that you take exercise or indulge in a hobby immediately after or around the time of a stressful event. Recreation can be as effective as drugs in treating stress-related illnesses.

- Take exercise. This doesn't need to be organised, structured or even especially strenuous. One study of ten elderly people suffering from stress-induced neuro-muscular tension measured electrical activity in the muscles to find out the tranquillising effect of exercise when: their heartbeats were at 100 beats a minute; their heartbeats were at 120 beats a minute; they were on a tranquilliser; they were taking a placebo. The best of all of these methods, as regards decreasing electrical activity in the muscles, was the mild exercise (taking their heartbeats to 100 a minute). Exercise at the higher pulse-rate level had an insignificant tranquillising effect, and the tranquilliser drug and the placebo had no effect on the electrical measurements at all. The researchers concluded that 'twenty minutes of walking would do the job nicely to reduce stress! With more rigorous exercise you start to release adrenaline and this fires you up more than it relaxes you.'

- Have a massage. Emotional and psychological stress produces physical tensions in certain muscle groups, especially those of the neck, back and shoulders. In most stressed people it is possible actually to feel the 'knots' in their muscles. In others the area feels 'gritty' when massaged. Learn how to massage your partner, or indeed your children. There are lots of good books on the subject. A shower head can be bought that 'injects' pulsed water at you and this, and a jacuzzi or similar bath can be very soothing too.

Undoubtedly at least some of the benefit from a massage comes from simply relaxing and being stroked, but there is also a strong possibility that the person doing the massage will transfer healing forces to your body. Many people have healing powers in their hands which can be transferred to another person by the 'laying on of hands' or by massage. This sort of statement used to be ridiculed until the demonstration of these healing fields by Kirlian photography.

- Have a hot bath. Warmth is almost always soothing but the bath should not be too hot – the water should be slightly above body temperature. Heat in any extreme is another stress – so don't overdo it. Have a short, relaxing soak. Lie back in the bath, put a rolled-up towel behind your head, close your eyes and relax.

- Breathe more slowly and deeply. We looked at this in some detail on page 76. Most of us breathe shallowly, especially when we are stressed. Practise breathing in (taking 7 seconds) and out (taking 8 seconds) for a couple of minutes at a time, *especially* when you feel stressed. With a little practice you can drop into your stress-reducing breathing very easily at the first sign of stress.

- Learn to relax. See page 87 for more details.

- Pray. Increasing numbers of people in the West are turning to prayer as a way of de-stressing themselves but prayers that are said off by heart and with little thought are useless, according to the author of a book on the subject. You have to be conscious of the meaning of the words if prayer is to have a de-stressing effect. Better still, the author suggests, 'construct your own prayers when under stress'. He finds that the most effective prayers involve the body and the mind as well as the spirit. 'Don't just talk to God – write a letter to him. If you are angry with some-one, tell God you are angry by putting the person's picture on the floor and dancing around it.' The author of the book, *Prayer-ways* (Harper & Row 1980), feels that people need physical as well as spiritual outlets for stress if they are to avoid building up physical symptoms of stress. 'If you play the piano, guitar or other musical instrument, make a prayer song, then play and sing it to God.' It is a great stress discharger, he says.

- Talk to your friends. Many people feel they have no one to whom they can turn when they are stressed and so bottle up all their stress, with harmful effects. Few of us have more than a handful of people to whom we are this close and often it is not our partners or family – they are too involved in our lives in other ways. Social support is a vital element in combating stress yet it is a commodity that is fast being lost in many urban communities. Listening to your friends, as well as talking to them, will also help. Hearing other people's problems can often help put yours into perspective, and turning your thoughts outwards can itself be a valuable de-stressing manoeuvre.

SUFFOCATION AND CHOKING

What are they?

Conditions that lead to a blockage of the air passages and death if not handled quickly. Suffocation occurs when something shuts off the mouth and nostrils, and choking when something goes down the windpipe so that the person cannot breathe. It is mostly children who are affected by both of these conditions.

Children usually choke on pieces of food and sweets, but also on foreign bodies such as coins and buttons. The child chokes, coughs and possibly turns blue. Adults usually choke on food.

What causes them?

Suffocation

- Babies can be suffocated by a pillow in bed.

- Older children can suffocate by putting polythene or similar bags over their heads while playing.

- Older children can suffocate when they climb into a disused refrigerator and shut the door.

- Babies can suffocate by inhaling talcum powder – it clogs their lungs.

Choking

- A baby can choke on vomit in its cot if it is lying on its back.

- Babies or young children can choke on a piece of lumpy food when they are just getting used to eating solids. An older child can choke on a piece of food which has 'gone down the wrong way'.

- Choking on things other than food is a common occurrence in childhood. Beads, small toys and the like are really dangerous.

Prevention

Suffocation

- Don't use a pillow with a very young baby (under a year), unless it is a specially made baby pillow that cannot suffocate the child.

- Keep polythene bags and record sleeves away from young children and babies.

- Take doors off disused refrigerators.

- Keep talcum powder away from babies and young children.

Choking

- Lay a baby on its side or face-down to sleep.

- Mash up food small or put it through a processor until the baby is really ready to cope with lumps.

- Discourage children from throwing sweets, peanuts, and so on, into the air and catching them in their mouths.

- Never let children run around eating–especially sweets.

- Keep beads, coins, buttons, boiled sweets, small toys and marbles away from young children and babies.

If a child (or an adult for that matter) does begin to choke, here's what to do:

If a child begins to choke:

1. A very small baby can be held upside down and smacked on the back.
2. For an older child, lay him over your knee or over a chair and slap him hard on the back with the flat of your hand between the shoulder blades. This should dislodge the object and make him cough it up. If this doesn't work at once, try the Heimlich method:

Get behind the child and place your arms around his or her waist.

Clench one of your hands into a fist over the child's stomach between the navel and the rib cage.

Grip the clenched fist with the other hand.

Press your hands strongly against the abdominal wall, pressing slightly upwards. This sharp pressure drives the air out of the lungs suddenly and carries the obstructing object up through the windpipe.

If an adult begins to choke:

If you choke yourself it can be very difficult to explain what is wrong simply because you can't speak. Point to your throat repeatedly–someone will soon get the message. If an adult choking on something is simply coughing and spluttering, slap him or her on the back if he or she wants help but otherwise leave the cough reflex to cope–it usually does. Get him or her to try to breathe slowly and deeply–this reduces the spasm of the windpipe and will release the choking object.

If the person is so obstructed that he or she is going blue:

1. Open the mouth to see if you can hook out the object with your finger. It is usually too far back for this but it is worth taking a quick look.

2. Get him or her on the floor, lying on the side.

3. Slap him or her firmly on the back between the shoulder blades. This will almost always dislodge the foreign body.

4 If this doesn't work, use the Heimlich method (see above).

If a fishbone sticks in the throat:

If the person is choking really seriously, treat as adult choking above.

It is often difficult to know whether or not you are really in trouble with a bone as fishbones often simply scratch the lining of the throat, giving an impression of being stuck there when in fact they are not. If all is well after an hour or two, the chances are that it was simply a scratch. If things seem to be getting worse, go to hospital so that a doctor can look down your throat.

Do not try to reach into the throat to pick the bone out. Do not give cotton wool sandwiches or other bulky remedies to swallow. Neither of these procedures works.

SUGAR ADDICTION

What is it?

A condition in which an individual becomes 'hooked' on sugar-containing foods so that life without them becomes a misery or virtually impossible. Sugar addiction is worth worrying about because it makes people fat (with all the resultant health risks this entails) and causes tooth decay. It may also, via its action on insulin metabolism, have something to do with the causation of diabetes.

What causes it?

- There is little doubt that most higher animals find sugar a pleasant taste and many of nature's fruits and vegetables contain sugars. Although most western-ers with their sweet tooth don't realise it, vegetables such as carrots and onions are very sweet. So it appears that it is natural for us to like sweet-tasting things.

- Upbringing is undoubtedly the prime reason why so many people in the West are sugar addicts. From the very earliest days mothers give their babies dummies filled with sugar solutions or coated in honey to suck to keep them quiet. This sort of habit sets the body's sugar 'thermostat' so high that anything that is not extremely sweet is perceived as less palatable.

- A cultural acceptance of the myth that dietary rewards must involve sugar. The woman who feels low premenstrually or the unhappy child on the way home from school both opt for sweet, sugar-containing slugs of confectionary.

Prevention

- The best starting point is total and on-demand breastfeeding. Breast milk contains its own sugars and tastes very sweet. However, these sugars are balanced with other constituents and don't have the harmful effects that sucrose (table sugar) has. A baby nourished in this way will not crave sugary drinks and sweets.

- Don't have sugar on the table as your childen grow up. Teach them to find sweetness elsewhere–in vegetables or fruits.

- Once you are a sugar eater and want to change your ways, keep a sugar diary for a week or two. It is very difficult to appreciate just how much sugar you actually eat unless you do this. Statistics show that sugar added to food accounts for 25 per cent of all the calories eaten by the average adult. For teenagers this figure can be as high as 50 per cent. Get used to reading labels on foods and steer away from those that are rich in sugar or have anything ending in *ose*, (malt*ose*, dextr*ose*, sucr*ose*, etc.) on the label.

- Shop more wisely. This will mean buying few or none at all of the following: sweets and chocolates; cream-filled and iced biscuits; cakes and sweet pastries; jams, honey, marmalade and spreads; tinned fruit in syrup; sweetened yoghurts; jellies and ready-made desserts; sweet pickles; fruit sauces; tomato ketchup; and fizzy drinks and squashes containing sugar.

- Ban all sugar and sweets from the house. Feeding your craving is much more difficult if the things are not there to be eaten. In spite of all the publicity about the dangers of sugar consumption, in 1980 in the UK the use of sugars and sweeteners was up 50 per cent from 91 lb a year per person at the turn of the century to 143 lb a year.

- Get into the habit of nibbling only healthy foods in between meals. Chew nuts, raw vegetables (you will be surprised how sweet many of these are), seeds, fruit, cheese or even hard-boiled eggs. This will stop you feeling you have to reach for the sweet things. In the early days of weaning yourself off sugar, it is a good idea to have fruit, for example, in the car.

The trouble with sugar addiction is that, like any other addiction, it makes your body produce abnormal physical reactions–in this case a rise in insulin to combat the rise in blood sugar. Unfortunately, a rapid release of insulin produced in too large an amount in a sugar addict causes the blood sugar to fall about an hour later, producing the classical effects of hypoglycaemia (see page 248). These are so unpleasant that it often does not take much will power to stop this self-destructive behaviour. Don't see nibbling in between meals as bad–make it a virtue by nibbling at the right sort of foods. If you are eating healthily at mealtimes you will probably find you need fewer in-between meals snacks anyway. It is far better to eat six bulky, high-fibre meals a day than two or three energy-rich, sugary blow-outs.

- Eat more high-fibre foods and complex carbohydrates. Unfortunately, the majority of sugar addicts like these foods least of all so this could take a few weeks to get used to.

- Take more exercise – in particular, do something physical when you feel you would like to binge on sweets. When you crave sugar get down on the floor and do some push-ups or some other strenuous exercises.

- Use artificial sweeteners if you have to as a crutch while you wean yourself off sugar, but don't substitute one for the other permanently. A cloud hangs over the safety of all the artificial sweeteners and using them to overcome your addiction simply substitutes one form of sweetener with another. Aim to be off all sweeteners within a couple of months of getting rid of your addiction for sugar.

- Keep well away from confectionary vending machines. They are disastrous for the sugar addict.

- Research has found that the B vitamins, especially nicotinamide, help kill the hunger in sugar addicts. Whole grains, fresh vegetables and wheatgerm are all sources of this vitamin.

- Eat more chromium, manganese and zinc. The trace element chromium is known to be vital in sugar metabolism, and zinc and manganese help stabilise blood sugar. Zinc has a vital role in taste generally and a recent study found that it can help control a

sweet tooth. Ten healthy people were fed zinc supplements for fifteen weeks to see how it would affect their senses of sweet, sour and saltiness. The most dramatic finding was that they could all get by with less sugar.

SUICIDE

What is it?

There are two forms of suicide. True suicide is when a person kills themselves; para-suicide occurs when someone makes an 'attempt' to commit suicide but does not succeed.

Suicide is as old as the human race, and over the centuries has been condemned by Church and State. It is, however, an uncommon form of death, causing only about 1 per cent of deaths in the UK. In the under 20 age group, though, it is the second most common cause of death – after accidents. Suicide is still a crime in several US states but in the UK it stopped being illegal in 1961.

Although the actual number of suicides is falling in the UK and the US there is no room for complacency. Suicide is still twice as common in the US as is homicide and the figures for homicide are not low. Overall, in the US and UK, suicide is the fifth most common cause of death.

Why do people do it?

- If three or more of the following

factors apply to an individual, he or she must be considered to be at risk of committing suicide and should have professional help:

1. Depression (undoubtedly the major cause).

2. Severe insomnia.

3. Severe hypochrondriacal preoccupations.

4. A previous attempt at suicide.

5. A history of alcohol or drug abuse.

6. Schizophrenia.

7. A disabling painful disease or serious physical illness.

8. Social isolation.

9. Repeated suicidal thoughts.

10. A history of suicide in the family.

11. A history of bereavement, or recent bereavement.

12. Unemployment or financial problems.

13. Recovery from depression.

- Suicide is three times more common among divorced people than among the married and is also more common in the single than the married. Minority racial groups have higher suicide rates in almost every country that has been studied.

- Although at least twice as many women suffer from overt depression as do men, far more men than women kill themselves. In the 80–84-year-old group seven times as many men kill themselves as do women.

- For a quarter of a century professionals and executives have headed the list of successful suicides and among these health professionals come high up. Twice as many doctors kill themselves as do other professionals, for example.

- 'Why go on living?' is a common thought when depressed people contemplate suicide. Life for them has reached a point where it appears to have little meaning and they can see no end to their problems or a future for themselves. These thoughts are especially indicative of trouble if they are out of character for the individual concerned.

- A sudden impulse after a disappointment or a row can lead to spur-of-the-moment suicide. This is relatively uncommon and the suicide is usually unsuccessful. Sometimes a person who has just learned of their partner's infidelity or serious illness walks around in a daze of rage or distress and falls under a car, oblivious to its presence. Such 'suicides' are preventable if the individual is protected from him- or herself during this 'at risk' stage.

- Physical or mental exhaustion can trigger suicidal thoughts, even in non-depressed people. Repeated loss of sleep with endless mental and emotional trauma can wear down the most normal of people. This can happen, for example, in young mothers – the world simply gets on top of them temporarily. If they are not depressed, such people rarely want to die, and the opportunity to vent their feeling – perhaps by a good cry, a holiday, or the solving of practical problems – often alleviates their distress.

- Some people who try to commit suicide but are unsuccessful are trying to communicate something to those around them, and often to one person in particular. A husband or wife begging his or her partner to be faithful, a teenager trying to get some love and attention, are but two of the many examples. Such people rarely kill themselves, except accidentally as a result of dicing with death.

Prevention

It will be clear from the above that preventing suicide can be difficult. However, almost anyone who is close to or connected with a suicide victim blames themselves to some extent, feels guilty and wonders what they could have done to prevent it. Some ideas for prevention have been mentioned above. Here are some more that have been found to work.

- If someone you know is depressed, watch out for suicidal signs.

Most successful suicides have been planning it for some time. They often give subtle clues like tidying up their desk, ensuring that their papers are in order, giving away significant objects to special people, and so on.

Do not believe the dangerous old wives' tale that if a person talks about suicide it means he or she will never actually do it. This is not true – as thousands of distraught families can testify. Eighty per cent of successful suicides have talked about it before, sometimes even to their doctors. Talk about suicide should always be taken seriously. Seek medical help.

- Someone who has tried to kill themselves before is at special risk, so be very much more aware of the danger. It has been estimated that 2 million Americans who are alive today have tried to kill themselves. This is a vast pool of potential suicides.

- Don't assume that intelligent, highly moral or religious-minded people will not commit suicide – they are just as likely as anyone else to do so.

- Be aware of how people do it so you can protect those around you as far as possible. In the UK the vast majority of suicides occur with drugs; in the US guns feature prominently. Men by and large go for more bravado whilst women nearly always take tablets.

Most suicides occur in the spring (six months after the most common month for the onset of depression–September). May is the peak month for suicides. Many people also commit suicide near Christmas. Traditionally, Monday has been a prominent day for suicides–possibly something to do with the Monday Blues. Though treatment for depression can prevent suicide, the four months after release from hospital are the most dangerous period for potentially suicidal people. They feel more active now that their depression is better, and have the energy to kill themselves. Most people commit suicide at home, mainly in the morning.

- The Samaritans, a nationwide telephone help organisation for those in crisis, has probably been responsible for preventing more suicides than anything else. People who feel depressed can talk to a compassionate, yet disinterested, person down the telephone line, and this undoubtedly stops many from actively doing anything. The telephone number is in the local directory and they can be phoned twenty-four hours a day.

- Researchers have tried to develop blood tests that could predict a suicidal tendency in 'at risk' populations but these efforts have not met with much success. Several studies have linked the severity of depression with the urine output of various natural body steroids and others have looked at blood changes. Unfortunately, there are no predictive tests available yet.

- Treating depression seriously and well is clearly the best overall practical preventive measure against suicide. For more details on this, see page 188.

Lastly, here are some basic rules for dealing with people who are talking about or threatening suicide:

1. Do take every suicidal threat or action seriously. Don't be afraid to ask if the depressed person is really serious about committing suicide. Don't worry about giving them ideas–on the contrary, it shows them that you are taking them and their problem seriously and proves that they are better understood than they expected.

2. *Don't* be flippant or dismissive. Never make remarks like, 'You won't kill yourself', 'You're not the type', or 'You don't really mean it'. These only act as a challenge to severely depressed, suicidal people. They might just do it–not to spite you, but to show you that their depression is deadly serious. Desperate individuals, no matter what their beliefs, morals, aspirations, or personality, can and just might commit suicide, especially if challenged in this way.

3. *Never* try to bluff your way through with comments like, 'OK, go ahead then!' They might take you up on it.

4.   *Don't* go in for any do-it-yourself psychoanalysis–this should be done later by a professional.

5.   *Don't* get drawn into arguments about whether they should live or die–you can't win that one. They are so low that nothing you say will convince them and it could in fact annoy them so much that they will be precipitated sooner into suicide.

6.   *Do* be prepared to listen. Let them talk themselves out of it, if possible, while you await professional help.

7.   *Even* if you get over the acute crisis, don't assume that things will necessarily improve–they don't. Any life crisis that has driven a previously normal person to threaten suicide needs to be examined carefully and the root causes attended to. Never accept a suicidal threat as an idle show of emotion–it always mirrors an underlying problem that demands attention. It comes very hard to most relatives (and especially spouses) to learn that they can't be of any great help in sorting out the root causes, but this is all too often the case. Outside help is usually needed if the suicidal threats are not to be repeated or acted upon.

SUNBURN

What is it?

A reddening, blistering and eventual burning of the skin when exposed to sunshine. Sunshine can also predispose to the formation of certain skin cancers (see page 326).

What causes it?

Most westerners perceive that they look better if their skin is brown rather than pale. This leads many millions purposefully to expose themselves to sunshine, usually when on holiday in warm, sunny climates.

The sun continually bombards the earth with all kinds of radiation. Direct exposure to the whole spectrum would be fatal but the earth has a protective layer called the ozone layer which encircles the globe at high altitude. This layer lets through only the relatively harmless long-wave radiation (UVA) and a little of the short-wave type (UVB) which is more dangerous. It is UVB that is the main culprit in sunburn, skin ageing and skin cancers caused by sunlight. Clouds further cut out a lot of the less harmful UVA waves but let through as much as 80 per cent of the UVBs that have got this far. This makes hazy and overcast days just as dangerous as sunny days.

Certain drugs can sensitise people to the sun. All the following make people burn more easily: antibiotics such as tetracyclines; diuretics; oral contraceptives; some anti-histamines and tranquillisers; and certain heart medications. Even some perfumes and aftershaves can do this.

Exposure to the sun triggers a chemical reaction to produce a pigment called melanin in the skin.

Melanin absorbs UVBs, and the more the skin is exposed to sunshine the more melanin is produced and the better the protection from the harmful effects of UVBs. Dark-skinned 'white' people and, of course, brown-skinned people, have more melanin in their skin anyway and so tan with less sunburn. No tan offers total protection from the sun though.

Recent research has found that sun can weaken the body's immune systems. A group of fair-skinned people were exposed to artificial sunlight for half an hour daily over a two-week period. Tests showed a weakening of the immune system, including a slight reduction in white-blood-cell numbers. In some people these changes remained for up to two weeks after the exposure to the sunlight.

Prevention

The secret of sunburn is to prevent it. Here's how:

- It takes several days to get used to the sun, so start slowly. Expose yourself for only two half-hour periods a day over the first few days. Increase this exposure as the days go by. Take it especially gently if you are a blonde or a redhead.

- Drink plenty of fluids (not alcoholic).

- Remember that sea-water makes you burn faster.

- Use an effective sunscreen lotion. Most suntan lotions don't protect you from the burning rays of the sun at all – they are simply fluids that help you 'cook'. A protective sunscreen will contain a B-complex vitamin called para-amino-benzoic acid (PABA). Tests have found this to be by far the most effective protection against ultraviolet light. PABA still lets some of the UVBs through so you still get a tan, but you don't burn. It is vital to keep topping up the sunscreen preparation throughout the day because it washes off in water. Experiments with rats found that feeding them vitamins E and C built up a substantial resistance to the burning effects of ultraviolet light but this has not yet been confirmed in humans.

- Remember that water, concrete and sand reflect sun that can burn you badly and quickly.

- The sun is at its most dangerous between the hours of 11 a.m. and 3 p.m. so avoid these times, at least at first.

- Wear a hat when you go sightseeing. The hours pass quickly and you can get a lot of sun without realising it.

- Wear good-quality sunglasses. US ophthalmologists are concerned because they are seeing increasing numbers of people with a condition called macular degeneration. Some believe that this is directly related to sun exposure. It used to be seen only in the elderly but now is occurring in people in their thirties and forties. Experts think that, to be safe, you should wear sunglasses if you are in the sun for more than thirty minutes, and that sun-bathers should not expose their eyes to strong sun for more than fifteen minutes. Polaroid lenses keep out the glare but do not necessarily contain UV filters, and some experts maintain that wearing dark glasses that do not filter out UV light can actually be more dangerous than wearing none at all.

THRUSH

What is it?

Thrush is a yeast infection that affects both men and women but mostly women. The organism that causes it lives on our skin and in the mouth and is often found in the bowel. Usually this yeast causes no harm but sometimes it multiplies and produces problems. In babies it can produce a nappy rash (see page 289).

Most commonly thrush causes a thick, white, very irritant vaginal discharge in women. There is sore-ness on intercourse and often pain on passing water.

What causes it?

- Pregnancy is a common cause. During pregnancy the raised level of oestrogen in the woman's body encourages the yeast to grow.

- The contraceptive pill produces it for the same reasons (most pills contain an oestrogen).

- Wearing tights, nylon panties or tight-fitting jeans or trousers seems to raise the temperature and humidity in the woman's vulval area and encourage the growth of the yeast .

- Antibiotics kill off other or-ganisms in the bowel and in the body generally, leaving the yeasts free to multiply.

- Inflammation of the vulval area – caused by vaginal deodorants, bubble baths, talcum, perfumed soap, a scratch, etc. – can make thrush more likely.

- Poor health can make thrush more likely. Really run-down, overtired, and seriously ill women are more at risk.

- Sexual contact is an uncommon cause of thrush. In the vast major-ity of women the infection arises spontaneously but it can be transmitted sexually. Many doc-tors still think it is sensible to treat a woman's partner so that the two do not pass the infection back and forth between them.

- Refined carbohydrates act as 'food' for thrush in the gut and can produce increased bloating, flatulence, soreness, itching, disturbed bowel function and a general increase of the symptoms. Eat no refined carbohydrates. Restrict your total daily carbohydrate intake to 60–80 grams. It helps to go on to a low-refined carbohydrate, no yeasty-foods diet for two weeks before starting Nystatin from your doctor. Keep on the diet even when taking the Nystatin, until all your symptoms disappear. Slowly, you can loosen up on your diet. If symptoms reappear avoid these foods for good.

Prevention

- Avoid tights, nylon panties, and tight-fitting jeans and trousers. Wear skirts, cotton panties or no panties and stockings.

- Use pads rather than tampons during a period.

- Avoid perfumed soaps, vaginal deodorants, and other irritants such as bubble baths and disinfectants.

- After going to the lavatory, wipe yourself from front to back so as not to drag any yeasts from the bowel opening to the vaginal area.

- Use antibiotics only when absolutely necessary and then eat two or three natural yoghurts (live) a day to replace lost bacteria in the bowel.

- (For a man) never have casual sex with a woman unless you use a sheath.

- Keep generally healthy.

- Try a diet low in yeasts and refined carbohydrates for 2–4 weeks to see if there is any improvement. Yeasted foods include Marmite, frozen or concentrated orange juice, cheeses, bread made with yeast, alcoholic drinks, grapes and grape juices, unpeeled fruits, raisins, sultanas, food that has been 'left around' for some time, and B-vitamins (unless the label specifically says that they are yeast-free).

- Follow your doctor's advice about taking the drug Nystatin to kill the yeast and prevent its spread to your partner. As soon as you think you have thrush, stop having intercourse or you could infect your partner.

TIREDNESS

What is it?

A sense of fatigue, either mental or physical–a feeling that you never really have much energy. Chronic fatigue takes millions of people to their doctors yet in more than four out of five no physical cause is found.

What causes it?

- Overwork either at home or in your job.

- An undiagnosed underlying physical disease such as anaemia.

- An underlying emotional or

psychological problem such as depression, unhappiness, a sense of failure, sexual or marital tensions, and so on.

- A shortage of magnesium.

- A shortage of potassium.

- Iron-deficiency anaemia.

- A lack of folic acid in the diet.

- Vitamin C shortage.

- A shortage of good-quality sleep.

- Too little exercise.

- Being bored with your life and yourself.

Prevention

- Many people are overworked, especially those in stressful jobs and women who do a job as well as looking after a family. Many such people don't realise how tired they are getting because it all builds up slowly. The answer to this problem is to work less if at all possible, and to make a real effort to relax more. If you have a stressful job you should take up a hobby something totally different from your job and preferably something that is not goal-centred or competitive. If you have demanding responsibilities looking after a family, make sure that there are at least a couple of periods during the week that you spend doing something just for *you* and not for the family – go to an exercise class, or an evening class, or join a group of people who share an interest with you. Find labour-saving ways of running the house; get other members of the household to do more and to think more about you. Spread the load of heavier jobs among the family.

- Go to your doctor and ask for a blood test and a general check-up. You may be suffering from a treatable medical condition and it is a waste to walk around feeling under the weather with something that could be treated. This is what often happens with anaemia in women.

- If no physical cause is found, see a counsellor or other trained professional to try to sort out any emotional or psychological problems in your life. Many people find such conditions every bit as draining as true physical illness, yet often no notice is taken until they become a form of psychological illness that cannot be ignored. Mental and emotional wear and tear creeps up insidiously on us and makes the strongest person tired. Often, the help of a professional can make all the difference to knowing how to cope with what seems to the sufferer to be an impossible situation. Many things can't be changed but the way you deal with them can be.

- Magnesium is vital for many of the body's vital functions and gross deficiency signs are unlikely to go unnoticed. However, as with iron deficiency, most doctors are not trained to recognise *mild* magnesium deficiency. It has only one noticeable symptom – chronic fatigue. In one study of magnesium and fatigue 200 men and women who were tired during the day were given magnesium. In all but two the tiredness disappeared.

- Similarly, postassium can be in short supply. This deficiency is well recognised in long-distance runners and in those taking diuretic drugs (water tablets). In one study researchers took people at random and measured their potassium intakes. Those with a deficient intake (60 per cent of the men and 40 per cent of the women) had weaker grip strengths than those with a normal intake. As potassium intake fell, so did muscular strength. A study of 100 chronically fatigued people (84 women and 16 men) found that on a magnesium and potassium supplement 87 improved in 4–5 weeks.

- Iron deficiency is usually thought of by most doctors as being unimportant unless it produces anaemia. This is not so. Iron-deficiency fatigue can occur in people who have normal blood levels of the iron-containing red-blood-cell pigment called haemoglobin. Anaemia definitely makes people tired and easily fatigued and their heartbeats rise to higher levels on exercise than do those of the non-anaemic. Iron deficiency is,

of course, caused by a lack of iron but red blood cells need another nutrient too – folic acid.

- Too little folic acid can make a person tired and anaemic. Iron and folic acid given together appear to be more effective than either alone for many people. In a study in which women were given either iron or folate, or the two together, only 26 per cent of those who received a single nutrient had a rise in haemoglobin whilst 96 per cent of those who received both did so. But for folate to be used by the body you need to have enough vitamin B_{12}. In another study, twenty-eight men and women who complained of tiredness yet had no physical problems were given vitamin B_{12} and asked to evaluate its effect. For many of the twenty-eight the vitamin not only made them feel less fatigued but also improved their appetite, sleep and general well-being.

- Vitamin C too has been found to be of help in those who are always tired. Miners in Czechoslovakia were given 1 g of the vitamin a day and reported less fatigue and faster reaction times. Another study of 400 people found that those whose vitamin C intake was less than 400 mg a day had more fatigue than others who consumed more.

- Poor sleep can be a cause of constant tiredness. The value of sleep is discussed more on page 77, and how to promote sleep on page 266.

- Although it might seem strange, increasing the level of exercise you take can *reduce* feelings of tiredness. Many people who complain of tiredness, even if they are improved by the above regime, will still feel a lot better for having taken exercise. Whether this is because taking strenuous exercise raises endorphins which produce a sense of well-being, or whether it is because most such people have a sense of achievement after doing the exercise is not known. What *is* certain, though, is that even lethargic and 'tired' people who take exercise two or three times a week feel better in themselves and tend to feel less tired.

TOOTH DECAY

What is it?

Dental disease is the commonest disease in the western world. It consists of three interlinked problem areas:

1. Tooth decay.

2. Gum disease; and

3. The problems of those with no natural teeth.

We have looked at the second and third of these elsewhere. This entry deals with tooth decay.

The majority of tooth loss comes about because of tooth decay in early life and gum disease in adult life. Both start with plaque—a sticky substance that collects on teeth all the time. Plaque is laden with bacteria that live off the sugar in foods we eat. The bacteria produce acid and the acid erodes the bone-hard enamel of our teeth. The bacteria in plaque also play havoc with our gums (see page 224).

In 1984 25 per cent of the population of England and Wales over the age of 16 had no natural teeth. This is a great improvement on 1968 when the figure was 37 per cent, but the figure is still shocking.

But is the picture for children any better? Unfortunately not. In 1983 in England and Wales 48 per cent of children aged 5 had some experience of decay; and at the age of 14, the average number of decayed, missing or filled teeth was 4.6. Things have improved a little since then and there is increasing evidence that the level of dental decay in children is falling, for some unknown reason, even in areas that do not have fluoridated water. In areas where the drinking water *is* fluoridated the level of tooth decay in children is much lower than elsewhere.

Only about half of all people with natural teeth go to a dentist in any one year, and a quarter of schoolchildren and three-quarters of pre-school children fail to get regular dental care.

More and better treatment of dental problems is not the answer to this situation—prevention is. Dental diseases are almost all preventable; indeed no area of preventive medicine has been so extensively studied and pursued as has the prevention of dental decay, and the wisdom of trying to treat, rather than prevent, dental disease in whole populations has been seriously questioned. The World Health Organisation has stated that, 'Dental caries cannot be controlled by treatment alone and the problem can be reduced to manageable proportions only by preventive measures aimed at decreasing the prevalence of the disease.'

What causes it?

Tooth decay is caused by the acids produced by bacteria in plaque, as we saw above. Plaque builds up on teeth for several reasons:

- Too much sugar and refined foods in the diet. All sugars are potentially harmful to teeth but sucrose (table sugar) appears to be the worst offender. Unfortunately, it is not just added sugar that is the problem–there is also the sugar that is put into drinks and foods during their manufacture and processing. Sugar from food passes into the plaque very quickly and then the trouble starts.

- Too little dietary fibre. A refined diet consisting of white flour and its products, sweets and refined-carbohydrate foods is very pappy and sticks to the teeth. A diet rich in fibre is more chewy, promotes

the production of more saliva to bathe the teeth and to dilute the acids produced by plaque, and also physically scrapes off some plaque during the prolonged chewing needed to eat these foods. Studies have shown that populations that eat unrefined foods have very little dental decay and that as soon as they start to eat sugar and white flour their levels of dental decay shoot up. In more than 200 years there have only been two periods during which caries (decay) has fallen in the UK–during the two World Wars, when sugar and refined white flour were scarce or unavailable. Gum disease too is more common among people who eat soft, pappy foods rather than chewy, fibre-rich foods. But fibre-rich foods cannot clean teeth completely and toothbrushing is still vital.

- Poor toothbrushing. There is little doubt that toothbrushing plays a vital role in the prevention of both tooth decay and gum disease. Effective removal of plaque from the surface of the teeth is enough to prevent most of the problems. Evidence suggests that the removal of plaque once a day is sufficient–provided it is properly done.

- Forgetting to clean *between* the teeth. Brushing easily cleans off the flat surfaces of the teeth if it is properly done, yet danger areas remain between the teeth because a brush can't get there.

These places need to be tackled with dental floss (a kind of waxed cotton). Flossing should be carried out daily too, especially in people who have 'food traps' where food collects between two teeth.

- Too little fluoride on the surface of the teeth. Toothbrushing of itself is only partially valuable in the fight against tooth decay. A vital aspect of brushing is that it is a way of applying fluoride to the teeth. The debate over fluoride and teeth is long and confused but the current wisdom is that the best way to use fluoride is to apply it to the teeth at least once a day. This seems to have the best caries-preventing effect of all. And it is not just children who benefit from this application but adults as well. Fluoride acts by encouraging new calcium to form on the tooth surface–to replace the calcium removed by the acids produced by the bacteria in plaque. Results of numerous trials around the world consistently show that decay can be reduced by up to 30 per cent by using fluoride toothpaste. This is non-controversial and provable. Provided that young children don't swallow the toothpaste regularly there is no proven hazard to using fluoride toothpaste in this way.

- Too little fluoride in drinking water. This subject, unlike that of fluoridated toothpaste, *is* highly controversial. Fluoride in drinking water gets incorporated into the developing tooth of a child, making it more resistant to decay. Fluoridation of water supplies cuts dental decay by about half but it has vocal opponents who claim that it is dangerous and pointless to give a whole population a medication when so few need it. In fluoridated areas tooth decay is becoming a thing of the past yet alarming, if unconfirmed, reports are appearing about the increase of certain cancers and other diseases in these same areas.

Almost every responsible health body right up to the World Health Organisation recommends the fluoridation of water, but still only a small proportion of people in the western world are actually receiving fluoridated water. Dentists ostensibly support the fluoridation of water but few are truly committed to the cause and this coupled with the power and influence of the anti-fluoride lobby has made the fluoridation of drinking water a slow business. Dentists have been slow too when it comes to making progress with the food industry and the government on the subject of sugar control.

- Poor health education. There are numerous myths about tooth decay and its causes, especially when it comes to sugar. Far too many people still think of sugar as healthy and essential for energy–it is neither, of course.

Most dentists acknowledge that sweets are harmful but say little about the harm done by sugar in other forms or the dangers of refined foods generally. Dentists have not banded together to stop sweet advertising or tried to ban it from TV during children's programmes, for example. They also seem not to be particularly conscientious about preventive measures. In 1978, for example, a study found that only just over a quarter of adults claimed to have had toothbrushing demonstrated to them by a dentist.

A 1980 study in the Netherlands found that dentists, dental hygienists and dental assistants simply didn't know enough about prevention. The team gave 142 dentists, 21 dental hygienists and 35 dental assistants a questionnaire consisting of forty questions on preventive dentistry – all common questions that patients ask all the time. The average percentage of questions answered correctly was 57 per cent for dentists, 58 per cent for hygienists and 37 per cent for assistants. These figures are disappointingly poor. Older dentists know more than younger ones but it was found that very few of the dentists answered 'I don't know', which was an available choice for each question.

A subject over which people are very confused and on which the dental professionals have been slow to offer evidence is how often individuals should have dental check-ups. Most people are told by their dentists to have twice yearly check-ups but there is no reason for this. Young children certainly benefit from this frequency of check-ups but after the age of 16 there is no evidence that it has much preventive value. Yearly check-ups are probably adequate over the age of 16, especially in someone who is running their dental health along the lines suggested in this article, but there will always be those who will need to go more frequently.

Careful studies have shown that the difference in consumer satisfaction between dental patients with good dental health and those with poor dental health is negligible. This reflects a situation in which the criteria by which patients judge their dentists are very different from the criteria dentists use (or ought to use) to guide their work. Pain was the sole and compelling reason for seeking dental treatment in 33.3 per cent of university graduates and 46 per cent of those with a lower educational level, according to a study in 1974. In general, dentists have not 'sold' themselves adequately as preventive practitioners, although there are obviously individual exceptions to this. A study of dentists' attitudes to prevention, carried out in 1976, does not make happy reading although it has to be said that things have improved somewhat in the last decade. Given that dental hygienists can and should do much to further prevention and health care it is not surprising that only in the south of England did this study find a willingness on the part of dentists to expand the role of their hygienists.

Most of the 358 dentists favoured some kind of National Health Service fee for preventive services. Throughout the study dentists showed themselves to be far more committed to the dental health of their immediate family than to that of their patients.

Why should there be so little real prevention going on in routine dental practice and why is it that dentists still see themselves mainly as people who treat disease rather than preventing it? The answer starts in dental training schools. A recent UK report on dental education said that 'Students are mainly taught a mechanistic and qualitative approach to dentistry and it is not surprising that many adopt a materialistic attitude to practice. We perceive a tendency in many dental schools to value more highly the teaching of the prescribed body of knowledge and technical skills than the inculcation of professional attitudes based on a broad-based education.' The report advocated that dental disease be studied in the context of general health and lifestyles of different groups. Little attention is paid to teaching dentists to be counsellors and the report found resistance to the idea that dental students be taught simple applied psychology. Is it surprising, then, that dentists are loath to act as educators, and agents of social and behavioural change?

But the greatest problem is the way dentists are paid. Various countries pay very different proportions of their health budgets to dentistry, with Germany at the top of the league spending 14.3 per cent of the total health budget on dental treatments. The figure for the UK is 3.8 per cent, and for the US 7 per cent. Preventive practices flourish in the free-enterprise systems but the National Health Service is a treatment service and dentists are not remunerated for prevention. Dental disease is a prime example of an area of health in which practitioners could be paid to help keep patients dentally fit (like in ancient China, where patients paid the doctor to keep them well and stopped paying when they were ill). At the moment most countries are spending vast sums 'picking up the pieces' of dental disease, the majority of which could and should have been prevented.

Prevention

- Breastfeed your children totally for at least the first six months. Wean them on to sugar-free, unrefined wholefoods right from the start of solids.

- Discourage a taste for sweet foods. Read labels carefully and avoid foods and drinks with added sugar. If you can't ban sweets altogether, give them in batches after meals rather than letting children eat them between meals; or have a 'sweet day' once a week when the children can eat sweets to their heart's content and then prohibit them during the rest of the week.

- Give them fruit or savoury foods for school snacks and discourage them from buying sweets at the tuckshop.

- As a family eat healthy, unrefined foods rich in dietary fibre (see page 70).

- Ensure that you have a toothbrush for every member of the family. A good brush should have a small head, with soft nylon bristles and a flat brushing surface, so that you can reach all parts of the mouth. As soon as the bristles begin to splay out, replace the brush.

- Teach your children to clean their teeth from a very early age. A toddler can play with a toothbrush to get used to it but until they are about 8 or 9 children need to have their teeth cleaned for them by an adult if it is to be done well. Get the child to do them first; then follow up with a proper clean.

- Teaching children to clean their teeth properly is greatly helped by using disclosing tablets or solutions. These are harmless food dyes that stain the plaque and show how ineffective the brushing has been at getting rid of it. Once the plaque has been disclosed (stained) get the child to try to brush it away–both of you will be surprised at just how sticky plaque is. Disclosing tablets can be obtained from chemists and dentists.

- Always use a flouride toothpaste, but discourage little children

from swallowing it. Never scrub the teeth across, always brush from gum to tooth, and remember to clean the inside surfaces of the teeth and the crinkly biting surfaces of the big back teeth.

- When your children are older (about 12 or 13) they can be shown how to use dental floss. Pull out about 10 in from the container and wrap it around the middle fingers of both hands and make a 'bridge' of floss across your two thumbs. Gently ease the floss between the two teeth (in front of a mirror is easiest) being very careful not to snap it down and cut the gum. Gently scrape it up and down the sides of the neighbouring teeth to remove plaque and food residues. Once you have done one gap go on to the next and work systematically from gap to gap. The whole thing takes about two minutes when you get good at it.

- Take your children to the dentist regularly every six months from the age of 3. This will enable him or her to pick up disease early, to prevent the unnecessary loss of valuable first teeth, and to use surface applications of fluoride which are valuable preventives against decay. Discuss with your dentist whether fluoride tablets would be beneficial to your child.

- If in doubt about anything ask your dentist, and encourage him or her to be interested in prevention. Show him that you think it is important for you and your children.

- Adults should follow the advice given above but don't need to go for regular check-ups nearly so often as children. Fluoride tooth-paste is still advisable and valuable.

TOXIC SHOCK SYNDROME (TSS)

What is it?

Although TSS was most in the news in the early eighties, it is still a real problem which causes death today. To date in the United States 2,700 women have suffered the condition with about ten new reports coming into the Centres for Diseases Control each week. And this is just in the USA. Of the total number reported, about 120 have died in the US alone – a fatality rate of nearly five per cent. Clearly it is a problem worth taking seriously.

TSS is a condition which occurs mainly in menstruating women. It has, however, occurred in non-menstruating women, and even in men and children.

What causes it?

TSS occurs when the bacterium *Staphylococcus aureus* proliferates in the vagina when menstrual blood is dammed up by a tampon. The more absorbent the tampon, the greater the risk of developing TSS. One theory is that super-absorbent tampons dry out the vaginal lining and cause minute cracks to appear in the vaginal wall. Bacteria may then enter the bloodstream through the cracks.

Once diagnosed, TSS can be treated with penicillin and the outlook is excellent. The signs and symptoms of the disease are a sudden high fever, vomiting, diarrhoea, a skin rash and a fall in blood pressure.

Recently the contraceptive sponge has been linked to TSS. Among 600,000 American women using the sponge there have been twelve confirmed cases of TSS. None has proved fatal. Understandably, those involved with this method of contraception point out that the chances of getting TSS when using it are less than being struck by lightning.

Prevention

- Use sanitary towels rather than tampons.

- If you decide to use tampons, change them frequently – at least 6-8 hourly – and

- Choose a low-absorbency tampon. Some of the regular brands of certain makes are as absorbent as the 'highly-absorbent' brands of others. There is a suggestion in the US that the FDA require tampons to be labelled with their absorbency.

- When inserting a tampon, do not scratch the vaginal lining. When you are not naturally lubricated, use a little KY jelly or something similar. Favour a tampon with a rounded end and possibly one without an applicator.

- If you use the contraceptive sponge, follow the manufacturer's directions. Don't use the sponge during a period or immediately after childbirth. Never leave it in place for more than 24 hours.

- If ever you develop a high fever with vomiting, diarrhoea and a rash, tell your family doctor at once.

TRAVEL DISEASES

What are they?

A mixed collection of ailments, most of which are not serious, that afflict travellers, usually to exotic places. Most people are on holiday abroad when they experience these illnesses, but the business traveller (though usually more cautious) is subject to them too, of course. Obviously people are at very different degrees of risk of suffering from sickness whilst abroad. At one end of the scale is the business traveller who stays only in first-class hotels. Such a person is hardly at greater risk than he would be staying at home. At the other extreme is the high-risk traveller who, for example, goes off to live in the bush for long periods.

Most of us go on holiday to do something different from our daily routine, and this is part of the problem – we are well aware of the hazards around us at home, and have learned to live with them, but holidays can present entirely new problems.

The most important preparation from the illness point of view is to be well covered by insurance. Illness and accident can strike abroad just as easily as at home, but outside the umbrella of the National Health Service the British traveller can find him- or herself in expensive trouble very easily. The countries of the European Economic Community provide reciprocal medical cover for each other's citizens, but outside it bills can mount up very quickly. In order to avail yourself of the reciprocal arrangements you will need to have obtained an E111 form from your local DHSS office because without it you may have difficulty claiming back the money you have paid out for treatment in the foreign country.

Holiday companies can often arrange insurance, but most tour operators offer cover for a sum which is much too small, so it is wise to take out extra cover – multiply your tour operator's figure by three to be on the safe side.

Prevention

Immunisations

(A useful booklet about these is *Notice to Travellers: Health Protection*, published by the Department of

Health and Social Security).

Many countries have immunisation requirements which have to be met before they will let you in. The diseases that you are most likely to have to be protected against are tetanus, polio, typhoid and yellow fever. Smallpox vaccination is required by very few countries as the disease has been eradicated worldwide. It is always difficult to know exactly which immunisations you should have for any given country, especially as the regulations constantly change. Any IATA accredited travel agent (which is most of the reputable ones) can consult a master list and tell you exactly what is required, or you can phone your airline or the embassy of the country to which you are going. If you are pregnant, have a baby or suffer from a skin complaint see your doctor for advice about immunisations. Allow yourself a good month to make any health arrangements before going away. Last-minute immunisations will not give you such effective protection and may spoil your holiday because of a reaction.

Illnesses abroad

The most common ailment suffered by holidaymakers is diarrhoea and vomiting. This comes about by consuming food and drink contaminated with food-poisoning bacteria and their toxic products. In this country we are very complacent about such bacterial infections because we have drinkable water and the climate does not favour rapid bacterial growth in foods. Most of these infections are simply 'holiday tummy' but you can also get more serious conditions such as dysentery or cholera. To be safe:

- Boil all drinking water (or use purifying tablets). It is a good idea even to use boiled water for cleaning your teeth.

- Boil all milk.

- Don't just wash fruit and vegetables under water and then eat them. Use cooled, boiled water to clean vegetables. Peel fresh fruit and avoid salads.

- Keep fresh and cooked food in a refrigerator.

- Drink mineral water or wine if you are unsure of the water and cannot boil it. Even with all these precautions you may still get diarrhoea simply because of the change of food (perhaps to a more spicy diet than you are used to) or because your bowel has not got used to the new, quite harmless bacteria that come to inhabit the bowel when you eat and drink in another country.

- Wash your hands before eating anything.

- It is probably a good idea to take an anti-diarrhoea medicine with you because it will cost much more abroad.

Malaria, often thought of as an exotic tropical disease, is being caught by increasing numbers of holidaymakers as package tours venture further afield. It is a very serious disease and can kill you. As there is no vaccination against malaria, you will have to cover yourself by taking anti-malaria tablets, even if you are only passing through an infected area. One mosquito bite is all it takes to get the disease. Anti-malaria tablets are available from chemist shops and airport chemists. You have to take the tablets before you go and keep taking them for six weeks after your return.

If you should get any illness at all after your return from holiday, tell your doctor at once where you have been and what health precautions you took before and while you were there.

Travel problems.

For details of motion sickness and how to cope with it see next entry. Tell your doctor before taking travel-sickness pills, if you are taking any other pills.

Most of us go on holiday abroad in an aircraft. A short plane journey presents no health problems at all but a longer one can have ill effects that may mar the start of your holiday.

Here are some tips for long air trips:

- Drink plenty of non-alcoholic fluid before and during your flight. The air-conditioning in the aircraft is very dehydrating and this, as much as anything else, is what makes people feel bad after a long flight.

- Get some good sleep before you go as this helps minimise the effects of jet lag.

- Take things to freshen up in your cabin luggage – you'll feel a lot better when you arrive.

- Don't overeat or overdrink (alcohol) – or you will pay for it for the next couple of days.

- If possible, don't plan to do anything too strenuous for the first couple of days after you arrive at your destination. Give your body a chance to get back its balance in the new time zone. Because this can take two days off each end of your holiday it makes sense to travel long distances only for long holidays. It is probably not sensible to go halfway round the world for less than two or three weeks.

Local hazards

Lastly, remember that there could well be local hazards in the area to which you are going. For example, more package tours now go to very exotic places with poisonous plants and fish. Be guided by what the locals do – or don't do!

TRAVEL SICKNESS

What is it?

Nausea or actual vomiting when travelling in moving and rolling vehicles. Children suffer from it especially. Planes and ships are the worst offenders but many children are travel-sick in cars and coaches. Anxiety makes things worse. Some children appear to be immune and others to suffer a lot. Most children grow out of the worst of it.

A child (or adult) who is motion sick looks pale (sometimes frankly green) and anxious, sweats a lot and may vomit.

What causes it?

- A sensitivity of the inner ear that controls balance.

- Anxiety.

- Others being motion sick around you.

- Large, fatty meals before travelling.

- A feeling of airlessness in an aircraft.

- Reading or other close work in cars.

- Hot, stuffy cars.

Prevention

- Take motion-sickness pills half an hour before the journey. Ginger root has been found to be good for this condition.

- Keep the child happy and occupied before the journey so he or she doesn't get worked up about it and apprehensive. Reassure him or her that you don't mind if he or she is sick.

- Have only a light, small meal before travelling.

- Direct the air-conditioning jet in an aircraft on to your face if you feel at all sick.

- Never do close work, reading or writing while in motion.

- Have a polythene bag inside a brown paper one (so the vomit can't be seen by others) ready just in case. This preparedness can so reassure a child that he or she is not sick.

- Keep a window open in cars so that the atmosphere is not hot and sticky.

- Play audio tapes or the radio to keep the child's attention on something other than feeling travel sick.

- Suggest that he or she look forward all the time and not out of the side windows.

- When on a car journey stop from time to time to let the child walk about.

- Don't be pressurised into letting a young child into the front seat (the best from a motion-sickness point of view) if he or she is too small for the seat-belt.

ULCERS

What are they?

An ulcer is any naturally occurring break in a lining surface of the body. Ulcers can, for example, occur in the mouth, on the skin, in the vagina and in the gastro-intestinal system. This section is about what are called peptic ulcers. They get their name from the digestive enzyme called pepsin which is found in the stomach. A combination of pepsin and gastric acid erodes the lining of the stomach or duodenum (the part of the intestine immediately after the stomach) to produce an ulcer. In hiatus hernia (see page 232) and gastro-oesophageal reflux (see page 233) these substances produce an ulceration of the lower end of the oesophagus (gullet) where food enters the stomach.

We all have acid in our stomach and some have more than others. There is a general tendency for those who produce more acid (whether this is inherited or in response to life's stresses) to be more likely to have ulcers.

About one in ten westerners will have peptic ulcers at some time in their lives–usually during middle age. Duodenal ulcers are about four times as common as gastric (stomach) ulcers and men are affected more than women. For some unknown reason duodenal ulcers are becoming much less common than they were twenty or thirty years go. A high proportion of duodenal ulcer patients are of blood group O and close relatives of these patients are more likely to have an ulcer than are others.

The most common symptom of duodenal ulcer is a gnawing pain, usually in the middle to upper abdomen. The pains come on 1–3 hours after a meal and some sufferers wake every night at about 2 or 3 a.m. with their pain.

Most ulcers heal themselves but treatment with simple antacids, newer gastric-acid blocking medications or even surgery may be needed.

Gastric ulcers are less well-defined in their symptoms.

What causes them?

- Heredity definitely plays a part (see above).

- Men are more likely than women to get a duodenal ulcer. This difference is becoming less marked as more women smoke and so raise their gastric-acid secretion.

- Stress produces more acid in the stomach and so makes duodenal ulcers more likely.

- The heavy use of coffee, tea and cola drinks increases gastric acid production.

- Aspirin in large doses (especially as non-soluble tablets) can produce gastric ulceration.

- Milk actually *raises* the production of gastric acid in some people though it has for years been erroneously used as a treatment and preventive for duodenal ulcers.

- Refined foods are harmful too (see below).

- Alcohol produces dramatic rises in gastric-acid production and should be avoided.

- Peptic ulcers are always more common in smokers than in non-smokers and a recent study found that smokers who continued even when taking the latest anti-ulcer medications (H2-antagonists) had higher relapse rates than non-smokers.

Prevention

- There is nothing one can do about one's family history of ulcers but if there *is* a history it makes all the more sense to adopt as many of these preventive measures as possible to try to reduce your chances of developing an ulcer.

- Stress is definitely a provoking factor in ulcers but not just the classical stress of the business executive. It is probably not the stress itself that is the problem but more how you react to it. Being a doctor is probably one of the more highly stressed occupations yet studies of doctors fail to find an excess of ulcers. Potential ulcer patients are usually highly strung and have been subjected to long periods of anxiety and emotional tension. Even children under such stress can get ulcers. One study of twenty-four teenage and pre-teen ulcer patients found that ten of them had lost or almost lost a close relative or personal friend within the year of the ulcer diagnosis.

    Stress produces high gastric-acid levels in everyone but in the very tense and emotional individual who seems to have to 'work' hard at everything in life there seems to be a perpetual overproduction of acid. Any signs of upper abdominal pains or heartburn in such people should be taken as a warning sign that an ulcer could be on the way.

    Ideas on how to cut down stress are to be found on pages 87–9. Don't take sedatives and tranquillisers – favour natural methods such as yoga, meditation, relaxation and exercise.

- Cut out all caffeine-containing drinks and medications. This includes cola drinks (see page 164).

- If you need a pain-reliever use soluble aspirin or paracetamol for the odd headache. If you need more serious long-term pain relief for a medical condition talk to your doctor if you have ever had ulcer symptoms or if there are ulcers in the family.

- For years milk and a bland diet were the mainstay of the treatment and prevention of duodenal ulcers. Today they are considered to be useless and even possibly harmful. There is no evidence that such a bland and unappetising diet is of any value and it deprives the ulcer patient of valuable vitamins and minerals he or she would otherwise be getting.

    Milk neutralises acid in the stomach for a while but kicks

back by increasing acid secretion later by as much as 20 per cent! In one study some men had more than 30 per cent more acid after drinking milk. Other foods high in calcium also increase acid production. These include cheese and other dairy products.

- Sugar and white flour appear to promote ulcers too. One study of forty-one people with chronic stomach problems (with and without ulcers) found that twenty-eight were better on a reduced carbohydrate diet. A study at the University of Manchester of white and wholemeal bread led the researchers to conclude that 'The substitution of wholemeal bread for white might be of benefit to patients with duodenal ulcers and non-ulcer dyspepsia.'

- Historically, ulcer patients have been advised to eat frequent, small meals. Recent research, however, shows that this makes more acid even though the food buffers some of it. The best eating pattern has now been found to be three main meals a day, rich in dietary fibre and low in refined flour and sugar. Something late at night is often helpful to soak up acid that could irritate the stomach or duodenum overnight. The best policy is to take antacids at this time.

How you eat could be more important than when. Most nervous, tense individuals (ulcer-type personalities) bolt their food. This is harmful because a substance called urogastrone which is produced by the salivary glands and protects the lining of the intestine is in short supply.

- Smoking should be stopped because it does three harmful things in the context of ulcers. First, it stimulates the stomach to produce more acid; second, it reduces the amount of acid-neutralising bicarbonate produced by the pancreas, and third, it lets liquid parts of a meal out of the stomach ahead of buffering solid parts so that more acidic fluids hit the duodenum than should be the case.

- Zinc has been shown to be of value in healing duodenal ulcers in humans, and given that it is of proven preventive value in animal experiments it is probably worth trying as a preventive.

- Various pieces of research suggest that vitamins A and E when taken together offer a degree of protection against ulcers which is greater than any other known preventive. Take 50,000 IU vitamin A and 100 IU vitamin E daily.

UNWANTED PREGNANCY

It is estimated that 200,000 of the 600,000 pregnancies that occur in the UK each year are 'unwanted', although it should be said that many of those who become pregnant in this way come to terms with the pregnancy and so the baby becomes at least to some extent 'wanted'.

We look on page 44 at the general background to such a massive toll of unwanted babies and clearly the subject is extremely complex. Most people imagine that all such babies result from 'bad luck' or contraceptive failure but those who work in the field of psychosexual medicine are convinced that most of the pregnancies in the so-called 'bad luck' women can be explained on more convincing grounds.

Human females over the age of the menarche (once they start having periods) can only get pregnant if they have intercourse within a few days of ovulation. Ovulation (the release of an egg from an ovary) occurs 14 days before the onset of a period irrespective of the length of the woman's menstrual cycle. In a 'typical' cycle this means that the woman ovulates on day 15. To be safe from unwanted pregnancies, therefore, she will have to abstain from penis-in-vagina intercourse or use a contraceptive for a few days around this time. As no woman has a completely predictable cycle, however, preventing unwanted pregnancy generally means using some method of contraceptives throughout the menstrual cycle.

There are many different forms of contraception, all of which have their advantages and disadvantages, but all are unsatisfactory in one way or another. It is these unsatisfactory aspects that lead to at least some unwanted pregnancies. Truly satisfactory and acceptable methods would leave less room for poor usage and other practices that lead to 'failures'.

Let's look briefly at each of the main types of contraception and see what the advantages and disadvantages are:

Male methods.

Although many women feel they want to take responsibility for contraception – mainly because they don't trust men to be sufficiently responsible and because it is they, the women, who will have to carry and bear the baby – in some relationships and especially in premarital teenage sex, the man is looked to as the provider of contraception.

The male pill

This is still at its development stage and does not look like being available for some years yet. There are formidable technical problems to be overcome and anyway there is serious doubt as to whether most women, especially in an extramarital or premarital relationship, would trust a man to have taken the Pill properly at all. Many experts think that the future for a male Pill looks bleak.

The sheath (condom, French letter, Durex, rubber)

Advantages
- Cheap.

- Effective when used properly.

- Can be used by all men.

- Gives at least some protection against VD.

- Good for men who ejaculate prematurely as it reduces penile sensation.

- Useful if the woman has a vaginal infection, enabling sex to continue if she wants it to.

- Can be textured or ribbed to give the woman more sensation.

- Widely available without visit to doctor or clinic.

- No medical side-effects.

Disadvantages

- It reduces sensation, at least to some extent, for the man.

- It has to be put on each time the man has sex and therefore has to be bought and remembered at any sexual session.

How to use it

- Always use a new sheath for each intercourse—*never re-use one*.

- Always ensure that the sheath is on before the penis comes near the vagina—sometimes the fluid that a man's penis leaks *before* ejaculation can contain sperms.

- Apply the sheath to the penis when fully erect, holding the teat between finger and thumb of the other hand, so that the air is squeezed out of the teat and it is left empty for the semen to fill.

- Unroll the sheath along the length of the penis using the other hand to ease it back slightly towards the head of the penis.

- When the sheath is totally unrolled it should still show the packing rings clearly.

- Have intercourse as normal, then grip the condom at the base of the penis and withdraw your penis. Be careful not to spill any semen.

- Ideally the woman should also use additional spermicide in her vagina. This can be in the form of foam, jelly, cream or film.

- Never use Vaseline or other grease as a lubricant as these can perish the rubber rapidly. Special lubricants are available.

- Never use a sheath that is from an out-of-date packet.

Vasectomy

The cutting and tying of the two sperm-carrying ducts that lead from the testes to the penis.

Advantages

- Almost 100 per cent effective.

- Sex drive is not affected in most men.

- Once done it needs no further thought.

- The man can be sure that he cannot father children he doesn't want.

- There is no chance of his partner 'making a mistake'.

Disadvantages

- It is permanent and virtually irreversible–a major disadvantage in a world of unstable marriages because the man might want children in a new relationship.

- In men who are psychosexually unstable, or when the relationship is not good, there is a danger of sexual problems afterwards.

- It is not immediately effective and other methods have to be used for the first four months after the operation or until tests show that there are no live sperms in the semen.

Coitus interruptus (withdrawal, 'being careful')

With this method the man withdraws his penis just before he is about to ejaculate so that no sperms enter the vagina. The failure rate is undoubtedly very high. It is a good idea to keep some spermicidal foam handy in case of an accident.

Advantages

- It doesn't cost anything.

- It has no medical side-effects.

Disadvantages

- It is very unsafe because many men find it difficult to withdraw when it comes to it, especially if they are 'carried away' with the sex act.

- It restricts positions of love-making to those in which the penis can be withdrawn instantaneously.

- If the woman is worried that the man will not withdraw in time she may not relax and so will not enjoy sex much.

- The man may need to withdraw his penis before his partner has had an orgasm because his is about to occur. This can leave the woman 'high and dry'. Obviously she can be brought to orgasm in other ways but many couples find this unsatisfactory.

- It is not a good method for the inexperienced couple, mainly because the man probably has not learned to recognise when his ejaculation is imminent.

Female methods

The Pill

This works by suppressing ovulation as if the woman were pregnant. The failure rate is almost nil if the Pill is taken every day at the same time. There are two basic types. The combined Pill is taken for twenty-one or twenty-two days and then stopped, at which point the woman has a withdrawal bleed like a period. The mini (progestogen only) Pill is taken all the month around.

Advantages

- One hundred per cent reliable if taken regularly. If you forget to take a Pill, take one as soon as you remember–even if it means taking one the next morning, followed by that day's Pill in the evening. If you ever go for more than thirty-six hours without taking your Pill you won't be safe and must use another contraceptive method as you continue the rest of the course of pills.

- You can have sex at any time without thinking about preparing anything.

- It is completely separate from the act of intercourse and so does not intrude on it.

- It reduces the risk of suffering from: certain diseases of the breast; cancer of the ovary; cancer of the lining of the womb; and rheumatoid arthritis.

- It improves the complexion of many women, especially those who normally have spots around period time.

- It enables a woman to plan her periods. If, for example, she is going on holiday and doesn't want to have a period she can simply carry on taking the Pill,rather than stopping after one packet of twenty-one (or twenty-two) Pills, and have a period when the second pack of Pills is finished.

- It reduces or abates period pains

in a substantial proportion of sufferers.

- It makes periods shorter and lighter than normal.

Disadvantages

- It cannot be taken safely by women who are prone to thrombosis and certain other medical conditions.

- It may increase the risk of certain cancers. Research on this is still confused.

- It can produce blood-clotting disorders, liver problems, gallbladder disease, and an inability to wear contact lenses. Some of these are made worse if you are a smoker. Stop taking the Pill and tell your doctor at once if you ever have: breathlessness; pain in the chest, abdomen or legs; vision changes; headaches; a breast lump; or depression.

Longer-acting methods (Depo Provera, Noristerat)

Depo Provera is a synthetic progesterone which is given by injection, usually in the buttock muscle. It is slowly absorbed over the next three months and ovulation is stopped. Its use has been controversial but in 1984 in the UK it was granted a licence for long-term use and is slowly becoming more available. Most family-planning experts don't see this as a first-choice contraceptive.

Advantages

- A four-times-a-year injection renders the woman contraceptively safe.

- It is suitable for poorly-motivated women and those of low intelligence who would find other methods difficult to remember.

Disadvantages

- There are several side-effects including irregular and frequent bleeding, weight gain and delays in return to fertility.

Noristerat is a similar type of hormone that lasts for two months. It is used after a man's vasectomy to tide the woman over the vulnerable time while she needs contraceptive cover.

Intra-uterine devices (IUD, coil, loop)

An IUD works by preventing the newly-fertilised egg from implanting in the uterus. There are several types and your doctor or clinic will advise you which is best for you. Plastic types can be left in indefinitely but copper-containing ones should be changed every 2–3 years. IUDs used to be suitable only for women who had had children but today versions are available even for those that have not.

Advantages

- Once in place it can be forgotten, except for feeling inside each month after a period to ensure that the tail or string coming out

of the cervix is still there. If you can't feel it see your doctor at once and use another method of contraception in the meantime.

- It doesn't interfere with love-making and you don't have to buy replacements.

- IUDs have no bad effects on hormones or on the body generally. They do, however, have local side-effects – see below.

- It can, if inserted in the first few days after unprotected intercourse, act as an abortion-producing agent. It is used in this way as a post-coital contraceptive.

Disadvantages

- Subclinical pelvic infections can cause infertility in a proportion of women.

- During insertion there is a danger of the device being pushed through the uterine wall into the abdominal cavity.

- It can be expelled without the woman knowing it.

- The long-term effects of many years of irritation to the lining of the uterus are not known.

- Tubal (ectopic) pregnancies are more common in IUD users. The IUD should be removed immediately a pregnancy is confirmed.

- Heavy periods and 'spotting' are not uncommon.

- Some men complain of feeling

the tail or string during inter-course.

- It has to be put in by an expert in the first place and there can be quite a lot of pain for a few hours after its insertion.

- You have to go back 2–4 weeks after insertion to see your doctor.

Vaginal spermicides (foams, jellies, creams, film)

These substances kill sperms on their way to meet an egg and must be put into the vagina before intercourse. They are unsafe as a sole method of contraception and should be used along with a sheath or a diaphragm. Follow the instructions for the brand you intend to use. Most are active for only 1–3 hours.

Advantages

- Easy to use.

- Can be bought without a prescription.

- Work well if used together with a barrier method.

Disadvantages

- Not reliable except when com-bined with a barrier method.

- Can be messy as they melt and run out of the vagina.

- Put some men off oral sex. If this is a problem insert the spermicide just before intercourse.

- May have medical side-effects.

Research shows that liver func-tion is altered and blood pressure lowered in some women using spermicides. They are absorbed from the vagina, especially if left in place for long periods.

- You can't bath or have a wash on a bidet for six hours after sex.

The cap (diaphragm)

This is a dome-shaped barrier made of latex rather like a sheath. It has to be used with a spermicide to be safe. It is a good method for many women but it has to be supplied by a doctor, who will measure the woman for the correct size. For best results it must be used properly.

Advantages

- It is cheap and easy to use.

- It is nearly as safe as the Pill.

- There are no medical or health side-effects.

- It can be used to hold back menstrual flow to make for more pleasant love-making during a period.

Disadvantages

- It is not suitable for the woman who dislikes handling her geni-tals.

- It interferes with sensation in some women, especially those who enjoy the front wall of their vagina (around the G-spot) being stimulated during intercourse.

- It has to be put in well before sex and this removes the spontaneity for many women who find such 'premeditated' preparation un-sexy.

- It is easy to forget that it is in place for a day or two.

- It has to be supplied by a trained person in the first place.

- It should ideally be checked every six months by a trained person to see that the fit has not changed. This is especially important soon after a baby.

- It is easy for small holes, invisible to the naked eye, to develop which render the barrier ineffec-tive.

- It interferes with sensation in those men who like to feel their partner's cervix hitting against the tip of the penis.

How to use it

Place 3 or 4 inches of spermicidal jelly on the inside of the cap and spread some around the rim too. Insert the cap in the way that you have been taught and do so well in advance of intercourse. If you don't have sex within 3 hours use more spermicide in the vagina. Don't remove the cap for at least six hours after intercourse. If you have sex more than once during this six hours use more sperm-icide without removing the cap.

Look after the cap well. Remove it gently after intercourse ensuring that you don't damage the dome with your nails. Wash it with plain, warm water and leave it out to dry. Never use perfumed soap or detergent to wash it. Never use Vaseline or disin-fectant or you will spoil it. Hold it up to a good light every month and look for obvious holes. If there is any sign of damage, get a new one. Never wear a cap for more than twenty-four hours without removing and wash-ing it.

The sponge

This is a disc of spermicide-impreg-nated sponge that the woman places in the vagina before intercourse.

Advantages

- Fairly easy to use.

- A good, non-permanent, barrier method.

Disadvantages

- All the disadvantages of absorb-ing spermicides into the bloodstream.

- Must be left in place for six hours after intercourse.

- It has to be thrown away after a single use and so is expensive.

- It can be felt in the vagina by the man's penis or fingers.

- It is rather unreliable (75–85 per cent effective only) and so is really only suitable for couples who want to space their children rather than those who want to be absolutely sure about fertility control.

Natural methods (Calendar, sympto-thermal, Billings)

Calendar method

Using the onset of bleeding as day 1 and the day prior to the onset of bleeding as the last day of the cycle, map out your cycles for eight months. Find the longest and shortest and work out the times of ovulation in both cycles. This occurs fourteen days before the first day of bleeding in any one cycle. So if your cycle is 28–32 days long you will ovulate at some point on days 14–18 in any one month. Allow four days either side for safety. This means (continuing the example–the days will differ for different individuals) that you are *unsafe* from day 10 to day 21 in any month. Outside this time span you are *probably* safe.

Advantages

- Costs nothing.

- Gets around religious prohibitions on using 'artificial' methods of birth control.

- No medical side-effects.

- Makes couples more aware of the woman's reproductive cycle and the functioning of her body.

- Leads to couples finding alternatives to penis-in-vagina sex.

Disadvantages

- Very unreliable.

- Needs constant checking of cycle lengths to be sure that they are not changing.

- Rules out penis-in-vagina sex for twelve days a month unless you are absolutely regular. Couples who don't like making love during the woman's period will add at least four days during menstruation to this, making half the month either unsafe or unsuitable.

- Constant worry about timing can be unpleasant for both partners and probably leads to less sex overall.

Sympto-thermal method

A method which combines the taking of the woman's daily body temperature and an awareness of the state of her fertility cycle through charting her cervical mucus condition. The method is complicated to do well and needs practice. In principle it works as follows:

When the cervical mucus is relatively thick and cloudy in the early days of a cycle it may be safe to have sex unless your cycle is very short.

As the mucus becomes slippery, thin and clear, ovulation is about to occur. As soon as the mucus appears to stop being thick and cloudy stop having unprotected sex. Avoid intercourse until three full days after the 'peak' of slippery mucus. Obviously, this takes some experience at judging.

The safest time for sex using this method is from the fourth day after the peak slippery mucus day until the first day of a period.

Advantages

- Costs nothing.

- Good for religious groups for whom contraception is prohibited.

- No medical side-effects.

- Makes a woman (and her partner) much more aware of her reproductive cycle and the functioning of her body.

- Encourages the use of methods of love-making other than penis-in-vagina intercourse.

Disadvantages

- Unsafe. Studies have shown that in the best hands the reliability *can* be near to that of the diaphragm but this can only be achieved by restricting sex to a relatively few days of the month.

- As with the calendar method, travel, illness, drugs, stress infections and so on can all affect cycle length and so throw off the calculations. Women with irregular cycles find such methods tricky too.

- As with the calendar method, many days every month are unsafe, and others may be regarded as unsuitable because of menstruation. This can suit the couple with a low sex drive very well but for others it means using alternative methods of love-making, many or all of which are unacceptable to some.

Tubal sterilisation

This permanent method of contraception is ideal for the woman who definitely does not want to have any more children. The method involves some kind of interference with the fallopian tubes so that the eggs can no longer pass down into the uterus. There are five main types of procedure and almost all involve the removal of part of the tubes. The success rate is very high (with failure in only 4 in 1,000 cases).

Advantages

- It is permanent–no more worry about unwanted conceptions.

- It is virtually 100 per cent effective.

- It probably has no generalised effects on the woman's body– none have yet been recognised.

Disadvantages

- It means having an operation and there are dangers in this, albeit few. There is a small surgical complication rate (even in expert hands) but almost all of these get better quickly.

- It is irreversible to all intents and purposes, so you can't change your mind.

- It can result in heavy or irregular periods in some women and some have PMT for the first time ever.

Morning-after methods

Most people know of the morning-after Pill but there is also the post-coital IUD. Both are forms of very early abortion.

The morning-after Pill must be taken within seventy-two hours of intercourse and contains large doses of hormones. Fitting a coil (IUD) within five days of the unprotected intercourse is an alternative. These methods are only suitable for emergencies and are not used as routine forms of contraception.

Advantages

- They can be used in emergencies to ward off the possible consequences of a 'mistake' (i.e. unprotected intercourse). The IUD goes on to act as an on-going contraceptive.

Disadvantages

- The morning-after Pill can produce quite unpleasant side-effects – usually nausea and vomiting.

Contraceptive methods and their effectiveness

Method	Effectiveness (%)
The Pill	Almost 100
Mini-Pill	98
Depo Provera	Almost 100
IUD	96–98
Diaphragm*	97
Sponge*	75–85
Sheath*	97
Sympto-thermal	85–93
Sterilisation	100 (allowing for occasional failures)
Post-coital Pill	97–98
Post-coital IUD	Almost 100

*Spermicide ensures success.

VARICOSE VEINS

What are they?

Varicose veins are knotted, distended, twisted, leg veins in which the valves have ceased to function properly.

Approximately one in four North American women and one in ten North American men suffer from varicose veins, yet they are much less common in Third World countries. One survey found that over the age of 50 in the US 42 per cent of men and 64 per cent of women had them. In a survey of Egyptian women factory workers the figure was 6 per cent.

Not only do varicose veins look unsightly; they produce pain (a dull, aching heaviness); the ankles swell (especially in warm weather); there are painful calf cramps at night; the legs itch or burn; and more serious complications such as shin ulcers, inflammation of the veins, blood clots and bleeding can occur too. More than 100,000 Americans die each year from a blood clot which then lodges in the lung.

Treatment is traditionally with elastic stockings (hose) to apply pressure on the veins, injections of sclerosing agents to seal off the worst veins, and surgery to remove the offending veins. None of these is a very successful or pleasant treatment so once again prevention must be considered.

What causes them?

- Heredity. There is little doubt that varicose veins are more common in the families of those who already have them. Whether this is true heredity or due to an environmental factor (see below) is not yet clear.

- The erect posture of humans, constrictive clothing and repeated pregnancies have been discarded as primary causes of varicose veins because none of the theories stands up to scrutiny when examined in detail in other populations of the world.

- The probable cause of varicose veins is as follows. We in the West eat very little dietary fibre and strain at stool to pass a small number of hard, small 'sticky' stools in a seated position on a lavatory. Peoples around the world who have very few varicose veins eat plenty of fibre and pass large-volume, soft and easily evacuated stools in a squatting position.

Research has shown that the pressure produced when straining at stool is transmitted down the leg veins and it is postulated that this repeated downward pressure (against the blood flow) damages the valves in the veins. Normally the valves stop blood pooling in the leg veins under gravity as blood passes upwards against gravity propelled by the pumping action of the calf muscles as we walk. Once the valves have been rendered inoperative blood pools and distends the veins and blood flow becomes sluggish. Blood leaks out into the skin causing unsightly discolouration and other skin changes and the scene is set for the serious, even life-threatening complications listed above. In traditional peoples who squat to open their bowels the angle of the thighs to the abdomen is so acute that it shuts off the major leg veins in the groin, so preventing the pressure produced by straining at stool (which is very low anyway because of their high-fibre diet) from passing down into them.

- Standing for long periods definitely makes varicose veins worse because of the increased gravitational burden. Sitting, it appears, might also make things worse, as does crossing one's legs when seated.

- Female hormones may well have something to do with the problem. Indeed, something has to explain why it is that women are so much more likely to suffer from the condition than are men. Although they are more constipated than men this alone does not appear to answer all the questions. That a hormonal change during pregnancy could be involved is deduced from the fact that in some women inflamed leg veins are early signs of pregnancy–even before they miss a period. At this stage the fetus cannot possibly be compressing the large veins in the pelvis so perhaps it is the rising levels of the connective-tissue-relaxing hormone (relaxin) that make the vein walls relax too much and leads to varicosities.

Prevention

- Eat a high-fibre diet rich in fruit and vegetables, whole-grain breakfast cereals, and wholemeal bread and other wholemeal-flour products (including pasta), and cut down on refined sugar and refined flour.

- Drink more fluid to ensure that constipation is a thing of the past.

- Avoid long periods of sitting and standing if you have a history of varicose veins in your family or if you have early signs of them yourself. Do exercises frequently if you are in this group. Wiggle your toes a lot, raise and lower yourself on the balls of your feet while standing in a queue in the supermarket or at a bus stop. Raise your legs on to a table whenever you sit down (get them above heart level), break up long rail or car trips by walking every hour or so, and walk around on long plane journeys.

- Get more exercise. Swim, run, jog, walk or cycle to improve nature's muscle pump in your legs. Walking lowers the venous pressure to a third of standing pressure under normal conditions.

- Go barefoot at home as much as possible to exercise your foot muscles and improve your venous flow.

- If you have even a hint of varicose veins starting, shun tight boots, pants that are too tight at the groin and anything that restricts the legs such as self-supporting stockings.

- Make trips to the lavatory short and to the point–don't sit there reading for ages.

- Avoid very hot baths–these seem to encourage varicose veins.

- If you have a family history of varicose veins wear support stockings throughout pregnancy.

VENEREAL DISEASE (VD)

What is it?

Venereal disease is a family of infections involving the genital organs. They are, by definition, caught by having sexual contact with another person but in reality this is too narrow a way of looking at the problem, as we shall see.

VD (otherwise known as sexually transmitted diseases–STDs) is a fast-growing problem. Gonorrhoea, for example, is the second most common infectious illness in the world after measles.

VD is becoming more of a problem for several reasons. First, society's changed attitudes over the last twenty years or so have encouraged young people to have intercourse at a younger age. The babies born in the 1950s and 1960s are now teenagers and young adults and this group are exceptionally active sexually. Premarital sex is more commonplace than it used to be–a change particularly involving women. Most surveys show that over 90 per cent of women are not virgins when they go up the aisle. Half of all US women who have never been married have had more than one sex partner, compared with just over a third fifteen years ago. The divorce rate is rising steadily; more adults are choosing to remain single or are postponing marriage for various reasons; and so the list of changes goes on. All of this has led to increasing numbers of individuals having sex with larger numbers of partners than ever before.

Women and newborn babies bear the major brunt of this epidemic of venereal infections. One in every twenty babies born in the US has an infection with chlamydia, and of the infected group half will develop conjunctivitis and one in five pneumonia. Early syphilis, until recently a rare disease, is once more appearing in women of childbearing age. If early syphilis is untreated in pregnancy 40 per cent of the infants will be still-born, born prematurely or die prematurely. Another 40 per cent will have congenital syphilis. Such a woman has only a one in five chance of having a normal, healthy baby.

As many as three in every 10,000 babies are born with herpes. Half die very early in life and a quarter of those who survive will be damaged. Three in every 200 babies are affected with cytomegalovirus and one in seven of them will be deaf, retarded or suffer eye defects. Nearly 5,000 babies a year die from beta-haemolytic streptococcus–a proportion of these infections are probably sexually transmitted.

Pelvic inflammatory disease is the most common serious complication of chlamydial and gonococcal infections. These diseases cause 25,000 ectopic pregnancies (pregnancies that occur outside the womb in the fallopian tubes), 213,000 hospital admissions, 115,000 major surgical operations, and 900 deaths, per year in the US alone.

Let's now look briefly at each venereal disease in turn.

Gonorrhoea

This disease is caused by a bacterium that can be transferred from one person to another by oral sex, anal sex or normal intercourse. A large proportion of infected women have no symptoms and so don't know that they have the condition.

In women, symptoms include vaginal discharge, burning when passing water, fever and chills, abdominal pain and painful joints. In men there is pain on passing water and a yellow discharge from the penis. If you have any of these symptoms you should see your doctor or go to a special clinic at once.

Complications occur if the infection spreads to the fallopian tubes and ovaries of women and to the testes and prostate of men. Permanent damage can occur to the reproductive organs and joints. Cure rates are high if the condition is caught very early before it has spread.

Syphilis

This is now a curable condition if diagnosed early. It too can be caught by anal, oral or ordinary sex.

The first signs of infection appear from ten days to twelve weeks after infection. First, a painless sore appears on or near the sex organs. This can be inside the vagina or rectum where it can't be seen. In the second stage of the illness there is a rash (which may not itch), mouth sores, lumps, 'flu-like symptoms and a general feeling of ill health. The third stage has no symptoms – the disease is lying dormant. In the later stages of syphilis the heart, eyes, ears and central nervous system are affected.

Blood tests can pick up syphilis at the earliest stages and treatment cures the condition at this stage. Later on treatment can render the sufferer non-infectious but permanent damage may well have already occurred.

Herpes

This is discussed on page 239.

AIDS

This is discussed on page 130.

Non-specific urethritis (NSU)

This enormously common disease can be very difficult to treat. It is mainly a disease of men (women carry it but have few symptoms). There is considerable debate as to what causes it but an organism called chlamydia is certainly one culprit.

NSU develops ten days after having sex with an infected person and the symptoms are like those of gonorrhoea. The discharge may be white, yellow, green, grey or streaked with blood. The first sign is often pain on passing water. Tests will be done to rule out other forms of VD and you will be given a long course of antibiotics. It can take months to clear. It is possible for a man to get NSU even if he is having sex with only one partner. Such men must encourage their partners to go to the clinic to be examined and treated if necessary.

Pubic lice (crabs or nits)

These parasites live in pubic hair and suck human blood on which they live. Their eggs are called nits and look like small, white blobs attached to pubic hairs. They itch like fury. You can't wash off the eggs and need to get special chemical preparations from a clinic or a doctor. These kill off the crab-like nits and cure the condition.

Pubic lice can be caught not just from personal contact but also from bedding, clothes, towels or lavatory seats.

Scabies (the itch)

This is a similar infection but usually causes itching, often in the webs of the fingers, around the waist, on the wrists and under the armpits. It is not specifically a genital disease but occurs in people who have close bodily contact with one another.

Prevention

- The best prevention against venereal disease is to have as few sexual partners as possible. It is unusual for those who have sex with only one partner to catch a venereal disease but it is not impossible. Certain venereal infections can be caught from towels, sheets and lavatory seats, so it makes sense to avoid using other people's belongings. Some people avoid public lavatories for this reason. Thrush and certain other genital infections in women can be transmitted to their partners who need never have had sex outside the partnership. Needless to say, babies who catch herpes or other venereal infections have not had sexual contact with anyone – they have contact with the infected genitals of their mothers.

- If you are having sex with someone you don't know well (on a one-night stand, for example) it makes sense for the man to use a sheath. Women who have sex with strangers should always carry a sheath and insist that the man wear it. Likewise, men should carry a sheath against this eventuality. The diaphragm offers some small protection to a woman but not nearly as much as does a sheath. Spermicidal foam has some effect in killing off the organisms that cause VD.

- At the first sign of any of the above diseases seek help. This makes sense not only because you will be treated more quickly and more effectively but because the best form of prevention against VD is ensuring that anyone who knows he or she has the condition prevents themselves from passing it on to others. If you have any of the above symptoms *stop having sex* and get help.

- If you discover any of the above symptoms be ready to tell the clinic who your sex partners were so that they can trace them and treat them too. Absolute confidentiality is the rule at these clinics but unless your sexual contacts are traced and treated the infected people will go on to infect others.

- Prevention ideally starts early – at school and at home – by instructing children and teenagers about the dangers of sex with multiple partners. Many schools currently give such information but the quality is extremely variable and much of it takes the form of scare stories. This often has exactly the opposite effect as many children unconsciously turn away from such unpalatable information. There is a real need for professional sex educators, who would go round schools telling children about the many aspects of love and sex, among which would be a discussion of sexually transmitted diseases.

With the current scares over AIDS and herpes there are signs that VD is decreasing a little as people reduce their promiscuity somewhat. This started off among US homosexuals but is spreading to affect heterosexuals and other countries too.

WORMS

What are they?

There are several types of worms that can infest the human digestive tract. Most are found only in the tropics but a few can occur in the UK. The most common worms by far to be found in the US and UK are threadworms. Hook-worms are only seen in returning holidaymakers, and immigrant families, and tapeworms are usually found only in those who have eaten undercooked pork. The human roundworm is like an earthworm and produces stomach ache, fever, wheezing and even the coughing up of blood. Whipworms are the same size as threadworms (like tiny pieces of thread) and the only problem they cause is diarrhoea.

What causes them?

Worms enter the body in many different ways but most are eaten in the egg stage of their life-cycle as a result of poor food preparation conditions and poor hygiene generally.

Threadworms are 6–12 mm (½ in) long and look like pieces of sewing thread. They live in the bowel and at night the females come out of the child's back passage to lay eggs. The child scratches his or her itching bottom and transfers the eggs to his mouth. These are swallowed and the worm's life-cycle starts all over again.

Most children with threadworms have no symptoms except an itchy anus. Sometimes you can see the worms at night coming out of the child's anus but as you shine the torch on to them they dive back in.

Drugs can be used to kill the worms in the bowel. These are not unpleasant and do no harm–except to the worms!

Prevention

- If any member of the family has worms the whole family must be treated or the members will go on passing them around to one another.

- Threadworms can survive in a room for 2–3 weeks, so after starting treatment with the medicine strip the beds and wait for the dust to settle. Vacuum the carpet and damp-dust all the surfaces. Wash each person's bedclothes and bedding separately just in case any eggs survive the warm wash.

- Cut your child's fingernails and scrub them to remove any eggs.

- Put your child in knickers and cotton gloves at night to prevent scratching and wash these every day.

- If your child goes to a playgroup or school, tell the teacher as soon as the diagnosis has been made. There is probably another child in the class with them who has not been treated.

- Teach your children to wash their hands thoroughly after going to

the lavatory or touching anything in the lavatory at school. Disposable paper towels are better than cloth ones. Also teach them to wash their hands thoroughly before meals and before preparing food.

WOUND HEALING DIFFICULTY

What is it?

Wounds (cuts, abrasions, ulcers in the bowel, surgical incisions, and so on) heal naturally, restoring the surface or lining of the body to its undamaged state. The time taken for a wound to heal varies from place to place on the body from a few days to several weeks. Unfortunately, many people, especially those having operations, heal far less quickly than they should.

What causes it?

- Poor nutrition generally, especially a shortage of protein.
- Too little vitamin C in the diet.
- A shortage of vitamin A.
- Zinc deficiency.

Prevention

- Animal research shows that malnourished individuals suffer twice as many complications during healing, and that twice as many of them die from their wounds, as do normally nourished ones. The most common complication in human wound healing in hospitals is infection—in fact this is the single most common reason for post-operative patients to stay longer in hospital than they should have to. From this and other evidence it is clear that the person with a wound needs good-quality foods high in protein. Protein is the vital supplier of the raw materials necessary to rebuild damaged tissue. It does not, of course, have to be animal protein.

- Eat more vitamin C. Numerous studies have shown how valuable this vitamin is in normal wound healing. One study of over 1,000 patients with wounds found that wound infections worsened as blood vitamin C levels fell. Some of the people had white-blood-cell levels of vitamin C that were as low as those in people with scurvy. Similar studies have been done in patients with bed sores. Two 500 mg tablets of vitamin C a day healed the sores twice as fast as expected.

- Eat more vitamin A. Even minor wounds, it seems, increase the body's need for this vitamin. Animals fed vitamin A have stronger wounds (artificially created in a laboratory). Some severe burn or accident victims develop what are called 'stress ulcers' in their intestines. A study in Arizona found that giving such people 50,000–100,000 IU vitamin A twice daily reduced the stress ulcers to less than a third of what would be expected in an unsupplemented group.

Vitamin A is also valuable for anyone taking steroids for the relief of arthritis or other inflammatory conditions. Anti-inflammatory drugs and even aspirin retard open-wound healing, and vitamin A can help restore the balance. Zinc can also be protective against these effects of cortisone.

- Eat more zinc and zinc-containing foods. Zinc works alongside vitamin A in wound healing and helps mobilise stores of the vitamin. It is also essential for the production of new proteins and connective tissue. In a UK study, zinc accelerated the healing of leg ulcers, for example. For a list of zinc-containing foods, see page 314.

BIBLIOGRAPHY

A book such as this draws from many sources and learned papers too numerous to list. Many of the sources, especially those in specialist journals, are available only in the largest medical libraries.

What follows is a short list of some of the more interesting sources used.

In Part Three, entries have been grouped under three main headings: interesting papers or articles; key leaflets or booklets available free from the Health Education Council; and useful addresses for those who need more information about a condition—though not necessarily about its prevention.

General Books About Prevention

An Introduction to Preventive Medicine: John Simpson (William Heinemann, 1970)

Essentials of Preventive Medicine: J.A. Muir Gray & Godfrey Fowler (Blackwell Scientific Publications), 1985

'Practising Prevention', Articles from the *British Medical Journal* (Published by the BMA, Tavistock Square, London WC1H 9JR, 1983)

Prevention & Health: Everybody's Business (HMSO, 1976)

Public Health and Preventive Medicine: Ed. John M. Last. A very expensive, high-powered book for professionals. (Appleton-Century-Crofts, New York, 1980)

Some of the Sources Used in Parts One and Two

The Advance to Social Medicine, R. Sand (Staples Press, London, 1952)

'Aspects of Preventive Medicine', W. Thompson, *Public Health*, 96:pp 221-224, London, 1983

'Back to Methusela? Opportunities for Preventive Medicine', Sir R. Doll, *Irish Journal of Medical Science*, 1983, Vol. 152, No.1

'Behavioural Science & Prevention', E. Berkanovic, *Preventive Medicine*, 5: pp.92-105, 1976

'A Birth to Death Preventive Medicine/Periodic Health Screening Protocol', H.T. Milhorn, *Journal MSMA*, February 1982

'Child Health Supervision—is it Worth it?' A. Yankauer, *Pediatrics*, 52:pp 272-277, 1973

Chronic Illness in the United States, Vol. 1 (Published for the Commonwealth Fund by Harvard University Press, Cambridge, Mass., 1957)

'Concepts of Illness Causation and Responsibility: Some Preliminary Data From a Sample of Working Class Mothers', R. Pill and N. Stott, *Society of Science & Medicine*, 16: pp 43-52, 1982

'Contemporary Perspective on Prevention', Warren Winklestein, Jr, *Bulletin of the New York Academy of Medicine*, Vol. 51, No.1, January 1975

'Coronary Disease Among US Soldiers Killed in Action in Korea', W.F. Enos & J. Beyer, *JAMA*, 152: pp 1090-1093, 1953

'Cost-benefit Concepts in Health: Examination of Some Prevention Efforts', J. Lave and L. Lave, *Preventive Medicine*, 7: pp 414-423, 1978

'Disease Prevention: The Challenge of the Future', D.A. Hamburg, *American Journal of Public Health*, 69: pp 1026-1033, 1979

'The Emergence of the Concept of Screening for Disease', S.J. Reiser, *Milbank Memorial Fund Quarterly*, 56: pp 403-425, 1978

'Epidemiology & Prevention', J.N. Morris, *Milbank Memorial Fund Quarterly/Health & Society*, Vol.60, No.1, 1982

'Evaluating Well-women Clinics', G. Lloyd, *Practitioner*, Vol.277: pp 735-743, May 1983

'Factors Associated with the Maintenance of Positive Health Behaviour', D. Mechanic & P.D. Cleary, *Preventive Medicine*, 9: pp 805-814, 1980

'The Failure of Preventive Medicine', J.A. Muir-Gray,*Lancet*, 24 December 1977

'Health Care Costs & Preventive Medicine', M.M.Kristein, *Preventive Medicine*, 11: pp 729-732, 1982

'Health Economics and Preventive Care', M.M. Kristein, *Science*, Vol.195, No.4, 1977

'Health Education – The Key to Prevention', Editorial, *New York State Journal of Medicine*: 1171, July 1979

Health for All by the Year 2000 (World Health Organisation, 1981)

'Health Risk Appraisal: Some Methodologic Considerations', Axel Goetz and T. Mctyre, *Nursing Research*, Vol. 30, No.5, September/October 1981

Healthy People, The Surgeon General's Report on Health Promotion and Disease Prevention (US DHEW, Pub. No.79-55071, 1979)

'Historical Evolution of Primary Prevention', G. Rosen, *Bulletin of the New York Academy of Medicine*, Vol.51, No.1, January 1975

How to Practise Prospective Medicine: L.C. Robbins & J.H. Hall (Methodist Hospital of Indiana, Indianapolis, 1970

'How We Might Live Healthily and Enjoy It More', S. Katz, *Canadian Medical Association Journal*, Vol.11,21 December 1974

Inducing the Next Long Wave: I. Priban (Personal communication)

Inequalitities in Health. DHSS Report on a Recent Working Group: Sir Douglas Black, Chairman (HMSO, 1980)

'Interrelationships of Preventive Actions in Health and Other Areas', A.F. Williams and H. Wechsler, *Health Service Report*, Vol.87, No.10, December 1972

'A Life-time Health-monitoring Programme', L. Breslow & A. Somers, *New English Journal of Medicine*, 296: pp 601-608, 1977

'The Logic and Urgency of Primary Prevention', B.L. Bloom, *Hospital & Community Psychiatry*, Vol.32, No.12, December 1981

'Medical Evaluation of Healthy Persons', *JAMA*, Vol.249, No.12, 25 March 1983

The Medical Role of Environmental Health: H.A. Waldron (Oxford University Press, 1978)

'Medicine's Greatest Schism: Prevention vs Care' (An historical perspective), J.G. Frayman, *Medical Care*,Vol.XIII, No.7, July 1975

'Motivating Adolescents to Reduce Risk for Chronic Disease', C.L.Williams & E.L. Wynder, *Postgraduate Medical Journal* 54: pp 212-214, March 1978

'The Myths and Realities of Health Maintenance', D. Woods, *Canadian Medical Association Journal*, Vol.109: pp 1147-1155, 1 December 1973

'An Operational Classification of Disease Prevention', *Public Health Reports*, Vol.98, No.2, March-April 1983

'The People: Motivation, Education and Action', G.W.Steuart (Presented as part of the 1974 Annual Health Conference of the New York Academy of Medicine, Prevention & Health Maintenance Revisited), Published in *Bulletin of the New York Acadamy of Medicine*, Vol.51, No.1, January 1975

'Periodic Health Examination: A Guide for Designing Individualised Preventive Health Care in the Asymptomatic Patient', *Annals of Internal Medicine*, 95 (6): pp 729-732, December 1981

Personal Health Maintenance, Special Issue of the *Western Journal of Medicine*, Vol.141, No.6, 1984

'The Philosophy of Preventive Medicine', John E. Smith, *Minnesota Medicine*, March 1976

'A Policy Assessment of Preventive Health Practice', L. Breslow, *Preventive Medicine*, 6: pp 242-251, 1977

Poverty in the United Kingdom (Allen Lane, London, 1979)

'Present Status of Breast Cancer Screening', Editorial, *Canadian Medical Association Journal*, Vol.117: pp 845-846, 22 October 1977

'Prevention: An Idea Whose Time Has Come?', C. Holmes, *Western Journal of Medicine*, 132: pp 471-473, May 1980

'Prevention–A Political Choice', Georges Boileau, *Canadian Medical Association Journal*, Vol.125, 15 October 1981

'Prevention in Perspective: History, Concepts and Issues', A.D. Berg, *Journal of Family Practice*, 9: pp 37-46, 1979

'Prevention in the Canadian Health System': A.B. Morison, *Preventive Medicine* 7: pp 498-504, 1978

'Preventive: Rhetoric & Reality', N.A. Holtzman, *International Journal of Health Services*, Vol.9, No.1, 1979

'Prevention: Who Needs It?' N. Black and P.M. Strong, *British Medical Journal*, Vol.285, 27 November 1982

'Preventive Medicine', C. Sheps, *JAMA*, 241 (13), 30 March 1979

'Preventive Medicine & Natural Death', Editorial, *Acta Med Scand.*, 195: pp 441-442, 1974

Preventive Medicine in the United States 1900-1975, G. Rosen (New York Science History Publications, 1975)

'Preventive Medicine–Professes Much, Practises Little', A.B. Bergman, *American Journal of the Disabled Child*, Vol.131, June 1977

'Preventive Medicine: The Long Term Solution', Jesse L. Steinfield, *Preventive Medicine*, 1: pp 10-11, 1972

'Preventive Medicine USA'. Task Force Report, New York: PRODIST (Neale Watson Academic Publications, 1976)

Professed or Public Heath? Sociology in Health & Medicine (Nuffield Provincial Hospitals Trust, London, 1980)

'Public & Private Prevention', Editorial, *American Journal of Public Health*, Vol.73, No.9, September 1983

'Reducing the Cost of Medical Care: Prevention as a Cost-effective Measure', J. Brown, *Texan Medicine*, Vol.75, March 1979

'A Review of the Economic Evidence on Prevention', R.M. Scheffler & L. Parniger, *Medical Care*, Vol.XVIII, No.5, May 1980

The Role of Medicine: T.McKeown (Nuffield Provincial Hospitals Trust, 1976)

The Role of Voluntary Organisations in the Health and Personal Services System: B. Glanville (Personal communication)

'The Royal Commission and Prevention' P. Draper, *Lancet*, 25 August 1979

'Rustproofing people', D. Treffert, *Wellness*, Vol. 71, No.1, January 1982

'Screening for the Early Detection of Diseases in Great Britain', J. Chamberlain, *Preventive Medicine*, 4: pp 268-281, 1975

'Task Force Report: The Periodic Health Examination', *Canadian Medical Association Journal*, 121: pp 1193-1235, 1979

'Technology and Health Care', White Kerr, *New England Journal of Medicine*. Quoting Cochrane & Holland, 'Validation of Screening Procedures', *British Medical Bulletin*, 27: p 3, 1971

'Three Phases of Prevention in the United States', G. Pickett, *Bulletin of the Pan American Health Organisation*, 11: p 11, 1977

'Towards Prevention–An Outline Plan for the Development of Health Promotion Teams', John R. Ashton, *Community Medicine*, 4: p 231, 1981

'The Ups and Downs of Prevention', Editorial in *American Journal of Public Health*, Vol.71, No.1.

Western Diseases: Ed. H.C. Trowell & D.P. Burkitt (Edward Arnold, 1981)

'WHO Constitution', published in *Public Health Administration & Practice*, 6th edition, 1974

Part Three

Accidents

National Safety Council: Accident Facts (Chicago National Safety Council. 1980, No.55)

Danger from Fire (Free from council offices, local Fire Prevention Departments, & County Fire Brigade HQs)

Do You Have a Fire Escape Plan? (RoSPA, see below for address)

Help Yourself to Gas Safety (Dept SP, London W1A 2AZ)

Play it Safe–a guide to preventing children's accidents (Health Education Council)

Safe as Houses (RoSPA, see below for address)

Safety in the Home (From electricity showrooms)

Royal Society for the Prevention of Accidents (RoSPA): Cannon House, The Priory, Queensway, Birmingham B4 6BS (RoSPA has numerous helpful publications on all aspects of safety)

Aching Feet

'Solve your Foot and Heel Problems Now', *Prevention Magazine*, November 1983

'Why Stand for Aching Feet?' *Prevention Magazine*, June 1979

Acne

'Breaking out of Acne', *Medical Self-care*, Spring 1985

Ageing

'Preventive Gerontology', W. Hazzard, *Postgraduate Medicine*, Vol. 74, No.2, August 1983

'Preventive Health Care in the Elderly', M. Carnes, *Wisconsin Medical Journal*, Vol. 82, August 1983

'The Natural Reversal of Ageing', *Prevention Magazine*, September 1983

Age Concern England: 60 Pitcairn Road, Mitcham, Surrey CR4 3LL

Help the Aged: 32 Dover Street, London W1A 2AP

The Pre-Retirement Association: 19 Undine Street, London SW17 8PP

AIDS

'AIDS, the Facts, the Fears, the Future', *The Times*, 6 March 1985

Some Facts about AIDS (Health Education Council)

'Where Now with AIDS?', *Nature*, Vol.313, 24 January 1985

The Terence Higgins Trust: BM AIDS, London WC1

Alcoholism
'Alcohol and the Fetus–Is Zero the Only Option?', Leading article, *Lancet*, 26 March 1983

British Journal of Addiction, September 1977

'Nutrition: A Better Way to Fight Alcoholism', *Prevention Magazine*, August 1983

Health Education in the Prevention of Alcohol-related Problems (Scottish Health Education Council)

That's the Limit. A Guide to Sensible Drinking (Health Education Council)

Alcohol Concern: 3 Grosvenor Crescent, London SW1X 7EE

Alcoholics Anonymous: PO Box 514, 11 Redcliffe Gardens, London SW13

Asthma
'ABC of Asthma', Articles from the *British Medical Journal* (BMA 1984)

Action Against Allergy: 43 The Downs, London SW20 8HG

Allergy Support Service: 64a Marshalls Drive, St Albans, Herts

Asthma Society & Friends of the Asthma Research Council: St Thomas's Hospital, Lambeth Palace Road, London SE1 7EH

National Society for Research into Allergy: 60a Fox Lane, London N13 4AR

Arthritis
Arthritis and Rheumatism (Rodale Press, 1982)

The Arthritis & Rheumatism Council: 8 Charing Cross Road, London WC2H OHN (Publish several helpful booklets about all aspects of the condition)

Baby Battering
'Primary Prevention of Child Abuse–Focus on the Special Child', W. Friedrich & J. Boriskin, *Hospital and Community Psychiatrists*, Vol. 29, No. 4, April 1978

National Society for the Prevention of Cruelty to Children (NSPCC): 1 Riding House Street, London W1P 8AA

Parents Anonymous: (look in local telephone directory) or 6-9 Manor Gardens, London N7

Back Pain
Backache (Rodale Press, 1982)

Conquering Pain: Dr Sampson Lipton (Martin Dunitz, 1984)

Mind your Back (Health Education Council)

'Tips for a Healthy Back', *Prevention Magazine*, October 1983

The Back Pain Association: 31 Park Road, Teddington, Middx

Bedwetting
Bedwetting (Health Education Council)

Breast Abscess
Association of Breastfeeding Mothers: 131 Mayow Road, London SE26

Le Leche League: BM 3424, London WC1N 3XX

National Childbirth Trust: 9 Queensborough Terrace, London W2 3TB

Bronchitis and Emphysema
Bronchitis & Emphysema (Rodale Press, 1982)

The Chest, Heart & Stroke Association: Tavistock House North, Tavistock Square, London WC1H 9JE

Bruising
'What to Do Before You're Black and Blue', *Prevention Magazine,* July 1980

Cancer
'Blocking Cancer with Vitamin A',
Prevention Magazine, September 1979

Cancer Detection & Prevention, Vol.5, No.3,
1982

'Cancer Update–Fighting Back with
Nutrition', *Prevention Magazine*, October
1983

Carcinogenesis – A Comprehensive Survey, Vol.2
–Mechanism of Tumour Production &
Co-carcinogenesis. Ed. T.J. Slaga (Raven
Press, New York, 1978)

'Don't Wait until Cancer Strikes', *Prevention
Magazine*, November 1979

*Estimates of the Fractions of Cancer in the
United States Related to Occupational Factors*:
Bethesda Md. (National Cancer Institute,
1978)

'Familial Susceptibility to Cancer', leading
article, *British Medical Journal*, 14 May 1983

'Friendship Is a Good Health Diet', *New
Scientist*, p 42, 21 March 1984

Journal of the National Cancer Institute,
September 1978

'Missed Opportunities for Early Diagnosis
of Cancer of the Cervix', R. Fruchter, J.
Boyce & M. Hunt, *American Journal of Public
Health*, 70: pp 418-420

The No-cancer Lifestyle', *Prevention
Magazine*, July 1980

'Selenium–the Double-Duty Protector',
Prevention Magazine, June 1979

'Who is Being Screened for Cervical
Cancer?' J.C. Kleinman & A. Kapstein,
American Journal of Public Health, 71: pp
73-76, 1981

'The World Cancer Burden: Prevent or
Perish', Editorial, *British Medical Journal*,
Vol. 290, 5 January 1985

A Guide to Reducing Your Risks (Health
Education Council) (Also contains a useful
reading list)

Cancer Risk and Your Diet (Rodale Press,
1982)

The Association for New Approaches to
Cancer: 28 Blythe Road, London W14

Cancer Information Association: Marygold
House, Carfax, Oxford

Imperial Cancer Research Fund: PO Box
123, Lincoln's Inn Fields, London WC2A
3PX

Cholesterol: high blood levels
'12 Ways to Lower Your Cholesterol–
Naturally', *Prevention Magazine*, November
1982

Colds and 'Flu
Colds & Influenza (Rodale Press, 1982)

*Some Useful Tips for Fighting 'Flu and Common
Colds* (Health Education Council)

What to Do About 'Flu (Health Education
Council

Cot Death
The Foundation for the Study of Infant
Deaths: 5th Floor, 4 Grosvenor Place,
London SW1X 7HD

Cough
'Taming the Common Cough', *Prevention
Magazine*, March 1982

Cystitis
Cystitis and What to Do About It (Health
Education Council)

Denture Problems
'How to Keep Your Teeth Even After You
Lose Them', *Prevention Magazine*,
September 1979

Depression
Depressives Anonymous: 36 Chestnut
Avenue, Beverley, N.Humberside

National Association for Mental Health (MIND): 22 Harley Street, London W1

The Samaritans: (Look in local telephone directory for emergency number) or at 17 Uxbridge Road, Slough SL1 1GN

Diabetes
'Chromium Can Shine up Your Metabolism', *Prevention Magazine*, July 1980

'Fibre–Good for Everyone, Great for Diabetics', *Prevention Magazine*, November 1979

British Diabetic Association: 10 Queen Anne Street, London W1M OBD

Drug Abuse
Drug Misuse: A Basic Briefing (DHSS leaflet)

What Every Parent Should Know About Drugs (DHSS leaflet)

What Parents Can Do About Drugs (DHSS leaflet) (This and the two above are available from the DHSS Leaflets Unit, PO Box 21, Stanmore, Middx

What to Do About Glue Sniffing (Department M50, 13-29 Standard Road, London, NW10)

Families Anonymous: 88 Caledonian Road, London, N7

Institute for the Study of Drug Dependence: 1-4 Hatton Place, Hatton Garden, London EC1N 8ND

Dry Skin
'Moisturizing Dry Skins', *Prevention Magazine*, January 1982

Eczema
National Eczema Society: Tavistock House North, Tavistock Square, London WC1H 9SR

Episiotomies
Association for Improvements in the Maternity Services: 163 Liverpool Road, London N1 ORF

Association of Radical Midwives: 8a The Drive, Wimbledon, London SW20 8TG

Fits
British Epilepsy Association: Crowthorne House, Bigshotte, New Wokingham Road, Wokingham, Berks RG11 3AY

Food Allergies
Food Intolerance and Food Aversion: Royal College of Physicians (The British Nutrition Foundation, April 1984)

Food Poisoning
Germs Are a Dirty Business (Health Education Council)

Fluid Retention
'Natural Remedies for Fluid Retention', *Prevention Magazine,* December 1983

Gall-stones
'Dont Get Stuck with Gallstones, *Prevention Magazine,* 1982

Glaucoma
International Glaucoma Association: King's College Hospital, Denmark Hill, London SE5

Gum Disease
'A Nutritional Formula for Healthy Gums', *Prevention Magazine,* April 1983

Hair Problems
'Overcoming Common Hair Problems', *Prevention Magazine*, November 1979

Institute of Trichology: 38 St George's Road, Wimbledon, SW20

Hay Fever
See Asthma for useful addresses

Headaches
Conquering Pain: Dr Sampson Lipton (Martin Dunitz, 1984)

'Brush Your Headache Away', *Prevention Magazine*, November 1980

The Migraine Trust: 23 Queen Square, London WC1N 3AY

Heart Disease
'Fish Oil–a New Harpoon Against Heart Disease', *Prevention Magazine*, December 1982

General Practitioner, Supplement, 6 May 1983

'21 Ways to Prevent a Heart Attack', *Prevention Magazine*, April 1982

British Heart Foundation: 102 Gloucester Place, London W1H 4DH

The Chest, Heart & Stroke Association: Tavistock House North, Tavistock Square, London WC1H 9JE

The Coronary Prevention Group: Central Middlesex Hospital, London NW10 7NS

Herpes
Herpes. What It Is and How to Cope (Health Education Council)
The telephone number and address of your local VD clinic is in the telephone directory under 'Venereal Disease'.

High Blood Pressure
'Dietary Salt and Hypertension: Treatment & Prevention', Leader, *British Medical Journal*, Vol. 290: p 949

'Hypertension Detection and Follow-up Programme Co-operative Group', *JAMA* 237: p 2385, 1977

'Veterans Administration Co-operative Study Group on Anti-hypertensive Agents', *JAMA* 202: p 1028, 1980

High Blood Pressure, Cause, Effect and Prevention (Rodale Press, 1982)

Hypoglycaemia
'Sugar Neurosis', *Prevention Magazine*, April 1979

Hypothermia
'Staying Warm–Naturally', *Prevention Magazine*, December 1980

Warmth in Winter (Age Concern: Bernard Sunley House, 60 Pitcairn Road, Mitcham, Surrey CR4 3LL

Indigestion
'All About Digestive Aids', *Prevention Magazine*, January 1984

American Journal of Clinical Nutrition, July 1982

'Keeping Indigestion Out of Your Life', *Prevention Magazine*, October 1983

Infectious Diseases in Childhood
'The "Built-in Failure Rate" of Immunisation at Infant Health Clinics', A.E. Dugdale, *Lancet*, 1: pp 409-411, 1969

Immunisation (Health Education Council)

Immunisation: George Dick (Update Books, 1978)

Measles Is Misery (Health Education Council)

Is Your Daughter Between 10-14? (Health Education Council)

Association of Parents of Vaccine Damaged Children: 2 Church Street, Shipston-on-Stour, Warwickshire CV6 4AP

Impotence
See Sexual Boredom for useful addresses

Infertility
National Association for the Childless: 318 Summer Row, Birmingham

Infant Damage and Death
Healthy Mother, Healthy Baby (The Spastics Society, for address see below)

The Prevention of Cerebral Palsy–the Basic Facts (The Spastics Society, for address see below)

Contact a Family: 16 Strutton Ground, London SW1P 2HP

Foresight, Association for the Promotion of Preconceptual Care: Woodhurst, Hydestile, Godalming, Surrey GU9 4OY

The Spastics Society: Park Crescent, London W1N 4EQ

Stillbirth & Perinatal Death Association: 37 Christchurch Hill, London NW3 1LA

Voluntary Council for Handicapped Children: 8 Wakely Street, London EC1V 7QE

Inflammatory Bowel Disease
'Fire Down Below', *Prevention Magazine*, February 1980

National Association for Colitis and Crohn's Disease: 7 Thornfield Close, Marshalwick, St Albans, Herts AL4 9TJ

Kidney Stones
International Journal of Clinical Pharmacology Therapy & Toxicology, 1982

Journal of the American College of Nursing, Vol.1, No.2, 1982

Journal of Urology, January 1981

Loneliness
'How to Be Alone Without Being Lonely', *Prevention Magazine*, December 1979

Loneliness: Dr Tony Lake (Sheldon Press, London, 1979)

National Council for One-Parent Families: 255 Kentish Town Road, London NW5 2LX

National Federation of Solo Clubs: Room 8, Ruskin Chambers, 191 Corporation Street, Birmingham 4

Memory Loss
'Five Proven Ways to Sharpen Your Memory', *Prevention Magazine*, February 1982

Menopause Problems
'How Nutrition Helps Menopause', *Prevention Magazine*, May 1980

Miscarriages
Miscarriage Association: 2 West Vale, Thornhill Road, Dewsbury, W.Yorks SW12 9QH

Obesity
'A Little Body Fat May Not Hasten Death', *JAMA*, 244: p 1660, 1980

'Exercise–the Key to Weight Loss?', *Prevention Magazine*, December 1983

NACNE–A discussion paper on proposals for nutritional guidelines for health education in Britain (Health Education Council, September 1983).

Osteoporosis
'New Life for Old Bones', *Prevention Magazine*, November 1983

Poor Vision
'Look to Nutrition for Sharper Vision', *Prevention Magazine*, May 1982
'Switch to Better Vision', *Prevention Magazine*, December 1979

Post-Natal Depression
Association for Improvements in the Maternity Services: 163 Liverpool Road, London N1 ORF

Association for Post-Natal Illness: 7 Gowan Avenue, London SW6

Association of Radical Midwives: 8a The Drive, Wimbledon, London SW20 8TG

Meet-a-Mum Association: 26a Cumnor Hill, Oxford OX2 9HA

Premature Ejaculation
See Sexual Boredom for useful addresses

Premenstrual Tension
'There's New Help for Those Monthly Blues', *Prevention Magazine*, August 1983.

Pre-menstrual Tension Advisory Service: PO Box 268, Hove, Sussex BN13 1RW

Prostate Problems
Prostate Problems (Rodale Press, 1982)

Psoriasis
Psoriasis Association: 7 Milton Street, Northampton NN2 7JG

Rape
Rape Crisis Centre: PO Box 69, London WC1, Tel 01-837-1600 (24 hours)

Sexual Boredom
The Association of Sexual and Marital Therapists will send you the name of your nearest therapist. Write to Dr M. Duddle, Student Health Centre, University of Manchester M13 9QS

Brook Advisory Centres can be found in all major towns. Check with your local Citizens Advice Bureau for the nearest centre. The main London number is 01-323-1522

London Marriage Guidance Council: 76a New Cavendish Street, London W1

Smoking
'A Diet to Help Quit Smoking', *Prevention Magazine*, October 1979

'Effect of General Practioners' Advice Against Smoking', M.A.H. Russel, *British Medical Journal*, 2: pp 231-235, 1979

Smoking in Pregancy – a Review (The Spastics Society, 12 Park Crescent, London W1N 4EQ

Smoking Prevention – a Health Promotion Guide for the NHS (Published by Action on Smoking and Health, see below for address)

The Facts About Smoking (Health Education Council)

So You Want to Stop Smoking? (Health Education Council)

Action on Smoking and Health (ASH): 5-11 Mortimer Street, London W1N 7RH (Has many useful publications about the prevention of smoking and how to stop if you are a mother)

Stress
'10 Sure-Fire Stress Releasers', *Prevention Magazine*, December 1982

Your Complete Stress-proofing Programme: Leon Chaitow (Thorsons, 1983)

Sugar Addiction
'How to Overcome Sugar Addiction', *Prevention Magazine*, September 1983

Suicide
See Depression

Sunburn
'A Plague of Sunshine', *Prevention Magazine*, July 1983

Lancet, 12 March 1983

'Summer Sun Without the Burn', *Prevention Magazine*, June 1979

Thrush
A Self-help Guide to Thrush (Health Education Council)

Vaginal Thrush and Discomfort (Health Education Council)

Tiredness
'Cross Fatigue Off Your Schedule', *Prevention Magazine*, November 1979

Tooth Decay
'Answers from Dentists, Dental Hygienists and Dental Assistants to Questions Asked by Patients Concerning Preventive Dental Matters', M.A. Eijkman & C. De Witt, *Comm. Dentistry and Oral Epidemiology*, Vol. 8:7, 1980

'Cultural Barriers to Preventive Dentistry', D.C. Blaikie, *Australian Dental Journal*, Vol.24, No.6, December 1979.

'Is the Six-monthly Dental Examination Generally Necessary?', A. Sheiham, *British Dental Journal*, 148:4, 1980

Journal of the American Medical Association, 14 January 1983

Journal of Human Stress, December 1982

'The Role of Health Education in the Prevention of Dental Disease', H. Hodge, *Royal Society of Health Journal*, Vol. 101:5, 1981

The Scientific Basis of Dental Health Education, (A policy document) (Health Education Council)

Smile, Fluoridation Makes It Easy (Health Education Council)

Your Children's Teeth (Health Education Council)

British Dental Health Foundation: 26 Ravensdale Avenue, London N12 9HS

Travel Diseases
'A Doctor's Health Kit for Travellers', *Prevention Magazine*, February 1979

'Exotic Diseases – Ounce of Prevention or Pound of Cure?', M. Schultz, *Postgraduate Medicine*, Vol. 62, No. 2. 1977

'Preventing Illness While Abroad', *British Medical Journal*, Vol. 286, 19 March 1983

Unwanted Pregnancy
Brook Advisory Centres: 233 Tottenham Court Road, London W1P 9AE

Durex Contraception Information Service: North Circular Road, London E4 8QA

Family Planning Association: 27-35 Mortimer Street, London W1N 7RJ

Life: 7 Parade, Leamington Spa, Warwickshire CV32 4DG

Pregnancy Advisory Service: 11-13 Charlotte Street, London W1

Ulcers
Ulcers (Rodale Press, 1982)

Varicose Veins
'The Prevention and Treatment of Varicose Veins', *Prevention Magazine*, August 1980

Venereal Disease
'Sexually Transmitted Diseases: Meeting the 1990 Objectives – a Challenge for the 1980s', *Public Health Reports*, Vol. 97, No.5: p 409, Sept/Oct 1982

Sexually Transmitted Infections (Health Education Council)

Worms
What to Do About Threadworms (Health Education Council)

Wound Healing Difficulty
'Nutrients That Heal the Hurt Fast', *Prevention Magazine*, January 1980

Other books by the same author on which he has drawn in compiling this book:

Breast is Best (Pan)
Choices in Childbirth (Pan)
Overcoming Depression (Hamlyn)
Pears Encyclopaedia of Child Health (Sphere)
Taking the Rough with the Smooth (Pan)
The Baby and Child Book (Pan)
The Boots Book of First Aid
The Complete Book of Love & Sex (Century)
The Complete Book of Sexual Fulfilment (Century)
The Great British Diet (Century)
Trace Elements – A New Chapter in Nutrition (Van Dyke)
Why Us? A Commonsense Guide for the Childless (Thorsons)

INDEX